Maternal Obesity

Maternal Obesity

Edited by

Matthew W. Gillman
Professor and Director of the Obesity Prevention Program, Department of Population Medicine,
Harvard Medical School/Harvard Pilgrim Health Care Institute;
Professor, Department of Nutrition, Harvard School of Public Health, Boston, MA, USA

Lucilla Poston
Head of Division of Women's Health at King's College London and
Research Lead of the Women's Health Academic Centre of King's Health Partners;
Chair of Maternal and Fetal Health at King's College London, UK

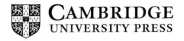

CAMBRIDGE UNIVERSITY PRESS
Cambridge, New York, Melbourne, Madrid, Cape Town,
Singapore, São Paulo, Delhi, Mexico City

Cambridge University Press
The Edinburgh Building, Cambridge CB2 8RU, UK

Published in the United States of America by Cambridge University Press, New York

www.cambridge.org
Information on this title: www.cambridge.org/9781107003965

First published 2012

Printed in the United Kingdom at the University Press, Cambridge

A catalogue record for this publication is available from the British Library

Library of Congress Cataloguing in Publication data
Maternal obesity / [edited by] Matthew W. Gillman, Lucilla Poston.
  p. ; cm.
Includes bibliographical references and index.
ISBN 978-1-107-00396-5 (hardback)
I. Gillman, Matthew W.   II. Poston, Lucilla. [DNLM: 1. Obesity.
2. Pregnancy Complications.   3. Pregnancy. WD 210]
618.92'398–dc23   2012011809

ISBN 978-1-107-00396-5 Hardback

Contents

Contributors

Kjersti M. Aagaard-Tillery, MD, PhD
Assistant Professor, Division of Maternal-Fetal
Medicine, Department of Obstetrics
and Gynecology, Baylor College of Medicine,
Houston, TX, USA

Ruth Bell, MBBS, MSc, MD, FFPH
Senior Lecturer/Honorary NHS
Consultant, Institute of Health and Society,
Newcastle University, Newcastle upon Tyne, UK

Ana Pilar Betrán, MD, PhD
Medical Officer, Department of Reproductive Health
and Research, World Health Organization, Geneva,
Switzerland

Lisa M. Bodnar, PhD, MPH, RD
Assistant Professor of Epidemiology and Obstetrics,
Gynecology and Reproductive Sciences,
Graduate School of Public Health and
School of Medicine, University of Pittsburgh,
Pittsburgh, PA, USA

Sebastien G. Bouret, PhD
Assistant Professor of Pediatrics, The Saban Research
Institute, Neuroscience Program, Children's Hospital
of Los Angeles, University of Southern California,
Los Angeles, CA, USA;
Inserm, Jean-Pierre Aubert Research Center,
University Lille 2, Lille, France

Helen Budge, MA, BM, BCh, MRCP, FRCPCH, PhD
Clinical Associate Professor in Neonatology,
The Early Life Nutrition Research Unit, Academic
Division of Child Health, School of Clinical Sciences,
University Hospital, Nottingham, UK

Jorge E. Chavarro, MD, ScD
Assistant Professor of Nutrition and Epidemiology,
Harvard School of Public Health; Assistant Professor
of Medicine, Brigham and Women's Hospital and
Harvard Medical School, Boston, MA, USA

Carolyn Chiswick, MRCOG, MBChB, BSc (Med Sci)
Clinical Research Fellow/Specialty Trainee
in Obstetrics and Gynaecology, MRC Centre for
Reproductive Health, Queen's Medical Research
Centre, University of Edinburgh, Edinburgh, UK

Helen Croker, BSc, RD
Clinical Research Dietician, Health Behaviour
Research Centre, Department of Epidemiology
and Public Health, University College London,
London, UK

Andrea Deierlein, PhD, MPH, MS
Pediatric Environmental Health Fellow,
Mount Sinai School of Medicine, New York,
NY, USA

**Fiona C. Denison, MD, MRCOG, MBChB,
BSc (Med Sci)**
Senior Lecturer and Honorary Consultant
in Maternal and Fetal Health, MRC Centre for
Reproductive Health, Queen's Medical Research
Centre, University of Edinburgh, Edinburgh, UK

Roland G. Devlieger, MD, PhD
Associate Professor, Faculty of Medicine,
Department of Development and Regeneration,
Catholic University Leuven, Leuven, Belgium

Pat Doyle, BSc, MSc, PhD
Professor of Public Health, London School
of Hygiene and Tropical Medicine, London, UK

Abigail Fraser, MPh, PhD
MRC Research Fellow, MRC CAiTE Centre,
School of Social and Community Medicine,
University of Bristol, Bristol, UK

Dilys J. Freeman, DiP, BSc, PhD
Senior Lecturer, Institute of Cardiovascular
and Medical Sciences, University of Glasgow,
Glasgow, UK

Matthew W. Gillman, MD, SM

Professor and Director of the Obesity Prevention Program, Department of Population Medicine, Harvard Medical School/Harvard Pilgrim Health Care Institute; Professor, Department of Nutrition, Harvard School of Public Health, Boston, MA, USA

Isabelle Guelinckx, MSc, PhD

Postdoctoral Fellow, Department of Public Health – Nutrition, Catholic University Leuven, Leuven, Belgium

Louise M. Howard, MBBS, PhD, MRCP, MRCPsych

Professor of Women's Health and Consultant Perinatal Psychiatrist, Institute of Psychiatry, King's College London, London, UK

Frank B. Hu, MD, PhD

Professor of Nutrition and Epidemiology, Harvard School of Public Health; Professor of Medicine, Harvard Medical School, Boston, MA, USA

Debbie A. Lawlor, MBChB, FFPH, MSc, PhD

Professor of Epidemiology, MRC CAiTE Centre, School of Social and Community Medicine, University of Bristol, Bristol, UK

Mario Merialdi, MD, MPH, PhD

Coordinator, Department of Reproductive Health and Research, World Health Organization, Geneva, Switzerland

Peter Nathanielsz, MD, PhD

Professor, Center for Pregnancy and Newborn Research, The University of Texas Health Science Center at San Antonio, San Antonio, TX, USA

Scott M. Nelson, BSc, PhD, MRCOG

Muirhead Professor of Obstetrics and Gynaecology, Centre for Population and Health Sciences, University of Glasgow, Glasgow, UK

Shalini Ojha, MBBS, MRCPCH

The Early Life Nutrition Research Unit, Academic Division of Child Health, School of Clinical Sciences, University Hospital, Nottingham, UK

Emily Oken, MD, MPH

Obesity Prevention Program, Department of Population Medicine, Harvard Medical School/Harvard Pilgrim Health Care Institute, Boston, MA, USA

Eugene Oteng-Ntim, MBBS, MRCOG, PGDip

Consultant Obstetrician, Guys and St. Thomas's Hosptials and The Portland Hospital, London, UK

Meredith S. Parrott, MD

Resident, Department Obstetrics, Gynecology and Reproductive Sciences, University of Pittsburgh, Pittsburgh, PA, USA

Lucilla Poston, PhD

Head of Division of Women's Health, King's College London; Research Lead, Women's Health Academic Centre of King's Health Partners; Chair of Maternal and Fetal Health, King's College London, UK

Judith Rankin, PhD

Professor of Maternal and Perinatal Epidemiology, Institute of Health and Society, Newcastle University, Newcastle upon Tyne, UK

Kathleen M. Rasmussen, ScD, RD

Professor of Nutrition, Division of Nutritional Sciences, Cornell University, Ithaca, NY, USA

Naveed Sattar, MBChB, MRCP

Professor of Metabolic Medicine, Institute of Cardiovascular and Medical Sciences, University of Glasgow, Glasgow, UK

Anna Maria Siega-Riz, PhD, RD

Professor of Epidemiology and Nutrition and Associate Dean of Academic Affairs, The University of North Carolina Gillings School of Global Public Health, Chapel Hill, NC, USA

Melissa A. Suter, PhD

Postdoctoral Research Fellow, Department of Obstetrics and Gynecology, Baylor College of Medicine, Houston, TX, USA

Michael E. Symonds, PhD

Professor of Developmental Physiology, The Early Life Nutrition Research Unit, Academic Division of Child Health, School of Clinical Sciences, University Hospital, Nottingham, UK

Paul D. Taylor, PhD, BSc
Senior Lecturer, Department of Women's Health,
School of Medicine, King's College London,
London, UK

Peter W. G. Tennant, MSc
Research Associate and PhD Student (Epidemiology),
Institute of Health and Society, Newcastle University,
Newcastle upon Tyne, UK

Maria Regina Torloni, MD, PhD
Clinical Researcher, Department of Obstetrics,
Sao Paulo Federal University, Sao Paulo, Brazil

Thomas L. Toth, MD
Associate Professor of Obstetrics, Gynecology
and Reproductive Biology; Director, MGH
In Vitro Fertilization Unit; Director, Reproductive
Endocrinology and Infertility Fellowship Training
Program, Massachusetts General Hospital and
Harvard Medical School, Boston, MA, USA

Cuilin Zhang, MD, PhD
Investigator, Epidemiology Branch, Division of
Epidemiology, Statistics and Prevention Research,
Eunice Kennedy Shriver National Institute of Child
Health and Human Development, Bethesda, MD, USA

Preface

The obesity pandemic has spread to every part of the globe, and women of reproductive age are not immune. Obese women have reduced fertility, but when they do become pregnant, the subsequent adverse effects accrue to both mother and child.

The obese mother may develop pregnancy complications such as gestational diabetes, she may present challenges to obstetric care, and especially if she gains excessive amounts of weight during pregnancy, may develop ever-increasing weight and its sequelae over her lifetime. Should she become pregnant again, the pattern is repeated. Her offspring have an increased risk of becoming obese themselves. If the offspring is female, she is likely to enter her own pregnancy at increased weight, thereby spawning an intergenerational vicious cycle of obesity and its complications. Interrupting these cycles is of utmost public health importance.

Maternal Obesity will take you through the evidence underlying these concepts. We have divided the book into five sections, starting with trends and determinants of obesity in women of reproductive age. The next two sections appraise the evidence for short- and long-term outcomes in both mother and child. The chapters in these sections include animal and human data, and they range from the basic science of adipose tissue to long-term epidemiologic observations. The fourth section reviews the burgeoning literature on interventions to reduce the complications associated with maternal obesity. The final section contains chapters on clinical management and public health policy.

Our goal was to craft this first book on maternal obesity book for a wide audience, including researchers, clinicians, and policy-makers. The breadth and depth of the chapters is a function of the superb contributing authors, to whom we are indebted. We also thank the Cambridge University Press for shepherding us through the publication process, and our colleagues and families who endured our literal and metaphorical absences.

Matthew W. Gillman
Lucilla Poston

Chapter

1

Demography of obesity

Maria Regina Torloni, Ana Pilar Betrán, and Mario Merialdi

Introduction

According to the World Health Organization (WHO), overweight and obesity are defined as abnormal or excessive fat accumulation that may impair health [1]. Overweight and obesity are usually diagnosed when weight normalized for height, or body mass index (BMI: weight in kilograms divided by the square of the height in meters, kg/m^2), exceeds a defined threshold. In 1995, the WHO proposed a BMI classification for adults as a form of diagnosing excess adiposity [2]. According to this classification, individuals are considered overweight when their BMI is ≥25; those between 25 and 29.9 are designated as pre-obese and they are classified as obese when their BMI reaches or exceeds 30 kg/m^2 (Table 1.1). Many authors also use the term "overweight" to designate pre-obese individuals (BMI 25–29.9), which gives rise to some confusion, unless the specific range of BMI is specified. Although BMI does not directly measure the percentage of body fat, it offers a more accurate assessment of excess adiposity than weight alone. Due to its simplicity, BMI categorization is the preferred obesity measurement for clinicians, public health specialists, and researchers, and is currently used worldwide to track adult overweight and obesity prevalence [3].

Although BMI categorization is widely used, it has several limitations. The proposed BMI classification is age and gender independent and it may not reflect the same degree of adiposity in different populations, due to different body proportions in different ethnicities. Therefore, since the health risks associated with increasing BMI are continuous, the interpretation of BMI gradings in relation to risk may differ for different populations. Due to a growing debate in recent years on the need to develop different BMI cut-off points for different ethnic groups, the WHO convened

Table 1.1 The international classification of adult underweight, overweight, and obesity according to BMI: recommended reporting categories according to the WHO

| | | BMI (kg/m^2) | |
Main classifications	Main categories	Additional categories	Additional classifications
Underweight	<18.5	<16.0	Severe underweight
		16.0–16.9	Moderate underweight
		17.0–18.4	Mild underweight
Normal	18.5–24.9	18.5–22.9	Normal I
		23.0–24.9	Normal II
Overweight^a	≥25.0	–	–
Pre-obese^a	≥25.0–29.9	25.0–27.4	Pre-obese I
		27.5–29.9	Pre-obese II
Obese	≥30.0	–	–
Class I obesity	30.0–34.9	30.0–32.4	Mild class I obesity
		32.5–34.9	Moderate class I obesity
Class II obesity	35.0–39.9	35.0–37.4	Mild class II obesity
		37.5–39.9	Moderate class II obesity
Class III obesity	≥40.0		

Source: adapted from WHO, 1995 [2], WHO 2000 [1], and WHO 2004 [4].
^{a} In the USA, BMI 25.0–25.99 is often termed "overweight."

an expert consultation on BMI in Asian populations [4] to address this issue. Despite evidence that Asian individuals may be at higher than average risk at BMIs lower than the existing WHO cut-off point for overweight (25 kg/m^2), the experts observed that there is a large heterogeneity among the ideal cut-off points for

Maternal Obesity, ed. Matthew W. Gillman and Lucilla Poston. Published by Cambridge University Press. © Cambridge University Press 2012.

different Asian populations. Therefore, the panel maintained the recommendation that the current WHO BMI cut-off points should be retained as the international classification. However, they also suggested that the cut-off points of 23.0, 27.5, 32.5, and 37.5 kg/m^2 are to be added as points for public health action, to create different risk level subcategories within each current category (see Table 1.1). The WHO therefore recommends that countries should use all categories in Table 1.1 for reporting purposes.

To facilitate international comparisons and provide a global perspective on nutritional transition, the WHO created a database that provides survey information on adult BMI from almost one hundred countries covering approximately 80% of the world's adult population [3]. This database, available at http://apps.who.int/bmi/index.jsp, serves as an early warning system for the rapidly rising prevalence of obesity in adults worldwide.

The global race of obesity

Obesity is a chronic multifactorial disease caused by genetic, environmental, and behavioral factors that leads to serious health consequences. When compared to non-obese individuals with similar characteristics, obese adults are at significantly higher risk for cardiovascular and metabolic morbidity, ostheoarthritis, cancer, and mental disease, as well as overall mortality [5–9]. Besides the many individual physical and emotional costs of this disease, obesity also has important direct and indirect financial costs for government and society [10,11]. As the number of obese individuals in a population increases, the demands placed on the health resources of that population also increase [12,13].

The concept that obesity is a public health problem emerged in the second half of the twentieth century, as the prevalence of this condition started to increase in parallel with industrial development. The global nature of the obesity epidemic was officially recognized by the WHO in the late 1990s [1]. The current situation is described as a global pandemic ("globesity") that affects five of the six continents, sparing only sub-Saharan Africa. According to the latest WHO data [14], obesity has more than doubled since 1980 and in 2008 there were an estimated 1.5 billion overweight adults (BMI ≥ 25) in the world.

The prevalence of obesity is rising all over the world and is now recognized as an important public health problem that affects all age groups and both genders.

The global obesity pandemic is increasing at an alarming rate in both developed and developing countries and is considered one of the most important public health challenges of the twenty-first century.

Obesity in developing countries

Currently, 65% of the world's population lives in countries where overweight and obesity kill more people than underweight [15]. This includes all high-income and most middle-income countries. Although developed regions of the world have a higher prevalence of overweight and obesity [16] and the highest body mass indexes [17], the developing world faces a larger absolute burden because of larger population sizes [18,19].

There is a popular but erroneous belief that obesity is a problem of affluent societies and rich nations. This concept was generated in the early twentieth century, when most populations in which obesity became a public health problem were in the developed world, primarily the United States and Europe. In more recent decades, available data show that the most dramatic increases in obesity are occurring in developing countries such as Mexico, China, and Thailand [20].

In most developing countries, the prevalence of obesity is lower in rural compared to urban areas [20,21]. Rural inhabitants tend to eat traditional diets that are high in grains, fruits, and vegetables; when they move to the cities, they increasingly adopt a "Western-type" diet, high in fat and refined sugars. Rapid urbanization, accompanied by a significant reduction in fertility, aging of the population, receding famine patterns, and a marked increase in sedentary behavior, are the primary determinants for the explosive rise in obesity in developing countries. Obesity and all these factors, together with an increase in the consumption of tobacco and alcohol and stress-related ailments, contribute to the rising prevalence of non-communicable chronic diseases in these settings [22].

In the developing world, this nutrition transition is occurring more rapidly than previously seen in higher income countries that went through the same process [17,22]. It is difficult to assess obesity trends in developing countries because of the lack of nationally representative longitudinal data on BMI. Most of the available information in these countries comes from isolated cross-sectional surveys that used different sampling techniques and therefore are not necessarily representative of the country's population at the time of the survey. Despite these methodological limitations, the existing evidence indicates an unequivocal increase in the prevalence of obesity in most low- and middle-income countries starting in the late 1990s [23,24]. According to the few existing longitudinal studies, and to several cross-sectional surveys, the relative increase in the prevalence of obesity in middle-income countries has ranged from 30% to 100% over the past two decades [25]. In developing countries where data are available, the annual rate of increase in the prevalence of adult overweight is approximately 1% [17].

The rapidity of the changes in developing countries is such that a double burden of disease often co-exists: hunger and obesity can occur simultaneously in the same country, a phenomenon known as the nutrition paradox [26]. This paradox can occur not only in different geographical regions of a country, but within the same family. In low-income areas on the outskirts of many large cities in countries such as China, Brazil, and Indonesia, hungry children and obese adults often share the same household [27].

Yet, in many developing nations, the burden of overnutrition is greater than that of undernutrition [21]. In fact, the latest surveys indicate that over half of the adults are overweight and obese in many developing countries throughout the world [3].

Although increase in the prevalence of obesity is a population-wide phenomenon in most developing countries, there are substantial disparities between and within countries, especially when different ethnic and socioeconomic strata are analyzed. Initially, as happened in the rich nations of the world, obesity affected mostly the higher socioeconomic strata of the population in developing countries. However, more recently there has been a shift in prevalence from the higher to the lower socioeconomic level. For example, while in 1989 a national survey in Brazil reported that obesity was more prevalent in adults of higher socioeconomic status, ten years later the highest prevalence of obesity was observed among the lower socioeconomic status respondents [24].

The problem of obesity in developing nations is dramatic not only due to population size, but also to the proportionally smaller investments in public health programs in many of these countries. Additionally, due to technical, cultural, and political factors, health authorities in developing nations frequently employ their limited resources in less cost-effective interventions.

Female and maternal obesity

According to WHO data, of the 1.5 billion individuals with BMI ≥25 in 2008, nearly 300 million of these were obese women (BMI ≥30) [14]. Generally, in any population, men will have higher rates of overweight, while women will have higher rates of obesity [3]. Table 1.2 and Figure 1.1 present the prevalence of pre-obese and obese women in the world according to the latest available data.

Although the increasing prevalence of obesity among women of childbearing age is part of the larger worldwide epidemic, its consequences can be particularly devastating. As described in the later chapters of this book, the problems related to female obesity start in adolescence with amenorrhoea and dysovulation

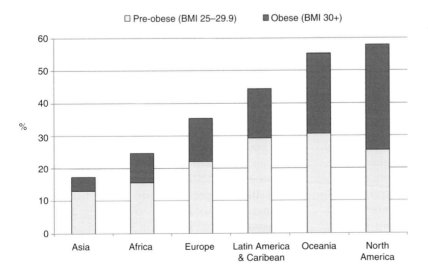

Figure 1.1. Prevalence of overweight women in the world.

Table 1.2 Regional distribution of female overweight

Region/ sub-region	Coverage of estimates (%)	Women with BMI 25.0–29.9 (%)	Women with BMI ≥30 (%)	Women with BMI ≥25 (%)
Africa	85.3	15.6	9.0	24.6
Eastern Africa	93.7	93.0	2.8	12.1
Middle Africa	84.5	11.3	3.5	14.8
Northern Africa	54.0	29.6	28.8	58.4
Southern Africa	96.6	28.9	25.0	53.8
Western Africa	98.7	14.8	5.4	20.2
Asia	92.9	13.1	4.2	17.3
Eastern Asia	88.3	15.4	3.4	18.8
Central Asia	100.0	15.2	5.9	21.0
Southern Asia	98.4	8.6	2.7	11.3
Southeastern Asia	91.4	15.2	4.5	19.7
Western Asia	86.7	28.6	21.4	50.0
Europe	98.4	22.1	13.2	35.2
Eastern Europe	96.7	24.5	16.8	41.3
Northern Europe	99.8	29.7	18.7	48.4
Southern Europe	99.6	20.8	8.1	28.9
Western Europe	99.7	14.9	8.4	23.3
Latin America and the Caribbean	91.9	29.2	15.2	44.3
Caribbean	81.4	22.3	8.5	30.8
Central America	96.8	35.6	25.7	61.3
South America	91.0	27.1	11.3	38.4
North America	100.0	25.6	32.3	57.8
Canada	100.0	26.1	16.9	43.0
USA	100.0	25.5	34.0	59.5
Oceania	79.3	30.6	24.6	55.2
Australia/New Zealand	100.0	30.7	24.3	55.0
Melanesia	19.1	31.4	25.1	56.6
Polynesia	63.5	22.8	44.3	67.1

Sources: latest Demographic and Health Surveys are available at www.measuredhs.com/ [39] or WHO database on BMI, available at www.who.int/bmi/index.jsp [3].

and continue throughout the reproductive period. Although there are no data available for a global assessment of obesity levels in pregnant women, this issue can be framed within the global weight increase among the female population. More women are entering pregnancy with excess weight, exposing them and their unborn child to increased risks of adverse gestational and perinatal outcomes, as well as long-term risks.

A body of evidence indicates that obesity in pregnancy is associated with increased risk for several clinical and obstetric complications, such as gestational diabetes, pre-eclampsia, preterm delivery, or fetal macrosomia [28–32]. Additionally, as detailed in Chapters 9 to 11 in Section 3, several longitudinal studies report that individuals exposed to maternal obesity during fetal life are at increased risks of

Table 1.3 Countries with the highest prevalence of female obesity and pre-obesity

Country	% female population with BMI >30
American Samoa	80
Nauru	78
Tokelau	68
Kiribati	59
French Polynesia	44
Saudi Arabia	44
Egypt	40
Iraq	38
Panama	36
Seychelles	35
Country	**% female population with BMI 25.0–29.9**
Mexico	37
Germany	36
Turkey	34
Portugal	34
Malta	34
United Kingdom	34
Panama	33
Colombia	33
Kuwait	33
Chile	33

Source: available at www.who.int/bmi/index.jsp [3].

becoming overweight or obese children and adults themselves [33], thus perpetuating the vicious cycle of obesity and creating an intergeneration effect.

Female obesity in developing countries is becoming very prevalent. In fact, the most recent data available on the WHO Global Database on BMI indicate that all ten countries with the highest prevalence of obese women are developing countries [3], as can be seen in Table 1.3. The striking representation of Polynesian islands in this list may be the result of genetic susceptibility fueled by geographical isolation and inbreeding, allied with environmental factors. Women of low socioeconomic status living in developing countries are at especially high risk for obesity [23,34,35].

Paradoxically, as a country's gross national product increases, the burden of obesity in that country tends to shift toward the lower socioeconomic groups. Thus, the increasing economic prosperity seen in many developing countries over the last decades may be contributing to the obesity epidemic among women of the lowest socioeconomic status in these nations. Moreover, the shift of obesity toward women of lower socioeconomic status apparently occurs at an earlier stage of economic development than it does for men [23,35].

Economic development is significantly related to a faster increase in the prevalence of overweight for women of lower socioeconomic strata and this relation varies by income inequality [36]. In the 1980s, the WHO initiated a ten-year study in 26 countries to monitor trends and determinants of cardiovascular disease, including obesity [37]. According to the data collected from over 50 million participants included in this study, there was a significant inverse association between educational level, used as a proxy for socioeconomic level, and BMI for women in almost all populations. Women with low education had higher BMIs than those with higher education. Additionally, the authors reported an increasing difference in BMI between educational levels over a ten-year period.

In developed as well as in developing countries, female obesity is clearly a problem associated with social class. However, it is also a problem related to income inequality: the prevalence of female obesity is higher in countries with the largest differences between the incomes of the rich and the poor [38]. In developing countries, the combination of rising national economies, persistent income inequalities, and increased "Westernization," will most likely lead to sustained increases of female obesity in the future.

As the number of women who are obese at the start of pregnancy continues to escalate worldwide, there is an urgent need to invest more resources on studies that analyze the determinants of this trend and that test population interventions to help curb this phenomenon.

Conclusion

In contrast to malnutrition and infectious diseases, which have always dominated the attention of public health specialists and organizations, the causes and consequences of obesity have only recently achieved global recognition. In fact, the WHO describes obesity as one of the most blatantly visible, yet most neglected, public-health problems that threatens to overwhelm both more and less developed countries [1].

With the increase in sedentary lifestyles and the availability and consumption of energy-dense foods, the incidence of obesity among women is rising globally. Health providers are expected to care for a growing number of obese reproductive-age women in the coming decades. Simultaneously, more and more women will enter pregnancy with higher BMIs, which will expose them and their unborn child to higher immediate and long-term risks.

The high and continuously accelerating rate of obesity among women living in developing countries is one of the darkest facets of this worldwide problem, since it involves an immense population and affects predominantly those in the lower socioeconomic strata. There is an urgent need for investments and studies on obesity in reproductive-age women, focused on understanding the determinants of this problem and the development of effective interventions to curb this trend while there is still time.

References

1. World Health Organization. Division of Noncommunicable Diseases. *Obesity: Preventing and Managing the Global Epidemic*. Report of a WHO consultation on obesity. (Geneva, Switzerland: World Health Organization, 2000).

2. World Health Organization. *Physical Status: the Use and Interpretation of Anthropometry*. Report of a WHO expert committee. (Geneva, Switzerland: World Health Organization, 1995).

3. World Health Organization. *Global Database on Body Mass Index: an Interactive Surveillance Tool for Monitoring Nutrition Transition*. 2011. www.who.int/bmi/index.jsp [Accessed January 4, 2012]

4. WHO Expert Consultation. Appropriate body-mass index for Asian populations and its implications for policy and intervention strategies. *Lancet* 2004;**363**(9403):157–63.

5. Allison D B, Fontaine K R, Manson J E, Stevens J & Van Itallie T B. Annual deaths attributable to obesity in the United States. *JAMA* 1999;**282**(16):1530–8.

6. Calle E E & Kaaks R. Overweight, obesity and cancer: epidemiological evidence and proposed mechanisms. *Nat Rev Cancer* 2004;**4**(8):579–91.

7. Friedman M A & Brownell K D. Psychological correlates of obesity: moving to the next research generation. *Psychol Bull* 1995;**117**(1):3–20.

8. Kenchaiah S, Evans J C, Levy D, Wilson P W, Benjamin E J, *et al.* Obesity and the risk of heart failure. *N Engl J Med* 2002;**347**(5):305–13.

9. Krauss R M, Winston M, Fletcher B J & Grundy S M. Obesity: impact on cardiovascular disease. *Circulation* 1998;**98**(14):1472–6.

10. Allison D B, Zannolli R & Narayan K M. The direct health care costs of obesity in the United States. *Am J Public Health* 1999;**89**(8):1194–9.

11. Kortt M A, Langley P C & Cox E R. A review of cost-of-illness studies on obesity. *Clin Ther* 1998;**20**(4):772–9.

12. Popkin B M, Horton S, Kim S, Mahal A & Shuigao J. Trends in diet, nutritional status, and diet-related noncommunicable diseases in China and India: the economic costs of the nutrition transition. *Nutr Rev* 2001;**59**(12):379–90.

13. Popkin B M. Will China's nutrition transition overwhelm its health care system and slow economic growth? *Health Aff (Millwood)* 2008;**27**(4):1064–76.

14. World Health Organization. *Obesity and Overweight. Fact sheet No. 311*. www.who int/mediacentre/factsheets/fs311/en/ [Accessed January 4, 2012]

15. World Health Organization. *Diet, Nutrition, and the Prevention of Chronic Diseases*. (Geneva, Switzerland: World Health Organization, 2003).

16. Haslam D W & James W P. Obesity. *Lancet* 2005;**366**(9492):1197–209.

17. Popkin B M. Recent dynamics suggest selected countries catching up to US obesity. *Am J Clin Nutr* 2010;**91**(1):284S–8S.

18. Gu D, Reynolds K, Wu X, Chen J, Duan X, *et al.* Prevalence of the metabolic syndrome and overweight among adults in China. *Lancet* 2005;**365**(9468):1398–405.

19. Reddy K S, Prabhakaran D, Shah P & Shah B. Differences in body mass index and waist: hip ratios in North Indian rural and urban populations. *Obes Rev* 2002;**3**(3):197–202.

20. Caballero B. The global epidemic of obesity: an overview. *Epidemiol Rev* 2007;**29**:1–5.

21. Mendez M A, Monteiro C A & Popkin B M. Overweight exceeds underweight among women in most developing countries. *Am J Clin Nutr* 2005;**81**(3):714–21.

22. Popkin B M. The nutrition transition in low-income countries: an emerging crisis. *Nutr Rev* 1994;**52**(9):285–98.

23. Monteiro C A, Moura E C, Conde W L & Popkin B M. Socioeconomic status and obesity in adult populations of developing countries: a review. *Bull World Health Organ* 2004;**82**(12):940–6.

24. Monteiro C A, Conde W L & Popkin B M. The burden of disease from undernutrition and overnutrition in countries undergoing rapid nutrition transition: a view from Brazil. *Am J Public Health* 2004;**94**(3):433–4.

25. Popkin B M. The nutrition transition: an overview of world patterns of change. *Nutr Rev* 2004;**62**(7 Pt 2):S140–S143.

26. Caballero B. A nutrition paradox – underweight and obesity in developing countries. *N Engl J Med* 2005;**352**(15):1514–16.

27. Doak C M, Adair L S, Bentley M, Monteiro C & Popkin B M. The dual burden household and the nutrition transition paradox. *Int J Obes (Lond)* 2005;**29**(1):129–36.

28. Sebire N J, Jolly M, Harris J P, Wadsworth J, Joffe M, *et al.* Maternal obesity and pregnancy outcome: a study of 287,213 pregnancies in London. *Int J Obes Relat Metab Disord* 2001;**25**(8):1175–82.

29. Siega-Riz A M & Laraia B. The implications of maternal overweight and obesity on the course of pregnancy and birth outcomes. *Matern Child Health J* 2006;**10**(5 Suppl):S153–S156.

30. Yu C K, Teoh T G & Robinson S. Obesity in pregnancy. *BJOG* 2006;**113**(10):1117–25.

31. Torloni M R, Betrán A P, Horta B L, Nakamura M U, Atallah A N, *et al.* Prepregnancy BMI and the risk of gestational diabetes: a systematic review of the literature with meta-analysis. *Obes Rev* 2009;**10**(2):194–203.

32. Torloni M R, Betrán A P, Daher S, Widmer M, Dolan S M, *et al.* Maternal BMI and preterm birth: a systematic review of the literature with meta-analysis. *J Matern Fetal Neonatal Med* 2009;**22**(11):957–70.

33. Parsons T J, Power C, Logan S & Summerbell C D. Childhood predictors of adult obesity: a systematic review. *Int J Obes Relat Metab Disord* 1999;**23**(Suppl 8):S1–S107.

34. Martorell R, Khan L K, Hughes M L & Grummer-Strawn L M. Obesity in women from developing countries. *Eur J Clin Nutr* 2000;**54**(3):247–52.

35. Monteiro C A, Conde W L, Lu B & Popkin B M. Obesity and inequities in health in the developing world. *Int J Obes Relat Metab Disord* 2004;**28**(9):1181–6.

36. Jones-Smith J C, Gordon-Larsen P, Siddiqi A & Popkin B M. Cross-national comparisons of time trends in overweight inequality by socioeconomic status among women using repeated cross-sectional surveys from 37 developing countries, 1989–2007. *Am J Epidemiol* 2011;**173**(6):667–75.

37. Molarius A, Seidell J C, Sans S, Tuomilehto J & Kuulasmaa K. Educational level, relative body weight, and changes in their association over 10 years: an international perspective from the WHO MONICA Project. *Am J Public Health* 2000;**90**(8):1260–8.

38. Wilkinson R & Pickett K. Obesity: wider income gaps, wider waists. In Wilkinson R & Pickett K (eds.) *The Spirit Level: Why More Equal Societies Almost Always Do Better*, 1st edn. (London, England: Penguin Books Ltd, 2009), pp. 89–102.

39. Measure DHS. Demographic and Health Surveys. www.measuredhs.com/ [Accessed January 27, 2012]

Chapter

2

Determinants of obesity

Cuilin Zhang and Frank B. Hu

Introduction

Obesity has become a global epidemic. The World Health Organization's (WHO) latest report [1] indicates that in 2008 approximately 1.5 billion adults 20 years or older worldwide were overweight, defined as having a body mass index (BMI) $\geq 25\,kg/m^2$ [1]. Of these, nearly 500 million were obese, BMI $\geq 30\,kg/m^2$, including 200 million males and nearly 300 million females. The numbers of those overweight and obese are projected to reach 2.3 billion and 700 million respectively by 2015 [1]. In the United States, the percentage of obese adults increased from 15% in the late 1970s to over 33% in 2007–2008, with the greatest increase among Mexican American women [2]. Similarly, in a number of developing countries such as China and India, where the Western lifestyle and diet are becoming more common, the prevalence of overnutrition, obesity, and obesity-related disorders is increasing rapidly. For instance, according to the WHO's Global Information Database, 45% of males and 32% of females aged 15 years or older in China were overweight, or an average of 38.5% of the 2010 population. This is a sharp increase from the 2002 estimate of 25% in China (27.5% of males and 22.7% of females) [3].

Women of reproductive age are no exception. Based on data from the National Health and Nutrition Examination Survey (NHANES) 2007–2008, US women of 20 to 39 years old are alarmingly heavy: 60% are overweight, 34% are obese, and 8% have a BMI $\geq 40\,kg/m^2$ (class III obesity) [4]. Moreover, a very high proportion of pregnant women, approximately 45%, were overweight or obese when becoming pregnant [5]. Furthermore, in the United States, the greatest increase in the prevalence of obesity in the past decade is among women aged 20 to 39 years, a jump from

28% during 1999–2000 to 34% during 2007–2008, as compared with a slight increase from 37.8% to 38.4% among women of 40 to 59 years old. Substantial increase in obesity burden among women at reproductive age was observed in other countries as well. For instance, in a nationally representative study of maternal obesity in England, UK, first trimester maternal obesity more than doubled from 7.6% in 1989 to 15.6% in 2007 (p < 0.001) [6]. In South Asian countries (Bangladesh, Nepal, and India), although the prevalence of underweight has remained high, the prevalence of overweight and obesity in women of reproductive age has increased substantially [7]. For example, between 1996 and 2006, in Bangladesh, the prevalence of overweight among women of 14 to 49 years old increased from 2.7% to 8.9%; in Nepal, from 1.6% to 10.1%; and in India, from 10.6% to 14.8%.

Obesity has adverse impacts on multiple aspects of the health of reproductive-age women. Obese women generally experience more difficulty in conceiving than lean women [8]. Among women who succeed in conceiving, pre-pregnancy BMI has long been known as a major determinant of adverse pregnancy outcomes [9]. For example, maternal obesity is strongly associated with an increased risk of a number of pregnancy complications for both women and their children, such as gestational diabetes [10], pre-eclampsia, macrosomia, premature deliveries, fetal injury during delivery, and intrauterine mortality [11,12]. Long-term adverse outcomes related to maternal obesity include chronic diseases, e.g., diabetes and cardiovascular disease, and certain cancers, premature death, and complications during the next pregnancy. See Chapter 8 for more details of these phenomena.

In view of the escalating burden of obesity among women of reproductive age and the detrimental

Maternal Obesity, ed. Matthew W. Gillman and Lucilla Poston. Published by Cambridge University Press. © Cambridge University Press 2012.

impacts of obesity on women's health overall, it becomes increasingly important to identify risk factors and determinants for obesity, in particular factors that may contribute to its prevention. Our aim for the present chapter is to provide readers with an overview of the determinants of obesity, in particular those relevant to women of reproductive age.

Determinants of obesity

Diet and lifestyle factors

Diet

Obesity and weight gain usually result from the cumulative effects of a small daily positive-energy balance. Excessive caloric intake is a major driving force behind the escalating obesity epidemic worldwide, but diet quality has also been demonstrated to have an independent impact on the risk of obesity. Over the past few decades, numerous observational studies and clinical trials have investigated the role of dietary factors in weight control and obesity prevention. In general, the impact of major dietary factors such as macronutrient amounts (i.e., fat, protein, carbohydrate) on body fatness remains uncertain, with the existing literature suggesting that altering macronutrient composition itself is unlikely to have a substantial impact on long-term weight control [13]. Moreover, the effects of popular diets designed to promote weight loss remain controversial. Clearly, there is no magic diet or nutrient that offers weight control. Rather, many individual dietary factors exert a modest effect on body weight and, over time, the cumulative effects of small changes in daily energy balance lead to weight gain and obesity [13].

Although dietary fat has long been considered the main culprit behind obesity, large prospective studies [14,15] and long-term randomized clinical trials [16] do not support a major role of fat consumption, either total fat or types of fat including saturated, mono-unsaturated, and polyunsaturated fat, in weight loss and obesity prevention. By contrast, emerging evidence suggests that restricting carbohydrates and reducing glycemic load (GL) may improve weight control [17–19]. Investigations of diet in terms of specific foods, food groups, and dietary patterns have yielded more conclusive findings than focusing on individual nutrients. In general, these findings indicate that increasing consumption of plant-based foods such as whole grains, fruits, and vegetables is associated with

less weight gain over time [13,19]. On the other hand, there is substantial evidence that higher consumption of sugar-sweetened beverages (SSB) induces greater weight gain. Indeed, the consistent increase in SSB intake over the past three decades parallels the growth of the obesity epidemic [20]. Findings from a systematic review of 30 studies including large cross-sectional investigations, well-powered prospective cohort studies with long follow-up and repeated measures of diet and weight, as well as clinical trials provide strong evidence for an independent role of SSBs, particularly soda, in the promotion of weight gain and obesity [21].

In a recent prospective study [19] based on data from three large prospective cohorts of males and females aged 24 to 74 years at baseline, the Nurses' Health Study, the Nurses' Health Study II, and the Health Professionals Follow-up Study, Mozaffarian et al., demonstrated that dietary quality, i.e., types of foods and beverages consumed, could have a strong impact on dietary quantity, i.e., the amount of food and total calories, and thus risk of long-term weight gain. Most of the foods that were significantly and positively associated with weight gain during each four-year follow-up period were those rich in refined carbohydrates or starch: for instance, sweets, desserts, and potato products (see Figure 2.1). By contrast, higher consumption of foods rich in fiber (for instance, vegetables, nuts, fruits, and whole grains) was associated with less weight gain. The inverse associations with weight gain could be because increasing the consumption of these foods reduced the intake of other foods to a greater extent, thereby decreasing the overall amount of energy consumed. Higher fiber content and slower digestion of these foods may also increase satiety, and their increased consumption would also displace other more highly processed foods in the diet, decreasing energy intake. Interestingly, in this study, greater yogurt consumption was also associated with less weight gain in both men and women, though the precise mechanisms underlying this association are unclear. Changes in colonic bacteria and the microbiome related to yogurt consumption might influence weight gain [22]. It is also possible that certain unmeasured factors that are highly correlated with yogurt consumption may minimize weight gain. For instance, individuals who increased their yogurt consumption may have other weight-influencing behaviors that were not measured in the study.

Most studies of dietary factors and obesity and weight control have been conducted in developed

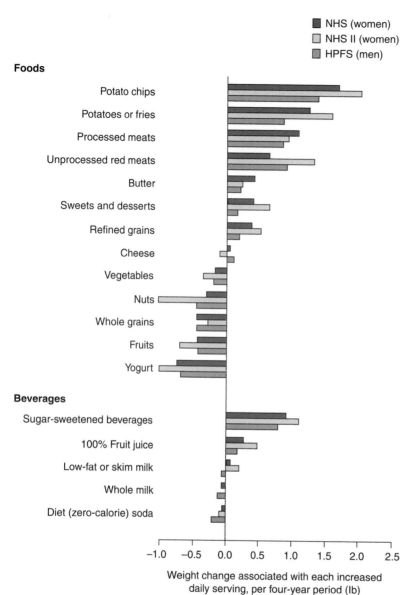

Figure 2.1. Associations between changes in food and beverage consumption and weight changes every four years, according to study cohort. Study participants included 50 422 women in the Nurses' Health Study (NHS), followed for 20 years (1986 to 2006); 47 898 women in the Nurses' Health Study II (NHS II), followed for 12 years (1991 to 2003); and 22 557 men in the Health Professionals Follow-up Study (HPFS), followed for 20 years (1986 to 2006). Weight changes are reported for each increase in the daily serving of the food or beverage; decreased intake would be associated with the inverse weight changes. There was little evidence of a significant interaction between diet and physical activity (p > 0.10 for the interaction in each cohort). All weight changes were adjusted simultaneously for age, baseline body mass index, sleep duration, and changes in smoking status, physical activity, television watching, alcohol use, and all of the dietary factors shown. The p value is less than 0.001 for all dietary factors with the exception of butter in the NHS II, cheese in the NHS and NHS II, low-fat or skim milk in the NHS and HPFS, diet soda in the NHS, and whole-fat milk in all three cohorts. Reproduced with permission from reference [19], © 2011, *New England Journal of Medicine*. (See figure in color plate section.)

countries. However, data from the developing world have begun to emerge. As discussed previously in the present chapter, in some developing countries such as China and India, where the Western lifestyle and diet are becoming more common, the prevalence of obesity and obesity-related disorders is increasing rapidly. Economic development and globalization have spurred nutritional transitions in these countries typically involving increased consumption of animal fat and energy-dense foods and SSBs, decreased consumption of fiber, and more frequent intake of fast foods, which are related to weight gain and obesity. At the same time,

a shift away from agricultural labor toward employment in manufacturing services has led to a dramatic decline in physical activity, the main determinant of variation in energy expenditure in the population [23]. The combination of excessive energy intake and drastically reduced energy expenditure is driving the increased obesity epidemic in these countries.

Physical activity and inactivity

In addition to diet, physical activity may play a pivotal role in maintaining energy balance and weight control. Numerous prospective studies have examined the association between physical activity, mostly vigorous exercise or high-intensity activities, and weight change over time [24]. Most studies, though not all, found that increasing physical activity attenuates weight gain during midlife [25]. In general, recent studies (published after 2000) showed more consistent findings on physical activity and weight gain than earlier studies. Overall, the effects of physical activity on the prevention of age-related weight gain appear to be modest.

The optimal amount of physical activity that is required to prevent obesity and weight gain in adults remains unclear. The effect of physical activity may vary by gender, age, and energy intake. In the Health Professionals Follow-up Study [26] of males aged 40 to 75 years, increasing physical activity by 1.5 hours/week decreased weight gain but was not sufficient to offset it completely. However, in combination with reduced TV watching, increasing exercise appeared to offset the expected weight gain after four years of follow-up. In a meta-analysis of data [19] from three large prospective cohorts including both females and males, Mozaffarian *et al.* demonstrated that, across quintiles, participants with greater increases in physical activity gained 1.76 fewer lbs (0.80 kg) within each four-year period. In the CARDIA study [27] among young adults of 15 to 30 years, increasing vigorous exercise by two hours/week was needed to offset weight gain. Overall, the young adults needed to exercise an average of four to five hours/week to completely prevent weight gain.

Physical activity reduces weight gain via multiple biological mechanisms, possibly depending on the type and intensity of activity. Increasing energy expenditure through physical activity may help maintain energy balance, but most activities consume only small amounts of energy, and it is unclear whether the added exercise is compensated for by a later decline in physical activity. In addition, physical activity tends to increase appetite and overall energy intake. Thus, exercise training without dietary intervention may have a relatively modest effect on weight control.

Independent of physical activity levels, sedentary behaviors such as TV watching are associated with risk of obesity and weight gain. During a six-year follow-up of 50 277 middle-aged and older women in the Nurses' Health Study [28], each two hour/day increment in TV watching was associated with a 23% (95% CI: 17%–30%) increase in obesity; and each two hour/day increment in sitting at work was associated with a 5% (95% CI: 0%–10%) increase in obesity. Prolonged TV watching was also associated with significantly elevated risk of

developing type 2 diabetes in women, whereas regular brisk walking was protective against the disease. The effects of TV watching on obesity are probably mainly mediated by diet. Prolonged TV watching was associated with greater food and total energy intake, most likely because of increased exposure to food and beverage advertisements. In addition, those who spend more time watching TV tend to have unhealthful eating patterns characterized by increased consumption of snacks, sugary beverages, and fast foods.

Sleep

Evidence has been steadily accumulating over the past decade that sleep curtailment is a risk factor for weight gain and obesity. This association is likely mediated through neural pathways such as the orexin system, which contributes to the regulation of both body weight and sleep [29]. Sleep deprivation is a growing trend in the United States. A 2008 survey found that 16% of US adults sleep less than six hours per week night [30]. This epidemic in sleep deprivation parallels the US obesity epidemic [29,31]. Data from both cross-sectional studies and some prospective studies support an association between shorter sleep duration and increased risk of obesity [31]. In short-term metabolic trials, reduced sleep altered leptin and ghrelin and increased subjective hunger and preferences for calorie-dense refined-carbohydrate foods [29]. Findings from a recent study [19] including three large prospective cohorts of men and women in the USA suggested that the association between sleep duration and long-term weight gain is characterized by a U-shaped curve; that is, weight gain was lowest among persons who slept for six to eight hours a night and higher among those who slept less than six hours or more than eight hours. That association persisted even after adjustment for dietary and other risk factors for obesity. Due to the rising prevalence of short sleep duration, any causal association between sleep habits and obesity will have important public health significance in obesity prevention. Behavioral interventions that effectively improve sleep habits need to be developed, and more accurate measurements of sleep habits are sorely needed.

Psychosocial factors

Accumulating evidence indicates that achieving reduction in population prevalence of obesity may also require an altering of the social factors that impact diet and lifestyle factors [32]. Social factors are tightly related to obesity at multiple levels. For example, socio-economic resources heavily influence dietary choices and both the accessibility and feasibility of physical activity. Chronic exposure to psychosocial stress may increase the likelihood of "comfort eating," such as consuming foods or beverages high in sugar, and/or lead to sleep deprivation. For instance, in an analysis of a nationally representative longitudinal cohort of 1355 men and women in the USA, multiple domains of psychosocial stress, such as job-related demands, perceived constraints in life, strain in relations with family, and difficulty paying bills, were significantly and positively associated with weight gain from 1995 to 2004 [33]. Depression might also substantially reduce one's interest in physical activity and leisure time activity. Obesity and depression appear to share a biological pathway; the HPA-axis plays a major role in the development of both conditions [34]. A wide range of social determinants such as social-economic status, neighborhood characteristics, educational level, racial discrimination, and acculturation has been implicated in the obesity epidemic [32]. It is becoming increasingly accepted that the epidemic rise in the burden of obesity is reflective of the condition's social origins. A clearer understanding of the interrelationships of social determinants and the diet and lifestyle factors relevant to obesity will be essential to the development of effective interventions.

Overall, it is well recognized that diet, physical activity, and related lifestyle factors that are induced by obesogenic social and physical environments, are the primary determinants of obesity in both men and women. Because of high rates of weight gain, these factors may be particularly important for women of reproductive age. Clearly, there is no "magic bullet" for weight control. Rather, many individual dietary and lifestyle factors each exert a modest effect on body weight and, over time, cumulative effects of small changes in daily energy balance lead to weight gain and obesity.

Genetic factors

The etiology of obesity also has a genetic component. The search for obesity genes began several decades ago, but efforts have intensified in recent years with the completion of the Human Genome Project and advances in molecular biology, genotyping technology, and genetic epidemiologic methods. To date, at least 20 genetic variants have been identified for the monogenic form of obesity [35], with almost all the variants on the leptin/melanocortin pathway in the central nervous system (CNS) that is critical in the regulation of whole-body energy homeostasis and balance [36].

Common obesity is also influenced by genetic factors. Heritability estimates were 0.4 to 0.7 for BMI [37,38] and approximately 0.6 for both waist circumference (WC) and subscapular skinfold thickness [39,40]. However, the classical heritability estimates for obesity based on concordance and discordance of obesity rates among monozygotic and dizygotic twins are likely to overestimate the genetic components of obesity because monozygotic twins, who share 100% of genes, also share more of *intrauterine* and early childhood environments than dizygotic twins. Evidence is accumulating suggestive that both *intrauterine* exposures and early life factors may influence the risk of obesity during childhood and later in life (see Chapters 9 to 13 in Section 3 for details).

Recent genome-wide association studies (GWAS) have led to major advances in the identification of common genetic variants of obesity and related anthropometric measures. The first substantial advances in the discovery of obesity susceptibility loci were made in 2007, when GWAS demonstrated the initial success of identifying the first robustly associated obesity susceptibility locus, *FTO* (fat mass and obesity associated) [37,41,42]. This genetic association is consistent between men and women and across different age groups. These initial studies revealed the small effect sizes of obesity genes and suggested that increasing the power and sample size of studies was necessary to identify further susceptibility loci. As a result, even larger and better powered studies have followed. Made possible by technical and analytical developments in population genetics, GWAS are based on the principle that common genetic markers can be inherited together as "blocks" due to linkage disequilibrium. This allowed investigators to capture about 80% of all common variations (>14 million variants using as few as 500 000 carefully chosen single nucleotide polymorphisms or SNPs) [43,44]. Recent GWAS have identified at least 54 common loci associated with BMI and related phenotypes [38] (Table 2.1). Overall, many genes within the associated regions have been reported to fall within two broad categories: those affecting CNS function and those that probably operate peripherally, often through adipose tissue. While the effects of BMI-related SNPs are largely consistent between men and women, several SNPs that are related to fat distribution measured

Table 2.1 Confirmed genes of obesity-related anthropometric measures

Position	Gene name	BMI	WHR	WC
1p12	TBX15-WARS2		+	
1p21.3	PTBP2	+		
1p31	NEGR1	+		
1p31.1	TNN13K	+		
1q24.3	DNM3-PIGC		+	
1q25	SEC16B, RASAL2	+		
1q41	LYPLAL1, ZC3H11B	+	+	
1q43-q44	SDCCAG8	+		
2p16.1	FANCL	+		
2p23.3	RBJ-ADCY3-POMC	+		
2p25	TMEM18	+		
2q12.1	ZNRF3-KREMEN1		+	
2q22.2	LRP1B	+		
2q24.3	GRB14		+	
3p14.1	ADAMTS9		+	
3p21.1	NISCH-STAB1		+	
3P21.1	CADM2	+		
3q27	Near ETV5	+		
4p13	Near GNPDA2	+		
4q24	SLC39A8	+		
5q13.3	FLJ35779	+		
5q23.2	ZNF608	+		
5q35.2	CPEB4		+	
6p12	TFAP2B	+		+
6p21	NCR3, AIF1, and BAT2	+		
6p21.1	VEGFA		+	
6p22.2-p21.3	PRL	+		
6q22.33	RSPOS		+	
6p25.1	LY86		+	
7p15.2	NFE2L3		+	
8p23.1	MSRA	+		+
9p21.3	LRRN6C	+		
10p12	PTER	+		
11p11.2	MTCH2	+		
11p14	BDNF	+		
11p15.4	RPL27A	+		
12p21.1	ITPR2-SSPN		+	
12q13	FAIM2, BCDIN2D	+		
12q13.13	HOXC13		+	

Table 2.1 (*cont.*)

Position	Gene name	BMI	WHR	WC
12q24	PTPN11/C12orf51	+	+	
13q12.2	MTIF3-GTF3A	+		
14q12	PRKD1	+		
14q31	NRXN3	+		+
15q23	MAP2K5	+		
16p11.2	SH2B1	+		
16p12.3	GPRC5B	+		
16q22-q23	MAF	+		
16q22,2	FTO	+		
18q11,2	NPC1	+		
18q22	MC4R	+		
19q13,11	KCTD15	+		
19q13.32	QPTCL-GIPR	+		
19q13.32	TMEM160	+		

BMI: body mass index; WC: waist circumference; WHR: waist-to-hip ratio.
Data as of July 2011.

by waist circumference or waist-to-hip ratio exhibit sexual dimorphism [31]. For instance, in a recent sex-specific meta-analysis of 108 979 women (42 735 in the discovery stage and 66 244 in the follow-up) and 82 483 men, Heid *et al.* observed significant associations with waist-to-hip ratio only among women but not men for seven genetic variants close to *RSPO3*, *VEGFA*, *GRB14*, *LYPLAL1*, *HOXC13*, *ITPR2-SSPN*, and *ADAMTS9*, which reflects the sex-specific effects driving body fat distribution [45].

Although GWAS have been successful in identifying loci for the determinants of common obesity, the established loci together explain less than 2% of inter-individual BMI variation [38]. In addition, these loci, individually or in combination, have little clinical utility in the prediction or diagnosis of common obesity. Clearly, changes in behavioral, social, and environmental factors, instead of changes in genetic factors, are the driving forces behind the obesity epidemic that is unfolding globally. However, given the same obesogenic environment, individuals with different genetic backgrounds may have different trajectories of weight gain during childhood or adulthood, suggesting that genetic susceptibility may modify the effects of diet and lifestyle on obesity risk.

Current strategies for identifying additional genetic influence of obesity are focused on less common variants and the interplay between genes and the environment. Ongoing studies are harnessing the resources of large, well-powered population-based studies for initial discovery, replication, whole-genome sequencing, and data mining of gene–gene and gene–environment interactions for common obesity. Fine mapping and functional studies following significant signals identified by GWAS are being conducted to identify causal variants. Additional genetic factors such as rare genetic variants, copy number variations, and heritable changes, which affect gene function but do not modify DNA sequence such as epigenetic modifications (see Chapter 13 for more details), and non-coding RNA await intensive investigation. In the coming years, animal models, gene expression studies, and advances in genomic technology will continue to provide insights into the biological mechanisms underlying obesity and reveal novel genetic determinants for obesity and related anthropometric measures.

Determinants related to childbearing

Parity

Normal pregnancy, in particular the third trimester, is characterized by profound metabolic stresses on maternal lipid and glucose homeostasis, including marked insulin resistance and hyperinsulinemia, favoring the transfer of nutrients to the fetus [46]. Most women gain substantial weight throughout adulthood, and for some women, pregnancy substantially alters their weight-gain trajectory. Pregnancy has been regarded as an example of natural weight cycling, itself a risk factor for weight gain [47]. An increase in the degree of obesity with each additional child has been observed [48]; on average, each successive birth adds approximately 1 kg of postpartum body weight above that normally gained with age [49]. For this reason, any effect of parity on weight may be influenced not only by maternal age but also by the interval between the index and a second or any other subsequent pregnancy [50].

To investigate the impact of pregnancy on long-term weight gain and weight loss, it is necessary to follow study participants for a sufficient length of time after delivery. Inferences from the majority of available studies on childbearing and weight cycling, however, have been limited by small sample size, short duration of follow-up, and low retention rate. Findings from available longitudinal studies generally support the positive association between parity and risk of being overweight or obesity after pregnancy. For instance, a longitudinal study of US women aged 25 to 45 years at baseline found a 60% to 110% greater risk of becoming overweight among women with one birth when compared with women without births during the ten-year follow-up period [51]. Similarly, in an analysis from the US National Longitudinal Survey of Youth cohort, the five-year risk of developing obesity among women giving birth to at least one child was 3.5 times higher than women who had never given birth; this risk was notably greater for African American, Mexican American, and socioeconomically disadvantaged women [52]. Moreover, in a population-based sample of 2070 women aged 18 to 30 years at baseline in the CARDIA study, an excess weight gain of 3 kg to 6 kg was associated with having one or more pregnancies, or a first birth during ten years of follow-up among overweight women who had previously never given birth [53].

Gestational weight gain and postpartum weight retention

In addition to parity, factors related to childbearing such as pre-pregnancy overweight, excessive pregnancy weight gain, and postpartum weight retention were associated with long-term overweight and obesity [54]. In particular, excessive gestational weight gain is the most important predictor of postpartum weight retention [52]. See Chapters 8, 14 and 19 for more details.

Postpartum weight is made up of several components including uterine and mammary tissues, body water (intracellular and extracellular water), and fat. Abrupt decreases in skin folds have been observed after delivery, with total measures decreasing by 6.5 mm in two to three days postpartum, indicating great anthropometric changes after pregnancy [55]. However, postpartum weight retention has been observed among many women. National Maternal and Infant Health Survey data of 1988 indicate that 44% of White and 63% of Black women retain ≥4 lbs (1.81 kg) after pregnancy [56]. A more recent review of the data from five pregnancy cohort studies showed that 13% to 20% of women experienced postpartum weight retention of ≥5 lbs (2.27 kg) one year after pregnancy [51]. In addition to effects of retained gestational weight gain, postpartum weight retention is most likely due to a combination of factors occurring in the postpartum period, such as diet, physical activity, duration

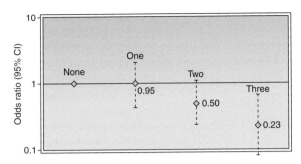

Figure 2.2. Odds ratios of retaining at least 5 kg at one year postpartum according to the number of beneficial postpartum behaviors. Beneficial behaviors defined as [1] being below the median for trans fat intake, [2] watching less than two hours of television daily, and [3] walking at least 30 minutes daily (p for trend across categories <0.001). Reproduced with permission from reference [59], © 2007, *American Journal of Preventive Medicine*.

of lactation, and depression [57–59]. For instance, in a prospective cohort study of 902 pregnant women enrolled in Project Viva, television viewing and trans fat intake in the early postpartum period were positively associated, and walking inversely associated, with substantial weight retention at one year postpartum [59]. Effects of these three behaviors were additive; women who watched less than two hours of television, walked at least 30 minutes, and consumed below the median amount of trans fat daily had an estimated 77% reduced odds of retaining at least 5 kg compared with women who reported none of the beneficial behaviors (Figure 2.2). Relatively few studies have investigated weight retention beyond two years postpartum. In a US study following women after pregnancy, pregnancy weight gain and failure to lose weight in an appreciable time were found to be the most significant predictors of obesity up to 15 years after pregnancy [49,60]; excessive postpartum weight retention at six months postpartum was associated with a weight increase of 10 kg 15 years after the index pregnancy [60].

Lactation

The role of breastfeeding/lactation in postpartum weight management has recently begun to draw greater attention. As discussed previously in the present chapter, during pregnancy, dramatic changes occur in a woman's metabolism to accommodate the demands of "metabolizing for two." These changes not only support the development of the fetus but also facilitate the accumulation of energy stores in anticipation of lactation [61]. The metabolic change is characterized by increases in visceral fat, insulin production, insulin

resistance, and circulating lipid levels [46]. Lactation may play a central role in mobilizing these accumulated fat stores and "resetting" maternal metabolism after delivery, and that is a significant dose–effect association; the longer a woman lactates, the more completely she loses these accumulated stores [61].

Epidemiological studies on the association between lactation and weight change after pregnancy, however, yield conflicting results [61]. The inconsistency in findings could result from heterogeneity in measures of lactation duration and intensity, duration of follow-up, statistical power due to sample sizes, retention rates, and in characteristics of study population, e.g., inclusion of dieters in the non-breastfeeding group, as well as analytical approach, e.g., whether confounding factors were sufficiently controlled for. In early studies of Dutch and Swedish women [62,63], formula-feeding mothers consumed fewer calories than breastfeeding mothers and lost substantially more weight in the first two to three months postpartum. From three to six months postpartum, however, weight loss among breastfeeding women increased substantially. Similar results were obtained in a longitudinal study of 85 US women followed up for 24 months [64]. There were no significant differences in weight loss in the first three months, but thereafter, women who breastfed for 12 months or more lost 2 kg more than women who breastfed for three months or less. These differences persisted at 24 months postpartum. Moreover, data from two randomized trials of low-income primiparous women [65] in Honduras indicated that greater frequency of breastfeeding from four to six months postpartum led to greater weight loss among mothers of normal birthweight infants. Studies evaluating the role of breastfeeding in long-term weight management (beyond two years) are sparse and, in general, there is modest evidence that breastfeeding-associated differences in adiposity persist beyond 24 months postpartum [61]. As in other stages of life, weight changes after delivery are dependent on many factors other than lactation status, such as reduced physical activity after delivery. An ideal cohort study of the role of breastfeeding in postpartum weight loss and weight management should include data on pre-pregnancy diet, lifestyle, and weight; gestational weight gain; and breastfeeding duration and intensity; as well as postpartum diet, energy expenditure, and intentional weight loss.

Given the potential impact of diet and lifestyle on managing weight gain, the escalating burden of obesity among women of reproductive age, and the detrimental impact of maternal overweight and obesity on reproductive and pregnancy outcomes, in 2009 the American Dietetic Association and the American Society for Nutrition recommended that "all overweight and obese women of reproductive age should receive counseling prior to pregnancy, during pregnancy and in the interconception period on the roles of diet and physical activity in reproductive health" [66].

Thus far, intervention studies aimed at preventing excessive weight gain during pregnancy are sparse and findings are inconclusive (see Chapter 14). A few studies focusing on weight loss during the first year postpartum have yielded promising results [49,67–71]. Taken together, available data appear to suggest that an intervention combining calorie restriction and exercise promotion appears to be more effective than diet alone in weight management after childbirth. The combination was shown to improve weight loss postpartum and maternal cardiovascular fitness level, and preserve fat-free mass, while the diet-alone intervention reduced only fat-free mass [72].

Summary

There is no doubt that obesity has become a global epidemic. Obesity among women of reproductive age is particularly detrimental, given its high prevalence and short-term and long-term adverse health impacts on both the women themselves and their offspring. Identification of modifiable risk factors for prevention efforts is of paramount importance. In this chapter, we provide readers with an overview of major risk factors of obesity, including those that are specifically relevant to women of reproductive age. Available data support the roles of unhealthful food choices, a sedentary lifestyle, and inadequate sleep duration in the occurrence of weight gain and obesity. Childbearing-related factors such as parity, lactation, breastfeeding, gestational weight gain, and postpartum weight retention also play an important role in long-term weight gain among women. Although genetic factors also contribute to the common form of obesity, their effects are modest and explain only a small fraction of obesity in the population. Research is needed in the most effective ways to prevent weight gain through improving diet and lifestyle and promoting breastfeeding among women of reproductive age, including individual behavioral changes and creation of a supportive social environment. Minimizing gestational weight gain and reducing weight retention after pregnancy appear to be attractive public health interventions to reduce weight gain or obesity for women. Reproductive age may represent an ideal time to improve behaviors that lead to less weight gain and reduced obesity.

References

1. World Health Organization. *Obesity and Overweight. Fact sheet No. 311.* www.who.int/mediacentre/factsheets/fs311/en/index.html [Accessed January 4, 2012].

2. Flegal K M, Carroll M D, Ogden C L & Curtin L R. Prevalence and trends in obesity among US adults, 1999–2008. *JAMA* 2010;**303**:235–41.

3. World Health Organization. WHO Global Infobase: Data for Saving Lives. http/apps.who.int/infobase [Accessed January 4, 2012].

4. Ogden C L, Carroll M D, Curtin L R, McDowell M A, Tabak C J, *et al.* Prevalence of overweight and obesity in the United States, 1999–2004. *JAMA* 2006;**295**: 1549–55.

5. Gunderson E P. Childbearing and obesity in women: weight before, during, and after pregnancy. *Obstet Gynecol Clin North Am* 2009;**36**:317–32, ix.

6. Heslehurst N, Moore H, Rankin J, Ells L J, Wilkinson J R, *et al.* How can maternity services be developed to effectively address maternal obesity? A qualitative study. *Midwifery* 2010;**27**(5):e170–7.

7. Balarajan Y & Villamor E. Nationally representative surveys show recent increases in the prevalence of overweight and obesity among women of reproductive age in Bangladesh, Nepal, and India. *J Nutr* 2009;**139**:2139–44.

8. Ramlau-Hansen C H, Thulstrup A M, Nohr E A, Bonde J P, Sorensen T I, *et al.* Subfecundity in overweight and obese couples. *Hum Reprod* 2007;**22**:1634–7.

9. Nelson S M, Matthews P & Poston L. Maternal metabolism and obesity: modifiable determinants of pregnancy outcome. *Hum Reprod Update* 2010;**16**:255–75.

10. Zhang C & Ning Y. Effect of dietary and lifestyle factors on the risk of gestational diabetes: review of epidemiologic evidence. *Am J Clin Nutr* 2011;**94**(6):1975S–9S.

11. Siega-Riz A M, Viswanathan M, Moos M K, *et al.* A systematic review of outcomes of maternal weight gain according to the Institute of Medicine recommendations: birthweight, fetal growth, and postpartum weight retention. *Am J Obstet Gynecol* 2009;**20**:339–14.

12. Dietz P M, Callaghan W M, Cogswell M E, Morrow B, Ferre C, *et al.* Combined effects of prepregnancy body mass index and weight gain during pregnancy

on the risk of preterm delivery. *Epidemiology* 2006;**17**:170–7.

13. Hu F B. Diet, nutrition and obesity. In Hu F B (ed.) *Obesity Epidemiology*. (New York: Oxford University Press, 2008).

14. Field A E, Willett W C, Lissner L & Colditz G A. Dietary fat and weight gain among women in the Nurses' Health Study. *Obesity (Silver Spring)* 2007;**15**: 967–76.

15. Heitmann B L, Lissner L, Sorensen T I & Bengtsson C. Dietary fat intake and weight gain in women genetically predisposed for obesity. *Am J Clin Nutr* 1995;**61**: 1213–17.

16. Howard B V, Manson J E, Stefanick M L, *et al.* Low-fat dietary pattern and weight change over 7 years: the Women's Health Initiative Dietary Modification Trial. *JAMA* 2006;**295**:39–49.

17. Hu F B & Willett W C. Optimal diets for prevention of coronary heart disease. *JAMA* 2002;**288**:2569–78.

18. Ma Y, Li Y, Chiriboga D E, *et al.* Association between carbohydrate intake and serum lipids. *J Am Coll Nutr* 2006;**25**:155–63.

19. Mozaffarian D, Hao T, Rimm E B, Willett W C & Hu F B. Changes in diet and lifestyle and long-term weight gain in women and men. *N Engl J Med* 2011;**364**:2392–404.

20. Duffey K J & Popkin B M. Shifts in patterns and consumption of beverages between 1965 and 2002. *Obesity (Silver Spring)* 2007;**15**:2739–47.

21. Malik V S, Schulze M B & Hu F B. Intake of sugar-sweetened beverages and weight gain: a systematic review. *Am J Clin Nutr* 2006;**84**:274–88.

22. Kinross J M, von Roon A C, Holmes E, Darzi A & Nicholson J K. The human gut microbiome: implications for future health care. *Curr Gastroenterol Rep* 2008;**10**:396–403.

23. Popkin B M. Nutrition in transition: the changing global nutrition challenge. *Asia Pac J Clin Nutr* 2001;**10**(Suppl):S13–S18.

24. Hu F B. Physical activity, sedentary behaviors, and obesity. In Hu F B (ed.) *Obesity Epidemiology*. (New York: Oxford University Press, 2008).

25. Wareham N J, van Sluijs E M & Ekelund U. Physical activity and obesity prevention: a review of the current evidence. *Proc Nutr Soc* 2005;**64**:229–47.

26. Coakley E H, Rimm E B, Colditz G, Kawachi I & Willett W. Predictors of weight change in men: results from the Health Professionals Follow-up Study. *Int J Obes Relat Metab Disord* 1998;**22**:89–96.

27. Schmitz K H, Jacobs D R, Jr., Leon A S, Schreiner P J & Sternfeld B. Physical activity and body weight: associations over ten years in the CARDIA study.

Coronary Artery Risk Development in Young Adults. *Int J Obes Relat Metab Disord* 2000;**24**:1475–87.

28. Hu F B, Li T Y, Colditz G A, Willett W C & Manson J E. Television watching and other sedentary behaviors in relation to risk of obesity and type 2 diabetes mellitus in women. *JAMA* 2003;**289**:1785–91.

29. Van C E, Spiegel K, Tasali E & Leproult R. Metabolic consequences of sleep and sleep loss. *Sleep Med* 2008;**9**(Suppl 1): S23–S28.

30. Spiegel K, Tasali E, Leproult R & Van C E. Effects of poor and short sleep on glucose metabolism and obesity risk. *Nat Rev Endocrinol* 2009;**5**:253–61.

31. Patel S R & Hu F B. Short sleep duration and weight gain: a systematic review. *Obesity (Silver Spring)* 2008;**16**:643–53.

32. Bennett, G G. Social determinants of obesity. In Hu F B (ed.) *Obesity Epidemiology*. (New York: Oxford University Press, 2008).

33. Block J P, He Y, Zaslavsky A M, Ding L & Ayanian J Z. Psychosocial stress and change in weight among US adults. *Am J Epidemiol* 2009;**170**:181–92.

34. Bornstein S R, Schuppenies A, Wong M L & Licinio J. Approaching the shared biology of obesity and depression: the stress axis as the locus of gene–environment interactions. *Mol Psychiatry* 2006;**11**:892–902.

35. O'Rahilly S. Human genetics illuminates the paths to metabolic disease. *Nature* 2009;**462**:307–14.

36. O'Rahilly S & Farooqi I S. Human obesity: a heritable neurobehavioral disorder that is highly sensitive to environmental conditions. *Diabetes* 2008;**57**:2905–10.

37. Herrera B M & Lindgren C M. The genetics of obesity. *Curr Diab Rep* 2010;**10**:498–505.

38. Herrera B M, Keildson S & Lindgren C M. Genetics and epigenetics of obesity. *Maturitas* 2011;**69**:41–9.

39. Selby J V, Newman B, Quesenberry C P, Jr., Fabsitz R R, King M C, *et al.* Evidence of genetic influence on central body fat in middle-aged twins. *Hum Biol* 1989;**61**:179–94.

40. Rose K M, Newman B, Mayer-Davis E J & Selby J V. Genetic and behavioral determinants of waist-hip ratio and waist circumference in women twins. *Obes Res* 1998;**6**:383–92.

41. Frayling T M, Timpson N J, Weedon M N, *et al.* A common variant in the FTO gene is associated with body mass index and predisposes to childhood and adult obesity. *Science* 2007;**316**:889–94.

42. Scuteri A, Sanna S, Chen W M, *et al.* Genome-wide association scan shows genetic variants in the FTO gene are associated with obesity-related traits. *PLoS Genet* 2007;**3**:e115.

43. Barrett J C & Cardon L R. Evaluating coverage of genome-wide association studies. *Nat Genet* 2006;**38**:659–62.

44. Pe'er I, de Bakker P I, Maller J, Yelensky R, Altshuler D, *et al.* Evaluating and improving power in whole-genome association studies using fixed marker sets. *Nat Genet* 2006;**38**:663–7.

45. Heid I M, Jackson A U, Randall J C, *et al.* Meta-analysis identifies 13 new loci associated with waist-hip ratio and reveals sexual dimorphism in the genetic basis of fat distribution. *Nat Genet* 2010;**42**:949–60.

46. Knopp R H, Bergelin R O, Wahl P W, Walden C E, Chapman M, *et al.* Population-based lipoprotein lipid reference values for pregnant women compared to nonpregnant women classified by sex hormone usage. *Am J Obstet Gynecol* 1982;**143**:626–37.

47. Kim S A, Stein A D & Martorell R. Country development and the association between parity and overweight. *Int J Obes (Lond)* 2007;**31**:805–12.

48. Weng H H, Bastian L A, Taylor D H, Jr., Moser B K & Ostbye T. Number of children associated with obesity in middle-aged women and men: results from the health and retirement study. *J Womens Health (Larchmt.)* 2004;**13**:85–91.

49. Melzer K & Schutz Y. Pre-pregnancy and pregnancy predictors of obesity. *Int J Obes (Lond)* 2010;**34**(Suppl 2):S44–S52.

50. Billewicz W Z. Body weight in parous women. *Br J Prev Soc Med* 1970;**24**:97–104.

51. Rooney B L & Schauberger C W. Excess pregnancy weight gain and long-term obesity: one decade later. *Obstet Gynecol* 2002;**100**: 245–52.

52. Davis E M, Zyzanski S J, Olson C M, Stange K C & Horwitz R I. Racial, ethnic, and socioeconomic differences in the incidence of obesity related to childbirth. *Am J Public Health* 2009;**99**:294–9.

53. Gunderson E P, Murtaugh M A, Lewis C E, Quesenberry C P, West D S, *et al.* Excess gains in weight and waist circumference associated with childbearing: The Coronary Artery Risk Development in Young Adults Study (CARDIA). *Int J Obes Relat Metab Disord* 2004;**28**:525–35.

54. Gunderson E P. Childbearing and obesity in women: weight before, during, and after pregnancy. *Obstet Gynecol Clin North Am* 2009;**36**:317–32, ix.

55. Taggart N R, Holliday R M, Billewicz W Z, Hytten F E & Thomson A M. Changes in skinfolds during pregnancy. *Br J Nutr* 1967;**21**:439–51.

56. Keppel K G & Taffel S M. Pregnancy-related weight gain and retention: implications of the 1990 Institute of Medicine guidelines. *Am J Public Health* 1993;**83**:1100–3.

57. Stuebe A M, Kleinman K, Gillman M W, Rifas-Shiman S L, Gunderson E P, *et al.* Duration of lactation and maternal metabolism at 3 years postpartum. *J Womens Health (Larchmt.)* 2010;**19**:941–50.

58. Herring S J, Rich-Edwards J W, Oken E, Rifas-Shiman S L, Kleinman K P, *et al.* Association of postpartum depression with weight retention 1 year after childbirth. *Obesity (Silver Spring)* 2008;**16**: 1296–301.

59. Oken E, Taveras E M, Popoola F A, Rich-Edwards J W & Gillman M W. Television, walking, and diet: associations with postpartum weight retention. *Am J Prev Med* 2007;**32**:305–11.

60. Rooney B L, Schauberger C W & Mathiason M A. Impact of perinatal weight change on long-term obesity and obesity-related illnesses. *Obstet Gynecol* 2005;**106**:1349–56.

61. Stuebe A M & Rich-Edwards J W. The reset hypothesis: lactation and maternal metabolism. *Am J Perinatol* 2009;**26**:81–8.

62. van Raaij J M, Schonk C M, Vermaat-Miedema S H, Peek M E & Hautvast J G. Energy cost of lactation, and energy balances of well-nourished Dutch lactating women: reappraisal of the extra energy requirements of lactation. *Am J Clin Nutr* 1991;**53**:612–19.

63. Sadurskis A, Kabir N, Wager J & Forsum E. Energy metabolism, body composition, and milk production in healthy Swedish women during lactation. *Am J Clin Nutr* 1988;**48**:44–9.

64. Dewey K G, Heinig M J & Nommsen L A. Maternal weight-loss patterns during prolonged lactation. *Am J Clin Nutr* 1993;**58**:162–6.

65. Dewey K G, Cohen R J, Brown K H & Rivera L L. Effects of exclusive breastfeeding for four versus six months on maternal nutritional status and infant motor development: results of two randomized trials in Honduras. *J Nutr* 2001;**131**:262–7.

66. Siega-Riz A M & King J C. Position of the American Dietetic Association and American Society for Nutrition: obesity, reproduction, and pregnancy outcomes. *J Am Diet Assoc* 2009;**109**:918–27.

67. Walker L O. Managing excessive weight gain during pregnancy and the postpartum period. *J Obstet Gynecol Neonatal Nurs* 2007;**36**:490–500.

68. Leermakers E A, Anglin K & Wing R R. Reducing postpartum weight retention through a correspondence intervention. *Int J Obes Relat Metab Disord* 1998;**22**:1103–9.

69. Lovelady C A, Garner K E, Moreno K L & Williams J P. The effect of weight loss in overweight, lactating women on the growth of their infants. *N Engl J Med* 2000;**342**:449–53.

70. O'Toole M L, Sawicki M A & Artal R. Structured diet and physical activity prevent postpartum weight retention. *J Womens Health (Larchmt.)* 2003;**12**:991–8.

71. Dusdieker L B, Hemingway D L & Stumbo P J. Is milk production impaired by dieting during lactation? *Am J Clin Nutr* 1994;**59**:833–40.

72. Amorim A R, Linne Y M & Lourenco P M. Diet or exercise, or both, for weight reduction in women after childbirth. *Cochrane Database Syst Rev* 2007;CD005627.

Chapter

3

Obesity and fertility

Jorge E. Chavarro and Thomas L. Toth

Introduction

The role of body weight on human reproductive function and fertility has received considerable attention in the medical literature. A multitude of studies have documented the effects of underweight on fertility in a variety of populations. These include studies of seasonal patterns in fertility rates associated with food availability in agricultural societies and studies documenting menstrual cycle abnormalities among lean women in Western populations either engaging in extremely demanding physical activities (such as competitive sports or professional ballet) or suffering from eating disorders [1,2]. Cumulatively, these data led to the identification that the adipose tissue plays a critical role in regulating female reproductive function. Frish was the first to propose that a certain minimum amount of adipose tissue was necessary for the initiation and maintenance of menstrual function and fertility [2]. It is currently known that the effects of undernutrition on infertility are caused by hypothalamic dysfunction and decreased gonadotropin secretion possibly due to decreased signaling of leptin to the hypothalamus [3].

The opposite end of the body weight spectrum has only recently gained attention on its potential role on fertility due in part to the rapidly increasing prevalence of overweight and obesity worldwide. Even though polycystic ovary syndrome (PCOS), the most common cause of anovulation and a frequent cause of infertility, was first described in 1935 [4] and that some clinicians might have been aware of a connection between obesity and lower chances of conception as early as the fourteenth century [5], systematic investigations of the role of overweight and obesity did not take place until the 1980s and the biological mechanisms underlying this association are still being disentangled.

Obesity and spontaneous fertility

Overweight, obesity, and overall fertility

Several studies have attempted to estimate the overall effect of excess body weight on female fertility. Jokela and collaborators found that among a nationally representative group of American women born between 1957 and 1964, being overweight or obese at age 17 to 24 was associated with a lower cumulative probability of having one or more children by age 47 [6]. Being overweight was associated with a 3% (CI: 2%–3%) lower chance of having a first child and being obese was associated with a 13% (4%–21%) lower chance of having a first child by age 47 after taking into account differences in marital status, suggesting a true biological effect of excess body weight on fertility [6].

Time-to-pregnancy studies, where the time taken to achieve a conception is compared among women who have recently become pregnant (retrospective) or among couples prospectively followed as they try to conceive (prospective), provide a more accurate estimate of the overall biological effect of excess body weight on female fertility. Some of the earliest time-to-pregnancy studies did not find an association between body weight and fecundability, the probability of conceiving in any given menstrual cycle [7,8]. The authors in these papers did not provide details of their findings but rather reported that the results were not significant [7,8]. However, several subsequent studies suggest that excess body weight has, in fact, a deleterious effect on fertility although there is substantial variation in the estimated magnitude of this relation. Jensen and collaborators examined retrospectively a group of 10 903 Danish women who had planned their pregnancies. They found that being overweight

---

or obese (BMI $\geq 25\,kg/m^2$) was associated with a 23% (16%–30%) lower chance of becoming pregnant in any given menstrual cycle and an 82% (50%–120%) increased risk of taking 12 months or more to conceive compared to women with a BMI between 20 and $25\,kg/m^2$ [9]. Studies where BMI has been categorized more finely suggest that the risk of decreased fecundity increases with higher body weight. In a study of 7327 American women who had planned their pregnancies, being overweight was not significantly associated to fecundity but being obese (BMI $\geq 30\,kg/m^2$) was associated with an 18% (5%–28%) lower chance of pregnancy in a given cycle when compared to women with a BMI between 18.5 and $24.9\,kg/m^2$ [10]. The association between obesity and decreased fecundity remained significant even after statistical adjustment for menstrual cycle regularity (fecundability ratio (FR) 95% CI = 0.85: 0.74–0.99). Likewise, Lake and collaborators found that being overweight (defined in this study as BMI $23.9–28.6\,kg/m^2$) at age 23 was unrelated to fecundability whereas being obese (BMI $>28.6\,kg/m^2$) was associated with a 33% (13%–48%) lower chance of conception per cycle in a group of 3327 women representative of the general UK population in comparison to lean women (BMI $18.8–23.8\,kg/m^2$) [11]. Similar results were reported by Bolumar and collaborators in a study of 4035 women recruited from five European countries. Women with a BMI between 20 and $24.9\,kg/m^2$ served as the reference category. In this study overweight was unrelated to fecundity [12]. Obese women, however, were 48% (17%–67%) less likely to conceive in any given cycle if they were also smokers but not if they were non-smokers. Interestingly, among women who had never been pregnant before, being obese was associated with a 72% (20%–90%) lower fecundability if they were also smokers [12]. The interaction between smoking and obesity documented in this study has not been replicated in other studies.

Other time-to-pregnancy studies have found evidence of decreased fecundity among both overweight and obese women. Hassan and colleagues found that, compared to women with a BMI between 19 and $24.9\,kg/m^2$, women who were either overweight, class I obese, or class II obese were more than twice as likely (relative risk [RR] 95% CI: 2.2 [1.6–3.2]) and women who were class III obese were nearly seven times more likely (RR 95% CI: 6.9 [2.9–16.8]) to take more than 12 months conceiving [13]. In the largest time-to-pregnancy study conducted to date (47 835 Danish couples), overweight women were 27% (18%–36%),

and obese women were 78% (63%–95%) more likely to take more than 12 months to conceive than normal weight women after taking into consideration their partner's BMI [14], which has also been related to a couple's fertility (see below). Likewise, in the largest prospective time-to-pregnancy study conducted to date (1651 Danish couples) fecundability decreased linearly with increasing BMI after taking into account their waist circumference, menstrual cycle regularity, their partner's BMI, and other risk factors for infertility (Figure 3.1) [15]. Of note, waist circumference and waist-to-hip ratio (WHR) were unrelated to fecundability in this study.

There is some suggestion, however, that the distribution of adipose tissue may also play a role in female fertility. Zaadstra and collaborators conducted a study among 489 women undergoing intracervical insemination without controlled ovarian hyperstimulation for male factor infertility. Women were inseminated with donor sperm and their BMI and WHR were related to their fecundability. In univariate analyses, both BMI and WHR were inversely related to the per-cycle probability of conception. The FR (95% CI) per one WHR unit increase was 0.70 (0.57–0.87) and the FR (95% CI) comparing obese women to women with a BMI between 20 and $24.9\,kg/m^2$ was 0.37 (0.15–0.89). When BMI and WHR were simultaneously included in the same regression model, the association between BMI and fecundability was slightly attenuated and failed to reach statistical significance (FR 95% CI: 0.43 [0.17–1.09]) whereas WHR remained associated with lower fecundability (FR 95% CI: 0.71 [0.56–0.89]) [16]. These findings suggest that central obesity may also be an important determinant of female fertility.

Time-to-pregnancy studies are very useful in determining the overall effects of any exposure on overall fertility. However, they do not provide much insight into what specific physiologic processes might be affecting fertility. From these types of studies it is not possible to determine whether obesity is affecting exclusively ovulation, fertilization, embryo development or implantation, or even if the apparent association is due to a male exposure that is strongly related to female obesity. The studies discussed above, particularly the ones that were able to account for male BMI [14–16], suggest that there is a true biological effect on female reproductive physiology. However, pointing to a specific pathology requires other types of studies.

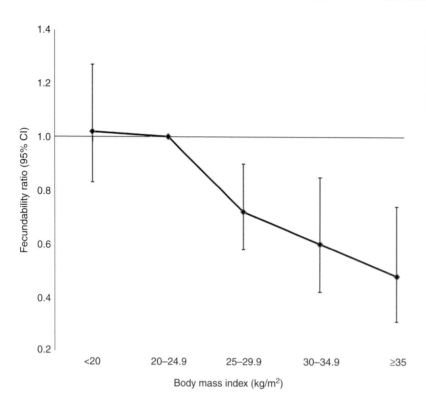

Figure 3.1. Fecundability ratios according to body mass index categories among Danish pregnancy planners. A fecundability ratio lower than one indicates a reduced probability of conception in a given menstrual cycle. Adapted from Wise *et al.* [15]

Overweight, obesity, and infertility due to specific causes

So far, disordered ovulation has been the underlying cause of infertility most commonly associated with overweight and obesity. Green and colleagues conducted a case-control study involving 308 cases of ovulatory infertility living in King County, WA. Ovulatory infertility was defined as infertility with evidence of ovulatory dysfunction by oligomenorrhea, amenorrhea, or abnormalities in basal body temperature charts consistent with anovulation. In this study, nulligravid women who were more than 120% of their ideal body weight according to the Metropolitan Life Insurance tables had twice the risk of ovulatory infertility than nulligravid women between 85% and 120% of their ideal body weight [17]. Body weight was not associated with ovulatory infertility among women experiencing secondary infertility (infertility following a successful spontaneous pregnancy). Similar results were observed by Grodstein and collaborators in a case-control study of 597 nulligravid women recruited from six fertility centers in the United States and Canada who received a diagnosis of ovulatory infertility (documented by abnormalities in basal body temperature charts,

endometrial biopsy, or hormonal measurements consistent with anovulation) as their first or second infertility diagnosis. Women with a BMI $\geq$27 kg/m² had three times the risk of ovulatory infertility than women with a BMI between 20 and 24.9 kg/m². When specific pathologies were examined, the association between BMI and ovulatory infertility was strongest for women with PCOS (six-fold greater risk) and women with hypogonadism (3.6-fold greater risk) [18].

Analyses of the Nurses' Health Study II cohort on ovulatory infertility have been consistent with the previous studies and provided additional insights into the relation between body weight and fertility. The initial report stemming from this cohort described that the risk of ovulatory infertility increased linearly with increasing BMI, even within the range of BMI considered normal. Women with a BMI at age 18 of 22 kg/m² or higher were at an increased risk of ovulatory infertility compared to women with a BMI between 20 and 21.9 kg/m², the lowest risk BMI category. Risk increased linearly with greater BMI levels at age 18, reaching a plateau at a BMI of 30 kg/m² or higher, which was associated with a 2.7-fold greater risk of this condition [19]. Body mass index at age 18 was also associated to a higher rate of long ($\geq$40 days) or irregular menstrual cycles [19].

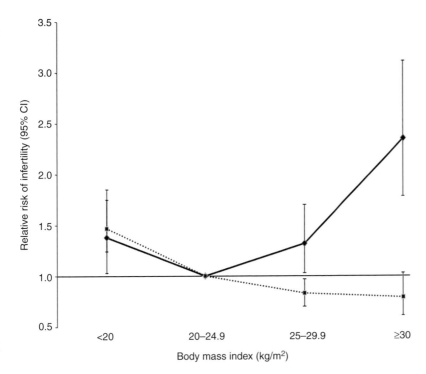

Figure 3.2. Body mass index in relation to infertility due to ovulation disorders (solid line) and other causes of infertility (dotted line). Adapted from Chavarro *et al.* [21]

Subsequent analyses of this cohort have found that the J-shape relation between adult BMI and risk of ovulatory infertility is similar to that described for BMI at age 18 [20,21]. However, for adult BMI the range associated with the lowest risk of infertility is slightly wider than for adolescent BMI, ranging from 20 to 24 kg/m², and the risk of infertility does not appear to plateau at any BMI level [20]. In addition, data from this study suggest that the association of overweight and obesity with ovulatory infertility is not modified by a woman's age or parity, and that overweight and obesity are not associated with infertility due to other common causes of infertility (Figure 3.2) [21]. Moreover, these data also suggest that the population burden of infertility due to obesity in the United States is more than double the population burden due to underweight [20].

There are additional data suggesting that obesity has deleterious effects on female fertility independent of its effects on ovulation. van der Steeg and colleagues followed a cohort of 3209 couples who had unsuccessfully tried to become pregnant and in whom normal ovulation, tubal patency, and no severe semen abnormalities were documented [22]. Couples with a high predicted probability of conception were advised to continue trying to become pregnant without treatment and were followed until they became pregnant or initiated infertility treatment. There were no significant differences in fecundability in the BMI range of 21 to 29 kg/m². In couples where the woman had a BMI >29 kg/m², fecundability decreased linearly with increasing BMI with the probability of conception decreasing by 4% (1%–9%) for every unit increase in BMI [22]. This study strongly suggests that there are aspects of reproductive physiology beyond ovulation, such as functional characteristics of gametes not routinely captured in clinical practice and early embryo development, which are affected by excess body weight and lead to decreased fertility. Consistent with this interpretation, Igosheva and colleagues found that, in a murine model of diet-induced obesity, oocytes of obese mice had altered mitochondrial distribution as well as increased mitochondrial activity, mitochondrial DNA, and oxidation of reactive oxygen species [23]. Furthermore, embryos of obese females were less likely to reach the blastocyst stage than embryos of lean mice [23].

Another potential mechanism explaining the association between female obesity and decreased fertility is that obese men have reduced reproductive capacity. Body mass index is positively correlated within a couple [24]. Therefore failure to account for male BMI in studies of the effects of female BMI on the couple's fertility could lead to an overestimation of the effects of female obesity on fertility. It is well known that obesity leads to alteration of reproductive hormone levels in men including increased circulating estradiol, decreased testosterone, SHBG, and inhibin B levels, and, in morbidly obese men, alterations in gonadotropin secretion [25–29]. The extent to which these endocrine changes lead to decreased fertility is not completely understood, however. Male overweight and obesity have been related to decreased fertility [30–33] and have been associated with deleterious effects on a number of semen analysis parameters including concentration [27,34–37], ejaculate volume [29,38], and total sperm count [27,29,36,38]. The most consistent positive finding across studies has been lower sperm concentration among overweight and obese men compared to normal weight men. In a recent meta-analysis including data from 14 studies and 9779 individuals, being overweight was associated with an 11% (1%–20%) greater risk of oligospermia and a 39% (–2%–97%) greater risk of azoospermia, while being obese was associated with a 42% (12%–79%) greater risk of oligospermia and an 81% (23%–166%) greater risk of azoospermia [39]. Also consistent, however, have been null findings on other semen quality parameters, including sperm motility [27–29,36,37,40,41], and morphology [27–29,36,40]. Conventional semen quality parameters (sperm concentration, motility, and morphology) may not fully characterize male fertility potential and additional functional measures may be necessary. Two studies have so far examined whether overweight and obesity is associated to measures of sperm DNA integrity. Although the studies used different techniques to assess sperm DNA damage, both concluded that obesity is associated with higher sperm DNA damage [29,42], which could translate into lower fertility [43]. Also, in a study among 305 couples undergoing assisted reproductive technology (ART) treatment for infertility, paternal BMI was associated with delayed blastocyst development and lower pregnancy and live birth rates [44]. Clearly more studies are needed in this area to clarify the independent effect of male body weight on a couple's fertility.

In summary, overweight and obese women have lower chances of spontaneous conception. There appear to be multiple mechanisms explaining this association. Anovulation, particularly as it relates to PCOS, appears to be one of the most important pathologies leading to decreased fertility. However, the effect of increased body weight on anovulation does not appear to be restricted

to women with PCOS. Moreover, several studies have shown that anovulation is not the only factor explaining the relation between obesity and decreased fertility. Defects in implantation, early embryonic development, and male contributions may also be at play. However, most of these factors are unobservable in couples attempting natural conception and it is therefore not possible to assess their individual contributions to overall fertility among couples attempting to conceive naturally.

Obesity and treatment outcomes among women undergoing assisted reproductive technology (ART) treatments

Studying the role of overweight and obesity among couples undergoing ART can serve multiple purposes. First, it provides clinically useful information addressing the specific needs of infertile couples and their clinicians as they attempt assisted conceptions. Second, ART provides a unique opportunity to study the role of obesity on reproductive physiology and pathology in a level of detail that is impossible to achieve among couples attempting natural conceptions (Figure 3.3). By externalizing the processes of fertilization and early embryonic development and closely monitoring the early development of a pregnancy, many of the steps involved in producing a viable pregnancy, including the ovarian response to gonadotropins, gamete quality, fertilization, early embryo development, implantation, and preclinical pregnancy outcomes, can be observed and evaluated.

Ovarian response to controlled ovarian hyperstimulation

Cycles involve stimulation of ovulation in order to retrieve multiple viable oocytes and the development of one or more embryos for subsequent transfer to the uterus. Spontaneous ovulation cannot, therefore, be studied in ART cycles. Nevertheless, since ovulation is achieved using supraphysiologic doses of the same hormones that naturally stimulate ovulation (or their analogues), it is possible to use the responses of the ovary to controlled hyperstimulation to gain insights into ovarian physiology.

The total dose of gonadotropins or the length of the stimulation protocol can serve as a marker of the

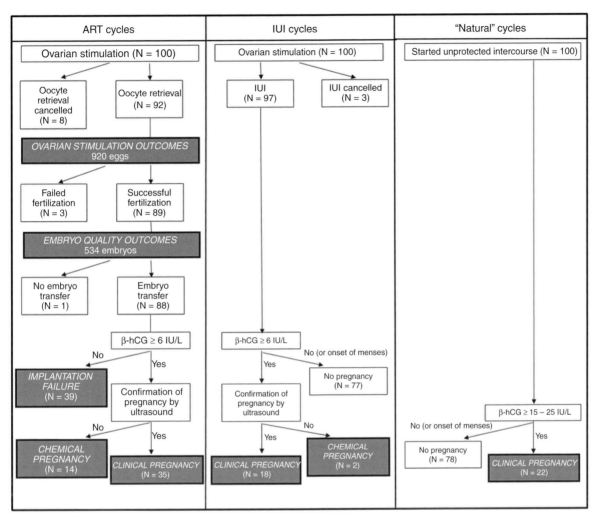

Figure 3.3. Comparison of observable outcomes prior to the recognition of a clinical pregnancy according to mode of conception. ART: assisted reproductive technology; IUI: intrauterine insemination. Numbers represent the number of women or observations that would be expected in one cycle of attempted conception in three hypothetical cohorts of 100 women regardless of BMI. Numbers for ART and IUI cycles are based on observed frequencies among participants of the EARTH Study at the Massachusetts General Hospital Fertility Center. Numbers for "natural" cycles are based on data from Wilcox *et al.* [73]

sensitivity of the ovary to FSH, which stimulates ovulation under physiologic conditions. Seventeen studies have examined to date the association between body weight and the dose of gonadotropins required to stimulate ovulation in in vitro fertilization (IVF) or intra-cytoplasmic sperm injection (ICSI) cycles. The majority of these studies have reported either a higher total dose of gonadotropins [45–49], a higher number of gonadotropin ampoules used [50–53], or a longer duration of stimulation protocol [46,51,54] with increasing BMI. For example, Bellver and colleagues analyzed the outcomes of 6500 cycles from a single clinic in Spain and found that the total dose

of FSH required to induce ovulation increased from 2184 IU for women with a BMI below 20 kg/m^2 to 2394 IU for obese women (BMI ≥30 kg/m^2) [45]. The effect of BMI on ovarian sensitivity to gonadotropins does not appear to reach a threshold among obese women, however. Awartani and colleagues compared class I obesity women to class II and class III obesity women undergoing IVF and found that, even among obese women, gonadotropin requirements increased with higher BMI [55]. The studies that have failed to find this association [56–60] are, with few exceptions [61], small studies usually involving no more than 500 ART cycles.

Despite the higher dose of gonadotropins required to stimulate ovulation in obese women, they appear to produce fewer oocytes and fewer mature oocytes than lean women. Of the 21 studies that have examined the relation between BMI and oocyte yield, 11 have found lower yield when comparing the leanest women to the most obese women in each study [46,47,51,52,55,59,62–66]. Among the 11 studies that have reported lower oocyte yield with increasing BMI, which collectively represent 8068 women undergoing 11,188 ART cycles, the magnitude of the association between BMI and oocyte yield ranges from a 7% lower yield [62] to a 25% lower yield [66] with the majority of studies reporting a reduction in oocyte yield of approximately 15% to 20%. Among these studies some have found that the association between BMI and oocyte yield appears to be limited to certain subgroups. Sneed and colleagues reported a significant interaction between BMI and age whereby BMI was associated to lower oocyte yield only among women younger than 35 years [65]. Interestingly, in many of the studies that do not report a statistically significant reduction in oocyte yield among obese women [57,61,67,68] the magnitude of the association is very similar to that reported in the studies reporting a statistically significant association.

There have been fewer studies reporting on the association between BMI and yield of MII oocytes (mature oocytes). Of the nine studies conducted to date [45,47,52,54,60,63–65,67], six have reported a statistically significant lower yield of MII oocytes when comparing the leanest women to the most obese women in each study [47,52,54,63–65]. The magnitude of the association in these six studies, as well as in one of the studies where the association failed to reach statistical significance [67], closely mirrors the association for total oocyte yield.

There are two important issues to consider in describing the relation between BMI and controlled ovarian hyperstimulation outcomes. First, there are substantial differences in the approach to ovarian stimulation across the globe. In general, European specialists tend to favor lower doses of gonadotropins for stimulation and thus recover fewer eggs than their American counterparts. Thus, it is possible that part of the discrepancies across studies is attributable to differences in clinical practice. Given a set sample size, studies conducted in centers using mild stimulation protocols may fail to detect associations between BMI and ovarian stimulation outcomes because the distribution of these outcomes will be narrower than in centers using conventional stimulation protocols. It is also important to consider the mitigating effect of PCOS. Overweight and obesity are common among women with PCOS [69]. However, women with PCOS often have a greater oocyte yield [63,70] and are at an increased risk of ovarian hyperstimulation [70–72]. Thus it is significant that the associations of BMI with markers of ovarian response to controlled ovarian hyperstimulation are still present in studies that have addressed this issue by either statistically adjusting the results for diagnosis of PCOS [63] or by restricting the analyses to women without PCOS [47].

Fertilization rate

In ART cycles it is also possible to examine whether female obesity has any impact on the chances that a mature egg is fertilized. Three studies have reported an association between BMI and fertilization rate [51,62,65]. The observed differences in fertilization rate between obese and non-obese women are of approximately 8% favoring leaner women [50,51], and in one case the association was restricted to women under 36 years of age [65]. Nevertheless, an additional 11 studies, collectively representing more than 25 000 ART cycles, have found no association between BMI and fertilization rate [45–49,54,55,57,61,63,64]. Of note, while most studies have combined IVF and ICSI cycles in their analyses of fertilization rate, studies where IVF and ICSI cycles are examined separately [46] and studies restricted to ICSI cycles [47] have not found an association between BMI and fertilization rate. In sum, the studies conducted to date do not suggest an association of female overweight or obesity with fertilization rate in the setting of ART.

Embryo quality

Embryo quality is usually evaluated by assigning scores to different embryos according to their morphological characteristics on day 2 or day 3 of development. Two studies have found that obese women have significantly lower embryo quality grades either on day 2 [49] or on the day of embryo transfer [67]. However, an additional five studies have not found any association between obesity and embryo quality scores [45,46,48,53,59]. One difficulty in assessing this evidence is the multitude of embryo grading systems available and the variability of the timing of embryo grading. In the seven studies conducted to date, six different embryo grading systems have been employed and the two studies using the same system are from investigators in the same group [46,59]. Nevertheless, the preponderance of the evidence suggests that BMI is not associated with early embryo development as assessed through morphology-based embryo quality scores.

Early pregnancy loss

The loss of a pregnancy before it is clinically recognized is one of the most common failure points in the road between conception and birth. Among couples conceiving spontaneously, 22% of pregnancies end before they can be detected clinically [73] and among couples undergoing ART between 5% and 10% of pregnancies are lost before they can be clinically confirmed by ultrasound at gestation week 6 or 7 (biochemical pregnancies) [45,46].

Of the four studies that have so far examined the association between obesity and early pregnancy loss, two have reported an association between BMI and increased frequency of this outcome. Fedorcsak and colleagues reported on a cohort of 383 women undergoing IVF or ICSI. In this study the frequency of early pregnancy loss was nearly double among overweight or obese women than among lean women [59]. A subsequent report from the same group, involving 2660 women who underwent 5019 IVF or ICSI cycles, also found a relation between BMI and early pregnancy loss although the magnitude of this association was not as pronounced. Early pregnancy loss was documented in 4.8% of pregnancies among normal weight women, 5.4% of pregnancies among overweight women, and 7.8% of pregnancies among obese women [46]. However, two large studies, collectively representing 7696 IVF/ICSI cycles, have failed to detect an association between BMI and early pregnancy loss [45,74]. Whether there is a relation between obesity and early pregnancy loss in women undergoing ART remains an open question.

Clinical pregnancy rates

Clinical pregnancies, defined as the confirmation of a pregnancy by ultrasound after a rise in human chorionic gonadotropin (hCG), are one of the most commonly assessed outcomes in studies of ART. Failure to achieve a clinical pregnancy may represent either a failure of the embryo to implant in the endometrium (implantation failure) or an early pregnancy loss. To date, 24 studies encompassing more than 78 000 ART cycles have assessed the relation between BMI and clinical pregnancy rate. Fourteen of these studies (14 131 ART cycles, collectively) did not find an association of overweight or obesity with clinical pregnancy rate [47, 49,50,52,54,57,60,61,63,64,68,75].

Nevertheless, the overwhelming majority of evidence suggests that overweight and obesity decrease clinical pregnancy rates among women undergoing ART. Of the studies reporting on 5000 ART cycles or more, only Thum and colleagues failed to detect an association between obesity and clinical pregnancy rate [61]. Among the 11 studies (64 156 ART cycles, collectively) reporting this association some are worth special mention. Wang and colleagues, reporting on 8822 ART cycles from a single center in Australia, found that the probability of achieving a clinical pregnancy decreased linearly with increasing BMI after accounting for differences in age, number of embryos transferred, number of previous ART cycles, treatment protocol, and infertility diagnosis [76]. The odds of conception were 19% (3%–32%) lower for overweight women, 27% (5%–43%) lower for class I obese women, and 50% (23%–68%) lower for class II or class III obese women when compared to women with a BMI between 20 and 24.9 kg/m^2 [76]. Similar results were reported by a Spanish group presenting data on 6500 IVF/ICSI cycles from a single center [45]. A study from Saudi Arabia limited to obese women undergoing IVF found that class II and class III obese women have significantly lower clinical pregnancy rates (20%) compared to class I obese women (29%) [55], suggesting that the association between BMI and pregnancy rate may not plateau within the range of BMI observed in fertility centers. The most compelling evidence of the association between excess body weight comes from a recent report by Luke and collaborators. This study analyzed data from the SART CORS, which contains standardized clinical reports from more than 90% of the clinics performing ART in the United States. Among 45 163 ART cycles that progressed through embryo transfer, the risk of failing to achieve a clinical pregnancy increased linearly with increasing BMI [77]. The increased frequency of failure to achieve a clinical pregnancy was more pronounced among women under 35 years using their own oocytes [77]. Overall, the data available to date suggests that overweight and obesity decrease clinical pregnancy rates among women undergoing ART.

Clinical pregnancy loss

The loss of a pregnancy between its clinical confirmation and prior to gestation week 20 is a common outcome among women undergoing ART. Metwally and collaborators recently conducted a meta-analysis on the association of overweight and obesity with clinical pregnancy losses in the setting of assisted conception including oocyte donor cycles, ovulation induction cycles, and ART cycles. When all the 16 studies were analyzed (16 696 women), women with a BMI ≥25 kg/m² had a 67% greater odds of miscarriage than women with a normal BMI [78]. When data were analyzed according to mode of conception, the association was strongest for ovulation induction cycles (OR = 5.1; 95% CI: 1.8–14.8). There was an estimated 52% greater odds of miscarriage for IVF/ICSI and donor oocyte cycles but the association for IVF/ICSI cycles (8503 women) failed to reach statistical significance [78]. Since the publication of this meta-analysis, eight additional studies involving 66 175 ART cycles have been reported in the literature [45,47,50,61,63,65,77,79]. Most of the recent publications are large studies involving more than 1000 ART cycles each. The two exceptions [50,63] did not find an association between overweight and miscarriage. Among the large studies, only Sneed and colleagues

failed to detect this association [65]. All the remaining studies, documented a dose–response relationship between BMI and miscarriage risk although it failed to reach statistical significance in two studies [45,47]. In the largest study conducted to date, the rate of clinical fetal loss increased linearly from 14% among underweight women to 22% among class III obese women [77]. The results of the meta-analysis together with the studies published thereafter strongly suggest that the risk of clinical pregnancy losses increases linearly with body weight.

Live birth rates

Live births are the goal of any infertility treatment. Eleven studies have examined to date the association between BMI and live birth rates among women undergoing ART. Of these, only the two smallest ones [50,63] did not document linear decrease in live births with increasing BMI. In all the remaining studies [45,46,52,54,59,61,65,77,80] there was an absolute difference in live birth rates of approximately 5% to 10% when the leanest and heaviest women within each study were compared, although this difference failed to reach statistical significance in two studies [52,54]. In the largest study conducted to date (Figure 3.4), Luke and colleagues reported that the odds of failing

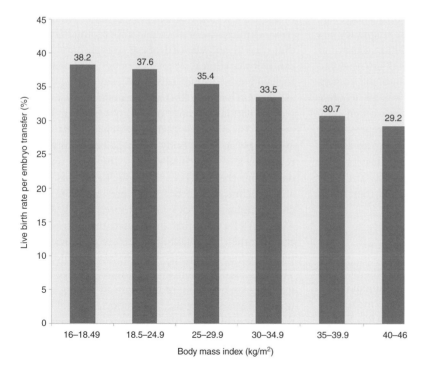

Figure 3.4. Live birth rates per embryo transfer according to BMI categories among 45 163 ART embryo transfers in the SART-CORS system. United States, 2007. Adapted from Luke *et al.* [77]

to achieve a live birth following the clinical confirmation of a pregnancy in an ART cycle was 18% higher in overweight women, 36% higher among class I and class II obese women, and 48% higher among class III obese women using their own eggs relative to normal weight women [77]. This association was slightly stronger among younger women (under 35 years) where the odds of failure to achieve a live birth were 64% greater in class III obese women compared to lean women [77].

In summary, overweight and obesity have a negative impact on ART outcomes. Overweight and obesity make the ovary more resistant to the action of gonadotropins as reflected in higher gonadotropin doses necessary in controlled ovarian hyperstimulation. In addition, it appears that the ovary is less responsive to gonadotropins as reflected by lower total and MII oocyte yields. Female overweight and obesity do not appear to influence fertilization or early embryonic development. However, overweight and obese women are less likely to have a live birth following an embryo transfer. The lower live birth rates appear to be due to a combination of a higher rate of implantation failure, early pregnancy losses, and clinical pregnancy losses.

Mechanisms

Obesity leads to a wide range of systemic alterations including changes in circulating levels of adipokines, reproductive hormones, markers of endothelial dysfunction and systemic inflammation, as well as metabolic disturbances in lipoprotein metabolism, glycemic control, and increased insulin resistance. A major challenge is to differentiate which of these obesity-induced changes are causally related to obesity's reproductive effects and which of them are epiphenomena. Although specific mechanisms for explaining the associations described in this chapter are still subject to active investigation, the strongest evidence to date suggest that obesity's effects on glycemic control and insulin resistance may be important mechanisms underlying these relations.

The strongest evidence available for a role of glycemic control on fertility stems from studies of the effects of antidiabetic medications on clinical manifestations of PCOS. Treatment of PCOS women with a wide range of oral antidiabetic medications including thiazolidinediones [81], metformin [81], d-chiro-inositol [82], and acarbose [83,84] improves ovulation rates and menstrual cycle regularity, clearly showing an effect of insulin resistance and glycemic control on ovulatory function. Furthermore, there is some evidence that antidiabetic medications may also improve fertility in PCOS women. In a recent randomized trial, PCOS women planning to undergo IVF for infertility treatment were allocated to metformin (2000 mg/day) or placebo [85]. Live birth rates were significantly higher in the treatment group (49%) than in the placebo group (32%), but this effect was due primarily to a doubling in the spontaneous pregnancy rate prior to initiation of IVF in the metformin group (20% metformin vs. 10% placebo) rather than to effects of metformin on live births among the women who underwent IVF (38% metformin vs. 29% placebo) [85]. The relations of glycemic control and insulin sensitivity with ovulatory function and fertility are also present in non-PCOS women. For example, oligomenorrheic non-PCOS infertile women are more likely to be insulin resistant and to have postprandial hyperinsulinemia than eumenorrheic infertile women [86]. Similarly, diabetic women in the general population have significantly lower fecundability than non-diabetic women [87]. Moreover, in a study of healthy pregnancy planners from the general population, HbA1c levels within the non-diabetic range were inversely related to fecundability and positively related to characteristics of PCOS (free testosterone levels and cycle irregularity) [88]. This mechanism may also explain some of the adverse outcomes of obesity observed in the context of ART. Follicular fluid and blood serum levels of advanced glycation end-products in a group of non-diabetic women undergoing ART were associated with lower oocyte yield, lower number of fertilized eggs, lower day 2 embryo quality scores, and lower ongoing pregnancy rates [89]. These data suggest that glycemia and insulin resistance are important determinants of ovulatory function even within non-pathologic ranges. Yet, it does not rule out the possibility that other mechanisms, such as alterations in oocyte mitochondrial function and developmental arrest of the embryo described in animal models [23], may also be involved in explaining the association between obesity and fertility.

Obesity management and fertility

The existing evidence on whether clinical management of obesity has any effects on fertility is mostly limited to women with PCOS. As mentioned above, pharmacotherapy with insulin-sensitizing agents in PCOS women improves ovulatory function [81] and fertility [85]. Modest weight loss (5% to 10% of initial body weight) also improves ovulatory function among women with PCOS [90]. Among women losing weight through diet, the absolute amount of weight loss appears to be more important than the specific macro-nutrient composition of weight loss diets in improving reproductive function [91]. Likewise, among morbidly obese PCOS women undergoing bariatric surgery, the amount of weight loss appears to be related to improvement in menstrual cyclicity [92–94]. Whether or not the findings on weight loss are applicable to non-PCOS overweight or obese women is unclear at this time. It is also uncertain at this time whether obese women who seek infertility treatment can benefit from losing weight prior to initiating treatment. As of the writing of this book there is an ongoing randomized trial whose goal is to address this issue [95].

Summary

Overweight and obesity can reduce fertility among women who try to conceive naturally as well as among women undergoing infertility treatment. Overweight and obesity are associated with decreased fecundability in the general population. This association appears to be driven to a large extent by obesity's effect on ovulation (including but not limited to PCOS), although defects in other reproductive processes are also present. Among couples undergoing ART, overweight and obesity lead to ovarian resistance to gonadotropins, decreased ovarian response to controlled hyperstimulation, and to lower live birth rates due to preclinical and clinical pregnancy losses. Of the many systemic consequences of excess body weight, insulin resistance and hyperglycemia appear to be important mechanisms underlying the relation between obesity and decreased fertility, although other mechanisms may also be at play. Weight loss and pharmacotherapy with insulin-sensitizing agents improve ovulatory function in women with PCOS. It is not clear, however, whether these treatment strategies can improve fertility in overweight or obese non-PCOS women trying to conceive naturally. It is also unclear whether weight loss prior to initiation of infertility treatment is beneficial.

References

1. Prentice A M, Rayco-Solon P, Moore S E. Insights from the developing world: thrifty genotypes and thrifty phenotypes. *Proc Nutr Soc* 2005;**64**(2):153–61.

2. Frisch R E. Body fat, menarche, fitness and fertility. *Hum Reprod* 1987;**2**:521–33.

3. ESHRE Capri Workshop Group. Nutrition and reproduction in women. *Hum Reprod Update* 2006;**12**:193–207.

4. Stein I F & Leventhal M L. Amenorrhea associated with bilateral polycystic ovaries. *Am J Obstet Gynecol* 1935;**29**:181–91.

5. Ben-Shlomo I, Grinbaum E & Levinger U. Obesity-associated infertility – the earliest known description. *Reprod Biomed Online* 2008;**17**(Suppl 1):5–6.

6. Jokela M, Elovainio M & Kivimaki M. Lower fertility associated with obesity and underweight: the US National Longitudinal Survey of Youth. *Am J Clin Nutr* 2008;**88**(4):886–93.

7. Wilcox A, Weinberg C & Baird D. Caffeinated beverages and decreased fertility. *Lancet* 1988;**332**:1453–6.

8. Howe G, Westhoff C, Vessey M & Yeates D. Effects of age, cigarette smoking, and other factors on fertility: findings in a large prospective study. *BMJ* 1985;**290**(6483):1697–700.

9. Jensen T K, Scheike T, Keiding N, Schaumburg I & Grandjean P. Fecundability in relation to body mass and menstrual cycle patterns. *Epidemiology* 1999;**10**(4):422–8.

10. Gesink Law D C, Maclehose R F & Longnecker M P. Obesity and time to pregnancy. *Hum Reprod* 2007;**22**(2):414–20.

11. Lake J K, Power C & Cole T J. Women's reproductive health: the role of body mass index in early and adult life. *Int J Obes Relat Metab Disord* 1997;**21**(6):432–8.

12. Bolumar F, Olsen J, Rebagliato M, Saez-Lloret I & Bisanti L. Body mass index and delayed conception: a European Multicenter Study on Infertility and Subfecundity. *Am J Epidemiol* 2000;**151**(11):1072–9.

13. Hassan M A & Killick S R. Negative lifestyle is associated with a significant reduction in fecundity. *Fertil Steril* 2004;**81**(2):384–92.

14. Ramlau-Hansen C H, Thulstrup A M, Nohr E A, *et al.* Subfecundity in overweight and obese couples. *Hum Reprod* 2007;**22**(6):1634–7.

15. Wise L A, Rothman K J, Mikkelsen E M, *et al.* An internet-based prospective study of body size and time-to-pregnancy. *Hum Reprod* 2010;**25**(1):253–64.

16. Zaadstra B M, Seidell J C, Van Noord P A, *et al.* Fat and female fecundity: prospective study of effect of body fat distribution on conception rates. *BMJ* 1993;**306**(6876):484–7.

17. Green B B, Weiss N S & Daling J R. Risk of ovulatory infertility in relation to body weight. *Fertil Steril* 1988;**50**(5):721–6.

18. Grodstein F, Goldman M B & Cramer D W. Body mass index and ovulatory infertility. *Epidemiology* 1994;**5**(2):247–50.

19. Rich-Edwards J W, Goldman M B, Willett W C, *et al*. Adolescent body mass index and infertility caused by ovulatory disorder. *Am J Obstet Gynecol* 1994;**171**:171–7.

20. Rich-Edwards J W, Spiegelman D, Garland M, *et al*. Physical activity, body mass index, and ovulatory disorder infertility. *Epidemiology* 2002;**13**:184–90.

21. Chavarro J E, Rich-Edwards J W, Rosner B A & Willett W C. Diet and lifestyle in the prevention of ovulatory disorder infertility. *Obstet Gynecol* 2007;**110**:1050–8.

22. van der Steeg J W, Steures P, Eijkemans M J, *et al*. Obesity affects spontaneous pregnancy chances in subfertile, ovulatory women. *Hum Reprod* 2008;**23**(2):324–8.

23. Igosheva N, Abramov A Y, Poston L, *et al*. Maternal diet-induced obesity alters mitochondrial activity and redox status in mouse oocytes and zygotes. *PLoS One* 2010;**5**(4):e10074.

24. Monden C. Partners in health? Exploring resemblance in health between partners in married and cohabiting couples. *Sociol Health Illn* 2007;**29**(3):391–411.

25. Pasquali R. Obesity and androgens: facts and perspectives. *Fertil Steril* 2006;**85**:1319–40.

26. Berga S L & Yen S S C. Reproductive failure due to central nervous system–hypothalamic–pituitary dysfunction. In Straus III J F & Baribieri R L (eds.) *Yen and Jaffe's Reproductive Endocrinology*, 5th edn. (Philadelphia: Elsevier, 2004).

27. Jensen T K, Andersson A-M, Jorgensen N, *et al*. Body mass index in relation to semen quality and reproductive hormones among 1,558 Danish men. *Fertil Steril* 2004;**82**(4):863–70.

28. Pauli E M, Legro R S, Demers L M, *et al*. Diminished paternity and gonadal function with increasing obesity in men. *Fertil Steril* 2008;**90**:346–51.

29. Chavarro J E, Toth T L, Wright D L, Meeker J D & Hauser R. Body mass index in relation to semen quality, sperm DNA integrity and serum reproductive hormone levels among men attending an infertility clinic. *Fertil Steril* 2010;**93**(7):2222–31.

30. Sallmen M, Sandler D P, Hoppin J A, Blair A & Baird D D. Reduced fertility among overweight and obese men. *Epidemiology* 2006;**17**(5):520–3.

31. Jokela M, Kibimaki M, Elovainio M, *et al*. Body mass index in adolescence and number of children in adulthood. *Epidemiology* 2007;**18**:599–606.

32. Nguyen R H N, Wilcox A, Skjaerven R & Baird D D. Men's body mass index and infertility. *Hum Reprod* 2007;**22**:2488–93.

33. Ramlau-Hansen C H, Thulsttrup A M, Nohr E A, *et al*. Subfecundity in overweight and obese couples. *Hum Reprod* 2007;**22**:1634–7.

34. Koloszar S, Fejes I, Zavaczki Z, *et al*. Effect of body weight on sperm concentration in normozoospermic males. *Arch Androl* 2005;**51**(4):299–304.

35. Hammoud A O, Wilde N, Gibson M, *et al*. Male obesity and alteration in sperm parameters. *Fertil Steril* 2008;**90**(6):2222–5.

36. Magnusdottir E V, Thorsteinsson T, Thorsteinsdottir S, Heimisdottir M & Olafsdottir K. Persistent organochlorines, sedentary occupation, obesity and human male subfertility. *Hum Reprod* 2005;**20**:208–15.

37. Fejes I, Koloszar S, Zavaczki Z, *et al*. Effect of body weight on testosterone/estradiol ratio in oligozoospermic patients. *Arch Androl* 2006;**52**(2):97–102.

38. Fejes I, Koloszar S, Szollosi J, Zavaczki Z & Pal A. Is semen quality affected by male body fat distribution? *Andrologia* 2005;**37**:155–9.

39. Sermondade N, Faure C, Fezeu L, *et al*. Obesity increases the risk of oligospermia and azoospermia. *Arch Intern Med*. In press.

40. Qin D D, Yuan E, Zhou W J, *et al*. Do reproductive hormones explain the association between body mass index and semen quality. *Asian J Androl* 2007;**9**:827–34.

41. Aggerholm A S, Thulstrup A M, Toft G, Ramlau-Hansen C H & Bonde J P. Is overweight a risk factor for reduced semen quality and altered serum sex hormone profile? *Fertil Steril* 2008;**90**(3):619–26.

42. Kort H I, Massey J B, Elsner C W, *et al*. Impact of body mass index values on sperm quantity and quality. *J Androl* 2006;**27**(3):450–2.

43. Spano M, Bonde J P, Hjollund H I, *et al*. Sperm chromatin damage impairs human fertility. *Fertil Steril* 2000;**73**:43–50.

44. Bakos H W, Henshaw R C, Mitchell M & Lane M. Paternal body mass index is associated with decreased blastocyst development and reduced live birth rates following assisted reproductive technology. *Fertil Steril* 2011;**95**(5):1700–4.

45. Bellver J, Ayllon Y, Ferrando M, *et al*. Female obesity impairs in vitro fertilization outcome without affecting embryo quality. *Fertil Steril* 2010;**93**(2):447–54.

46. Fedorcsak P, Dale P O, Storeng R, *et al*. Impact of overweight and underweight on assisted reproduction treatment. *Hum Reprod* 2004;**19**(11):2523–8.

47. Esinler I, Bozdag G & Yarali H. Impact of isolated obesity on ICSI outcome. *Reprod Biomed Online* 2008;**17**(4):583–7.

48. Dechaud H, Anahory T, Reyftmann L, *et al*. Obesity does not adversely affect results in patients who are undergoing in vitro fertilization and embryo transfer. *Eur J Obst Gynecol Reprod Biol* 2006;**127**(1):88–93.

49. Metwally M, Cutting R, Tipton A, *et al.* Effect of increased body mass index on oocyte and embryo quality in IVF patients. *Reprod Biomed Online* 2007;**15**(5):532–8.

50. Matalliotakis I, Cakmak H, Sakkas D, *et al.* Impact of body mass index on IVF and ICSI outcome: a retrospective study. *Reprod Biomed Online* 2008;**16**(6):778–83.

51. Orvieto R, Meltcer S, Nahum R, *et al.* The influence of body mass index on in vitro fertilization outcome. *Int J Gynaecol Obstet* 2009;**104**(1):53–5.

52. Wittemer C, Ohl J, Bailly M, Bettahar-Lebugle K & Nisand I. Does body mass index of infertile women have an impact on IVF procedure and outcome? *J Assist Reprod Genet* 2000;**17**(10):547–52.

53. Ku S-Y, Kim S D, Jee B C, *et al.* Clinical efficacy of body mass index as predictor of in vitro fertilization and embryo transfer outcomes. *J Korean Med Sci* 2006;**21**(2):300–3.

54. Dokras A, Baredziak L, Blaine J, *et al.* Obstetric outcomes after in vitro fertilization in obese and morbidly obese women. *Obstet Gynecol* 2006;**108**(1):61–9.

55. Awartani K, Nahas S, Al Hassan S, Al Deery M & Coskun S. Infertility treatment outcome in sub groups of obese population. *Reprod Biol Endocrinol* 2009;**7**(1):52.

56. Loveland J B, McClamrock H D, Malinow A M & Sharara F I. Clinical assisted reproduction: increased body mass index has a deleterious effect on in vitro fertilization outcome. *J Assist Reprod Genet* 2001;**18**(7):382–6.

57. Lashen H, Ledger W, Bernal A L & Barlow D. Extremes of body mass do not adversely affect the outcome of superovulation and in-vitro fertilization. *Hum Reprod* 1999;**14**(3):712–15.

58. Nichols J E, Crane M M, Higdon H L, Miller P B & Boone W R. Extremes of body mass index reduce in vitro fertilization pregnancy rates. *Fertil Steril* 2003;**79**(3):645–7.

59. Fedorcsak P, Storeng R, Dale P O, Tanbo T O M & ÅByholm T. Obesity is a risk factor for early pregnancy loss after IVF or ICSI. *Acta Obstet Gynecol Scand* 2000;**79**(1):43–8.

60. Frattarelli J L & Kodama C L. Impact of body mass index on in vitro fertilization outcomes. *J Assist Reprod Genet* 2004;**21**(6):211–15.

61. Thum M Y, El-Sheikhah A, Faris R, *et al.* The influence of body mass index to in-vitro fertilisation treatment outcome, risk of miscarriage and pregnancy outcome. *J Obstet Gynaecol* 2007;**27**(7):699–702.

62. Matalliotakis I, Cakmak H, Sakkas D, *et al.* Impact of body mass index on IVF and ICSI outcome: a retrospective study. *Reprod Biomed Online* 2008;**16**(6):778–83.

63. Beydoun H A, Stadtmauer L, Beydoun M A, *et al.* Polycystic ovary syndrome, body mass index and outcomes of assisted reproductive technologies. *Reprod Biomed Online* 2009;**18**(6):856–63.

64. Spandorfer S D, Kump L, Goldschlag D, *et al.* Obesity and in vitro fertilization: negative influences on outcome. *J Reprod Med* 2004;**49**(12):973–7.

65. Sneed M L, Uhler M L, Grotjan H E, *et al.* Body mass index: impact on IVF success appears age-related. *Hum Reprod* 2008;**23**(8):1835–9.

66. Lewis C G, Warnes G M, Wang X J & Matthews C D. Failure of body mass index or body weight to influence markedly the response to ovarian hyperstimulation in normal cycling women. *Fertil Steril* 1990;**53**(6):1097–9.

67. Carrell D T, Jones K P, Peterson C M, *et al.* Body mass index is inversely related to intrafollicular HCG concentrations, embryo quality and IVF outcome. *Reprod Biomed Online.* 2001;**3**(2):109–11.

68. Loh S, Wang J X & Matthews C D. The influence of body mass index, basal FSH and age on the response to gonadotrophin stimulation in non-polycystic ovarian syndrome patients. *Hum Reprod* 2002;**17**(5):1207–11.

69. Vrbikova J & Hainer V. Obesity and polycystic ovary syndrome. *Obes Facts* 2009;**2**(1):26–35.

70. Heijnen E M, Eijkemans M J, Hughes E G, *et al.* A meta-analysis of outcomes of conventional IVF in women with polycystic ovary syndrome. *Hum Reprod Update* 2006;**12**(1):13–21.

71. Swanton A, Storey L, McVeigh E & Child T. IVF outcome in women with PCOS, PCO and normal ovarian morphology. *Eur J Obstet Gynecol Reprod Biol* 2010;**149**(1):68–71.

72. Jabara S & Coutifaris C. In vitro fertilization in the PCOS patient: clinical considerations. *Semin Reprod Med* 2003;**21**(3):317–24.

73. Wilcox A J, Weinberg C R, O'Connor J F, *et al.* Incidence of early loss of pregnancy. *N Engl J Med* 1988;**319**(4):189–94.

74. Winter E, Wang J, Davies M J & Norman R. Early pregnancy loss following assisted reproductive technology treatment. *Hum Reprod* 2002;**17**(12):3220–3.

75. Matalliotakis I, Cakmak H, Arici A, *et al.* Epidemiological factors influencing IVF outcome: evidence from the Yale IVF program. *J Obstet Gynaecol* 2008;**28**(2):204–8.

76. Wang J X, Davies M & Norman R J. Body mass and probability of pregnancy during assisted reproduction treatment: retrospective study. *BMJ* 2000;**321**(7272):1320–1.

77. Luke B, Brown M B, Stern J E, *et al.* Female obesity adversely affects assisted reproductive technology (ART) pregnancy and live birth rates. *Hum Reprod* 2011;**26**(1):245–52.

78. Metwally M, Ong K J, Ledger W L & Li T C. Does high body mass index increase the risk of miscarriage after spontaneous and assisted conception? A meta-analysis of the evidence. *Fertil Steril* 2008;**90**(3):714–26.

79. Veleva Z, Tiitinen A, Vilska S, *et al.* High and low BMI increase the risk of miscarriage after IVF/ICSI and FET. *Hum Reprod* 2008;**23**(4):878–84.

80. Lintsen A M E, Pasker-de Jong P C M, de Boer E J, *et al.* Effects of subfertility cause, smoking and body weight on the success rate of IVF. *Hum Reprod* 2005;**20**(7):1867–75.

81. Tang T, Lord J M, Norman R J, Yasmin E & Balen A H. Insulin-sensitising drugs (metformin, rosiglitazone, pioglitazone, D-chiro-inositol) for women with polycystic ovary syndrome, oligo amenorrhoea and subfertility. *Cochrane Database Syst Rev* 2010;**1**:CD003053.

82. Galazis N, Galazi M & Atiomo W. d-Chiro-inositol and its significance in polycystic ovary syndrome: a systematic review. *Gynecol Endocrinol* 2011;**27**(4):256–62.

83. Sonmez A S, Yasar L, Savan K, *et al.* Comparison of the effects of acarbose and metformin use on ovulation rates in clomiphene citrate-resistant polycystic ovary syndrome. *Hum Reprod* 2005;**20**(1):175–9.

84. Penna I A, Canella P R, Reis R M, Silva de Sa M F & Ferriani R A. Acarbose in obese patients with polycystic ovarian syndrome: a double-blind, randomized, placebo-controlled study. *Hum Reprod* 2005;**20**(9):2396–401.

85. Kjøtrød S B, Carlsen S M, Rasmussen P E, *et al.* Use of metformin before and during assisted reproductive technology in non-obese young infertile women with polycystic ovary syndrome: a prospective, randomized, double-blind, multi-centre study. *Hum Reprod* 2011;**26**(8):2045–53.

86. Ohgi S, Nakagawa K, Kojima R, *et al.* Insulin resistance in oligomenorrheic infertile women with non-polycystic ovary syndrome. *Fertil Steril* 2008;**90**(2):373–7.

87. Whitworth K W, Baird D D, Stene L C, Skjaerven R & Longnecker M P. Fecundability among women with type 1 and type 2 diabetes in the Norwegian Mother and Child Cohort Study. *Diabetologia* 2011;**54**(3):516–22.

88. Hjollund N H I, Jensen T K, Bonde J P E, *et al.* Is glycosilated haemoglobin a marker of fertility? A follow-up study of first-pregnancy planners. *Hum Reprod* 1999;**14**:1478–82.

89. Jinno M, Takeuchi M, Watanabe A, *et al.* Advanced glycation end-products accumulation compromises embryonic development and achievement of pregnancy by assisted reproductive technology. *Hum Reprod* 2011;**26**(3):604–10.

90. Norman R J, Noakes M, Wu R, *et al.* Improving reproductive performance in overweight/obese women with effective weight management. *Hum Reprod Update* 2004;**10**(3):267–80.

91. Stamets K, Taylor D S, Kunselman A, *et al.* A randomized trial of the effects of two types of short-term hypocaloric diets on weight loss in women with polycystic ovary syndrome. *Fertil Steril* 2004;**81**:630–7.

92. Deitel M, Stone E, Kassam H A, Wilk E J & Sutherland D J. Gynecologic–obstetric changes after loss of massive excess weight following bariatric surgery. *J Am Coll Nutr* 1988;**7**(2):147–53.

93. Eid G M, Cottam D R, Velcu L M, *et al.* Effective treatment of polycystic ovarian syndrome with Roux-en-Y gastric bypass. *Surg Obes Relat Dis* 2005;**1**(2):77–80.

94. Teitelman M, Grotegut C A, Williams N N & Lewis J D. The impact of bariatric surgery on menstrual patterns. *Obes Surg* 2006;**16**(11):1457–63.

95. Mutsaerts M A, Groen H, ter Bogt NC, *et al.* The LIFESTYLE study: costs and effects of a structured lifestyle program in overweight and obese subfertile women to reduce the need for fertility treatment and improve reproductive outcome. A randomised controlled trial. *BMC Womens Health* 2010;**10**:22.

Chapter

4

Maternal outcomes in obese pregnancies

Eugene Oteng-Ntim and Pat Doyle

Introduction

The effect of obesity in pregnancy is wide ranging with potentially serious impacts on both the mother and the child. This chapter summarizes the current state of knowledge of the relationship between obesity and adverse maternal outcome, including effects on the health of the pregnant mother as well as complications at the time of delivery. We examine how obesity influences the risk of maternal death, gestational diabetes, hypertensive diseases of pregnancy, and infection. In regard to delivery we summarize evidence for effects on induction of labor, cesarean section (CS), postpartum hemorrhage, and other serious complications. This chapter draws together a considerable body of evidence to show that risks of adverse obstetric outcome may be doubled or even trebled in an obese woman compared to a woman with a healthy body mass index (BMI). The final section of the chapter looks at the impact of maternal obesity at a population, rather than an individual, level. We highlight the proportion of adverse obstetric outcome that is explained by obesity in the population and estimate that approximately one fifth of obstetric morbidity in developed countries could be avoided if maternal obesity was eliminated.

What is obesity in pregnancy?

Measurement and definition of obesity

Obesity is defined as "an accumulation of excess body fat to such an extent that may impair health" [1]. Total body fat can be measured by direct methods such as dual energy X-ray absorptiometry (DEXA) and magnetic resonance imaging (MRI) [2]. Both are expensive, cumbersome, and impractical to perform in most circumstances. Moreover, DEXA has

the added radiation risk [3]. Hence obesity is usually measured using indirect methods such as BMI, based on anthropometry. Body mass index is an expression of body weight-for-height using the formula weight (in kilograms) divided by height (in meters) squared (kg/m^2). Obesity in adults is defined by the World Health Organization (WHO), the US Institute of Medicine (IOM), and the UK National Institute for Health and Clinical Excellence (NICE) as BMI $\geq 30\,kg/m^2$. Table 1.1 of Chapter 1 describes the different classifications of obesity in common usage.

Body mass index has been shown by the WHO to correlate well with the accumulation of body fat and is a good reproducible indicator of metabolic risk [1,4]. The limitations are that it does not account for variation in body composition (for example in lean body mass or water) or the body distribution of fat [2].

Preconceptual BMI

Directly measured preconceptual BMI is the ideal measure when determining associations with pregnancy outcome. Since these data are not routinely available in most settings, clinicians and investigators often obtain this information by asking the pregnant woman to recall her pre-pregnancy weight, or use measured BMI at booking in the first trimester as a proxy. This is generally more feasible, since early pregnancy is when height and weight is, or should be, routinely measured and recorded (e.g., UK Royal College of Obstetricians and Gynaecologists recommendation 2010) [5]. But a limitation of using BMI during, rather than before, pregnancy is that changes in maternal body composition following conception, as well as the products of conception themselves, will be included in the weight measurement. This extra weight will result in an

Maternal Obesity, ed. Matthew W. Gillman and Lucilla Poston. Published by Cambridge University Press. © Cambridge University Press 2012.

increase in BMI and may enhance the likelihood of the pregnant woman being classified as obese. However, in early pregnancy, up to ten weeks gestation, this extra weight will average as little as 1.2 kg [6], which will increase maternal BMI by approximately 2% overall and will not have a major impact on the proportion of women wrongly classified as obese. As the pregnancy progresses and maternal weight increases, BMI will increase more markedly. For example, at 20 weeks, a maternal weight gain of 9 kg will increase the BMI of the average UK woman of reproductive age by 12% (authors' estimate). Using 20-week weight would lead to a higher proportion of false positive obese pregnant women using the standard definition of obesity, which would further increase as the pregnancy progresses. Body mass index or obesity in the second and third trimesters of pregnancy is thus not considered a useful index of preconceptual BMI.

Many use the term 'obese pregnancy' to describe a pregnancy in which the woman is obese at the start. In addition to obesity in early pregnancy, women who have excessive weight gain during pregnancy, with or without obesity in early pregnancy, are also at risk of adverse outcomes [7]. The influences of excessive weight gain on pregnancy outcome in women with a normal pre-pregnancy BMI and those who are overweight or obese form the basis of the US Institute of Medicine (IOM) guidelines for weight management in pregnancy and are addressed in Chapters 14 and 19.

Effects of obesity on the pregnant woman

Maternal mortality

Maternal obesity is overrepresented in maternal deaths in developed countries [8,9]. In the most recent Confidential Enquiry into Maternal Deaths in the UK, 27% of the 261 deaths occurring between 2006 and 2008 were in obese pregnant women [8]. This compares to an estimated background obesity prevalence of 15% in pregnant women in the UK at that time [10]. Similarly, a maternal death review from California reported that 30% of the 386 women who died in pregnancy during 2002 and 2003 were obese, compared to 16% of women having live births in California in the same time period. These findings reflect the fact that the leading direct and indirect causes of mortality such as thromboembolism, pre-eclampsia, and cardiovascular diseases have a higher prevalence in the obese, compared to

the lean, population. The UK maternal death enquiry reported that three quarters of the mothers who died from thromboembolism were overweight or obese, as were 61% of mothers dying from cardiac disease. For other causes, the percentage of women dying and who were overweight or obese was around 40%, except for those from suicide, hemorrhage, and sepsis where the rates were lower at 20% to 25% [8]. The importance of these findings has led to recommendations that obesity be recognized as a pre-existing medical condition requiring specific counseling and careful management from early pregnancy [5,8].

As detailed in Chapter 1, in some parts of the developing world too there is growing concern about rising BMI in women of childbearing age. Obesity is already a serious problem in Latin America, the Caribbean, the Middle East, and North Africa [11]. Rising national incomes in developing countries and increased "Westernization" will most likely lead to increased levels of obesity in the future with associated consequences for maternal mortality [12].

Gestational diabetes mellitus (GDM)

Endocrine changes make the pregnant woman more resistant to naturally produced insulin [13]. As discussed in Chapters 5 and 15, these changes confer some physiological advantage to the fetus, but in some pregnancies, particularly in obese women who demonstrate enhanced insulin resistance, they also increase the risk of hyperglycemia and frank GDM [13]. There is a strong correlation between obesity and GDM [14–16]; a systematic review by Torloni et al. [15], estimates that moderate obesity (BMI between 30 and <40 kg/m^2) in pregnancy results in a three-fold (OR = 3.01; CI = 2.34–3.87) increase in risk of GDM compared to women with healthy BMI (see Table 4.1). Morbid obesity (BMI ≥40 kg/m^2) is associated with over five times the increased risk of GDM (OR = 5.55; CI = 4.27–7.21). Based on the definitions, which until recently were widely used (see below), about 3% to 7% of women develop diabetes in pregnancy overall, ranging from 1% to 3% of women of normal weight compared to 14% to 17% of obese women [14,17]. Other than pre-pregnancy weight, risk factors related to the development of GDM include ethnicity, previous history of GDM, age, parity, and family history of diabetes [18].

Diabetes mellitus is a metabolic disorder characterized by persistent hyperglycemia, with disturbance of carbohydrate metabolism resulting from a defect in insulin secretion, insulin action, or both [19]. The early definitions of GDM were based on results from glucose tolerance tests (GTT), which predicted later diabetes in the mother, a definition endorsed by the WHO [19]. More recently it has become apparent that a definition of GDM would be more clinically relevant if it more precisely defined the degree of glycemia at which outcomes of pregnancy, such as neonatal health and CS, worsen. Two recently published studies, the Hyperglycemia and Pregnancy Outcome (HAPO) study [20] and the Australian Carbohydrate Intolerance Study (ACHOIS) have addressed this problem [21]. The HAPO study showed that with increasing hyperglycemia, there were increases in adverse outcomes in a continuous fashion. It also highlighted adverse outcome over a broader range of glycemia. However, the HAPO study does not yet contain long-term outcomes and it is an observational, not intervention, study. The ACHOIS, a randomized trial of standard antenatal care vs. a more rigorous regime for control of glycemia in women with GDM, showed that the rigorous protocol was associated with improved pregnancy outcomes. In a subset of the ACHOIS population, however, the intervention did not reduce offspring BMI at the age of 4 to 5 years [22].

Following HAPO and ACHOIS, the International Association of Diabetes in Pregnancy Study Group redefined GDM as fasting plasma glucose concentration >5.1 mM, one-hour plasma glucose concentration >10.0 mM, or two-hour plasma glucose concentration ≥8.5 mM following 75 g oral glucose challenge after fasting from midnight [20,23]. With the new HAPO definition about 30% of obese women will be classified as having GDM.

Women diagnosed with GDM have a higher risk of developing type 2 diabetes mellitus in later life. In a recent systematic review, Bellamy *et al.* [24] identified 20 studies that included over 675 000 women and 10 800 cases of type 2 diabetes. They found that women with GDM had seven-fold increased risk of developing type 2 diabetes compared to those who had normoglycemic pregnancies (RR = 7.43; CI = 4.79–11.51).

Also of importance is the recent hypothesis of the link between maternal diabetes and the child's risk of developing obesity in later life [25,26]. Thus obesity in pregnancy is not only a modifiable risk factor for gestational diabetes but may also play a role in childhood obesity. This issue is discussed further in Chapters 9 to 13.

Hypertensive disease in pregnancy

Hypertensive disease in pregnancy, or gestational hypertension, is defined as new onset hypertension (systolic blood pressure greater than 140 mmHg and/or diastolic blood pressure greater than 90 mmHg) after 20 weeks gestation [27,28]. If gestational hypertension is associated with proteinuria as shown by 1 (0.3 g/l) or more on proteinuria dipstick testing, or 300 mg or more per 24-hour urine collection, then the diagnosis is pre-eclampsia [14]. Many studies show that maternal obesity is associated with increased risk of gestational hypertension [29–32]. Two large population-based studies and a systematic review (see summary in Table 4.1) demonstrated clear and consistent strong positive associations between maternal pre-pregnancy BMI and the risk of pre-eclampsia [14,29,33]. The systematic review concluded that the risk of pre-eclampsia typically doubles with each 5 to 7 kg/m² increase in pre-pregnancy BMI [29]. Another recent study also addresses the dose–response effect of increasing BMI and the rise in the prevalence of pre-eclampsia [34]. With obesity prevalence rising throughout most countries [35], the role of pre-pregnancy BMI as an increasingly important independent risk factor for pre-eclampsia is apparent, and normalizing BMI becomes a target for preconceptual care. Moreover a systematic review concluded that mothers who develop pre-eclampsia are more likely to develop cardiovascular disease later in life [36], raising the possibility that any preventive measure is likely to benefit health later in life as well as the more immediate adverse maternal and neonatal outcomes.

Mechanistically, the association between the rise in BMI and increasing pre-eclampsia prevalence may be explained by increased insulin resistance, heightened inflammation, and, potentially, oxidative stress. Chapters 5 and 15 explore these mechanisms in more detail.

Thromboembolic complications

Venous thromboembolic (VTE) complications are a leading direct cause of maternal mortality in the UK and other developed countries [36,37]. Pregnancy-associated death from thromboembolism occurs in approximately 1 in 7000 pregnancies, a 12-fold increase compared to the non-pregnant state where the risk is around one in a million [38]. A small retrospective study in Denmark showed a strong association between venous thromboembolism in pregnancy and obesity, reporting an almost ten-fold increased risk for obese pregnant women compared to non-obese

Table 4.1 Risk of maternal outcomes in obese pregnant women: summary of evidence from systematic reviews and large observational studies

Outcome	Reference	Setting	Study design	Numbers in study	Estimated relative risk (95% CI)[a]
Gestational diabetes	Torloni et al. (2009) [15]	Worldwide	Systematic review of 59 cohort and 11 case-control studies published 1977 to 2007	70 studies involving 671 945 women	Overweight: 1.97 (1.77–2.19) Mild & moderate obesity: 3.01 (2.34–3.87) Morbid obesity: 5.55 (4.27–7.21)
Hypertensive disorders of pregnancy	O'Brien et al. (2003) [29]	Worldwide	Systematic review of cohort studies published 1980 to 2002	13 cohort studies comprising 1.4 million pregnant women	The risk of pre-eclampsia doubled with each 5 to 7 kg/m² increase in pre-pregnancy BMI
	Sebire et al. (2001) [14]	London, UK	Cross-sectional analysis of North West Thames maternity database	287 213 women with singleton pregnancies delivering 1989 to 1997	Overweight: 1.44 (1.28–1.62) Obese: 2.14 (1.85–2.47)
	Bhattacharya et al. (2007) [32]	Aberdeen, UK	Cohort study of singleton pregnancies delivering 1976 to 2005	24 241 nulliparous women with singleton pregnancies	Overweight: 1.6 (1.2–1.8) Mild & moderate obesity: 3.1 (2.8–3.5) Morbid obesity[b]: 7.2 (4.7–11.2)
Thromboembolism	Larsen et al. (2007) [39]	Denmark	Case-control study nested in a cohort	129 cases with VTE in pregnancy and 258 controls who are pregnant without VTE	Obese: 9.7 (3.1–30.8)
	Knight (2008) [40]	UK	Case-control study	143 women who had thromboembolism antenatally between 2005 to 2006	Obese: 2.65 (1.09–6.45)
Induction of labor	Sebire et al. (2001) [14]	London, UK	Cross-sectional analysis of North West Thames maternity database	287 213 women with singleton pregnancies delivering 1989 to 1997	Overweight: 2.14 (1.85–2.47) Obese: 1.70 (1.64–1.76)
	Zhang et al. (2007) [43]	Liverpool, UK	Cross-sectional study of deliveries in Liverpool Women's Hospital	3913 completed singleton pregnancies who delivered in 2002	Overweight: 1.41 (1.21–1.66) Obese: 2.10 (1.73–2.55)
Cesarean section	Poobalan et al. (2009) [47]	Aberdeen, UK	Systematic review and meta-analysis of publications 1996 to 2007	11 cohort studies involving 166 168 pregnant women	Overweight: 1.53 (1.48–1.58) Mild & moderate obesity: 2.26 (2.04–2.51) Morbid obesity[b]: 3.38 (2.49–4.57)

Postpartum hemorrhage	Sebire et al. (2001) [14]	London, UK	Cross-sectional analysis of North West Thames maternity database	287 213 women with singleton pregnancies delivering 1989 to 1997	Overweight: 1.16 (1.12–1.21) Obese: 1.39 (1.32–1.46)
	Usha et al. (2005) [46]	Wales, UK	A population-based birth survey between 1990 to 1999	60 167 women who delivered between 1990 to 1999	Obese: 1.5 (1.2–1.8)
	Heslehurst et al. (2008) [42]	Europe and USA	Systematic review of publications 1990 to 2007 on BMI in pregnancy and pregnancy outcomes	6 studies included in meta-analysis	Mild & moderate obesity: 1.20 (1.16–1.24) Morbid obesity: 1.43 (1.33–1.54)
Maternal infection	Heslehurst et al. (2008) [42]	Europe and USA	Systematic review of publications 1990 to 2007 on BMI in pregnancy and pregnancy outcomes	6 studies included in meta-analysis	Obesity: 3.34 (2.74–4.06)
Wound infection	Sebire et al. (2001) [14]	London, UK	Cross-sectional analysis of North West Thames maternity database	287 213 women with singleton pregnancies delivering 1989 to 1997	Overweight: 1.27 (1.09–1.48) Obese: 2.24 (1.9–2.64)
Length of hospital stay	Heslehurst et al. (2008) [42]	Worldwide	Systematic review of publications 1990 to 2007 on BMI in pregnancy and pregnancy outcomes	4 studies included in meta-analysis	Healthy BMI: 2.4 days Mild & moderate obesity: 2.71 days Morbid obesity: 3.28 days

[a] Comparison group women with healthy (normal) BMI
[b] This study defines morbid obesity as BMI ≥35.0 kg/m²

[39] (Table 4.1). A recent study from the UK Obstetric Surveillance System (UKOSS) found a more moderate effect, obese women were approximately two-and-a-half times more likely to develop thromboembolism compared to lean pregnant women [40] (Table 4.1). The possible mechanism underlying these observations may relate to elevated concentrations in the blood of procoagulant factors found in some studies [41]. Contributing to this may be heightened inflammatory damage to the venous endothelium and sedentary lifestyle in the obese.

Infection

Infection accounts for substantial morbidity during pregnancy. There is strong evidence of an association between maternal obesity and wound infection [20], genital tract infections, and urinary tract infections [14,32,42]. The risk of an obese woman having infection during pregnancy is almost three-and-a-half times higher than that for pregnant women with normal BMI (RR = 3.34, CI = 2.74–4.06). This finding is consistent in most studies [14,32,42].

Effects of obesity on labor and delivery

Induction and progress of labor

Obese pregnant women have an increased incidence of labor induction. The estimated increased risk is approximately two-fold (RR = 1.88, CI = 1.84–1.92), which remains largely unaltered after adjusting for associated antepartum complications [14,32,43] (Table 4.1). The evidence regarding labor duration is conflicting. Some investigators report higher incidences of prolonged labor and failure to progress but others do not [43,44]. A better understanding of the relationship between obesity and the mechanisms of labor is desirable to prevent the high rates of intervention during labor [42].

Cesarean section

Maternal obesity is an independent risk factor for CS. Sheiner et al. investigated the pregnancy outcome of obese patients not suffering from hypertensive disorders or diabetes mellitus in women who delivered at Soroka Medical Center in Israel between 1988 and 2002 [45]. They found that the unadjusted association between obesity and CS was three times higher compared to the lean (RR = 3.2; 95% CI: 2.9–3.5). After controlling for

each of several obstetrical variables that co-exist with obesity (but not for age), the relative risk was unchanged. The authors speculated that this remaining risk might be because of clinician–patient decision-making over and above clinical need. Similarly Sebire et al. showed that the CS rate for obese women was over 20% compared to nearer to 10% for normal weight women in London in the 1990s [14]. Usha et al. also reported the effect of maternal obesity on pregnancy complications with good control of confounding factors [46]. The study supported previous evidence that obese women had twice the risk of CS compared with non-obese women (RR = 1.6; CI = 1.4–2.0). These authors suggested that this increased risk may be an effect of the increased rate of large for gestational age (LGA) infants leading to disproportion during labor, suboptimal uterine contractility, or increased fat deposition in the soft tissues of the pelvis. A recent systematic review by Poobalan confirmed the consistency of this association and further showed that higher BMI is associated with increased likelihood of needing CS [47] (Table 4.1).

Postpartum hemorrhage

Overall the evidence indicates that obese women tend to have between 20% and 50% higher rates of postpartum hemorrhage than non-obese women [14,42,46] (Table 4.1). The increased incidence of CS among obese women has been implicated as a causal factor. However, Usha et al. showed the increased rate of CS might not be the only factor influencing blood loss in this group: obese women who had a vaginal delivery had a greater than 500 ml blood loss compared to those with a BMI of 20 to 30 kg/m² [46]. This study also noted a 44% increased risk for a major postpartum hemorrhage in primigravid obese women even after accounting for predisposing factors such as CS. They suggested this increased blood loss might be explained by excess bleeding from the larger surface area of implantation of the placenta usually associated with a large for gestational age (LGA) fetus [46]. Nuthalapaty and Rouse considered the possibility that a relatively larger volume of distribution for administered drugs, and the resultant decreased bioavailability of uterotonic agents, could be an additional factor related to the increased risk of postpartum hemorrhage in obese women [31].

Other postpartum complications

There is conflicting evidence regarding the relationship between obesity and failure to initiate lactation, and/or a decreased duration of lactation. Maternal obesity is implicated in alteration of the hypothalamic–pituitary–gonadal axis and fat metabolism, resulting in lactational dysfunction; however, the exact mechanism remains to be determined [44]. Physical discomfort may also play a role (see Chapter 8).

In the postpartum period obese women have longer hospitalization than non-obese women [42,48]. In a recent review [42], meta-analysis of four studies showed a gradual increase in mean length of hospital stay as BMI increased. The overall mean length of stay was 2.4 (CI = 2.4–2.6) days for those with a healthy BMI, 2.7 (CI = 2.6–2.8) days for women who were obese, and 3.3 (CI = 3.1–3.4) days for women who were morbidly obese. These disparities have substantial health resource implications [49].

The population impact of obese pregnancies on maternal outcome

The evidence presented thus far shows a marked increased risk of adverse obstetric events in obese pregnancies, including gestational diabetes, hypertensive diseases, thromboembolism, infection, CS, and postpartum hemorrhage. There are also clear indications that risks increase as BMI, or the levels of obesity, increase. This is vitally important information for an overweight or obese woman considering pregnancy, or

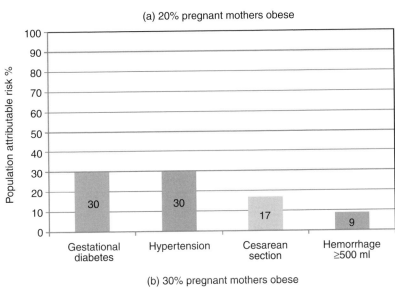

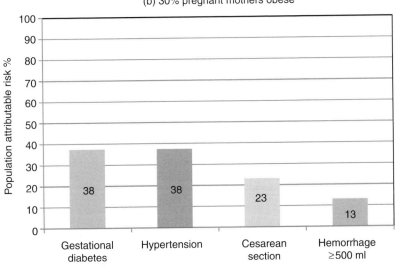

Figure 4.1. Proportion of selected obstetric events that could theoretically be avoided in the population if all pregnant women had a healthy BMI.

in the early stages of pregnancy, and for the clinician managing her pregnancy. The evidence is sufficiently robust to consider an obese pregnancy an "at-risk" pregnancy, as reflected by recent UK guidelines for the clinical management of women with obesity in pregnancy [5].

An important question to ask is what proportion of the adverse obstetric events seen in the population, rather than the individual, can be attributed to obesity. A useful measure is the population attributable risk (PAR) percent. This can be thought of as the proportion of obstetric morbidity attributable to maternal obesity in the population, and also as the proportion of "potentially avoidable" adverse outcome if obesity was eliminated in the population: that is, avoidable if all pregnant women were of healthy BMI.

The proportion of potentially avoidable adverse outcome increases with both the strength of association between obesity and the outcome, and the prevalence of maternal obesity in the population. For example, if maternal obesity is associated with an increased risk of 50% (relative risk 1.5), and the prevalence of maternal obesity in the population is low at 5%, the proportion of adverse obstetric events that could be avoided if obesity in the population was eliminated is only 2%. However, if obesity is linked to a five-times increased risk (relative risk of 5) of a particular outcome, and the prevalence of obesity in pregnancy is 50%, the proportion of potentially avoidable adverse outcome if obesity were eliminated is very high at 67%.

In most developed countries obesity is associated with two- to three-times increased risk and the prevalence of obesity is around 20%. The resulting PAR percents for four obesity-related pregnancy outcomes are depicted in Figure 4.1. Here we use the best available estimates of relative risk measures from the literature, after adjustment for potential confounding such as age and parity. Here, the contribution of maternal obesity on gestational diabetes and hypertension in pregnancy is around 30%, meaning that almost one third of these outcomes could be prevented in the population if maternal obesity were able to be prevented. For CS, the figure is around one fifth, and for postpartum hemorrhage, around 9%. If the prevalence of obesity were to increase to 30% sometime in the future the analogous PAR percents would be higher (Figure 4.1).

These are worrying estimates. They demonstrate the substantial impact of maternal obesity on obstetric health that currently exists in the population, which is likely to increase further if there is no reversal in the trend of increasing maternal obesity. The figures also point to potentially huge savings in health services expenditure if maternal obesity could be eliminated, or at least reduced, in the population.

Conclusion

Obesity is a strong determinant of obstetric morbidity and mortality. We have shown that obese pregnancies also represent a major public health issue in the UK and other developed countries with high impact on clinical obstetrics. Reducing the prevalence of obesity in pregnancy will almost surely reduce maternal morbidity and mortality. Interventions to address obesity pre-pregnancy, as well as during pregnancy, are now a public health priority in most developed countries and are becoming so in many developing countries as well.

References

1. World Health Organization. *Obesity: Preventing and Managing the Global Epidemic.* Report of a WHO Consultation. WHO Technical Report Series 894. 2000. www.who.int/nutrition/publications/obesity/WHO_TRS_894/en/index.html [Accessed January 4, 2012].

2. Despres J P, Lemieux I & Prud'homme D. Treatment of obesity: need to focus on high risk abdominally obese patients. *BMJ* 2001;**322**(7288):716–20.

3. Han T S, Sattar N, Lean M. ABC of obesity. Assessment of obesity and its clinical implications. *BMJ* 2006;**333**(7570):695–8.

4. Kopelman P. Obesity as a medical problem. *Nature* 2000;**404**:635–43.

5. CMACE/RCOG. *CMACE/RCOG Joint Guideline. Management of Women with Obesity in Pregnancy.* 2010. www.rcog.org.uk/files/rcog-corp/CMACERCOGJointGuidelineManagementWomenObesityPregnancya.pdf [Accessed January 4, 2012].

6. Rasmussen K M, Catalano P M & Yaktine A L. New guidelines for weight gain during pregnancy: what obstetrician/gynecologists should know. *Curr Opin Obstet Gynecol* 2009;**21**(6):521–6.

7. Rasmussen KM, Abrams B, Bodnar LM, *et al.* Recommendations for weight gain during pregnancy in the context of the obesity epidemic. *Obstet Gynecol* 2010;**116**(5):1191–5.

8. Cantwell R, Clutton-Brock T, Cooper G, *et al.* Saving Mothers' Lives: reviewing maternal deaths to make motherhood safer: 2006–2008. The Eighth Report of the Confidential Enquiries into Maternal Deaths in the United Kingdom. *BJOG* 2011;**118**(Suppl 1):1–203.

9. California Department of Public Health. *The California Pregnancy-associated Mortality Review. Report from 2002 and 2003 Maternal Death Reviews.* 2011. www.cdph.ca.gov/data/statistics/Pages/default.aspx [Accessed January 27, 2011].

10. Heslehurst N, Rankin J, Wilkinson J R, *et al.* A nationally representative study of maternal obesity in England, UK: trends in incidence and demographic inequalities in 619 323 births, 1989–2007. *Int J Obes (Lond)* 2010;**34**(3):420–8.

11. World Health Organization. *Global Database on Body Mass Index: an Interactive Surveillance Tool for Monitoring Nutrition Transition.* 2011. http://apps.who.int/bmi/index.jsp [Accessed January 4, 2012].

12. Campbell O M, Graham W J & Lancet Maternal Survival Series steering group. Strategies for reducing maternal mortality: getting on with what works. *Lancet* 2006;**368**(9543):1284–99.

13. Waugh N, Royle P, Clar C, *et al.* Screening for hyperglycaemia in pregnancy: a rapid update for the National Screening Committee. *Health Technol Assess* 2010;**14**:1–183.

14. Sebire N J, Jolly M, Harris J P, *et al.* Maternal obesity and pregnancy outcome: a study of 287,213 pregnancies in London. *Int J Obes Relat Metab Disord* 2001;**25**(8):1175–82.

15. Torloni M R, Betrán A P, Horta B L, *et al.* Prepregnancy BMI and the risk of gestational diabetes: a systematic review of the literature with meta-analysis. *Obes Rev* 2009;**10**(2):194–203.

16. Chu S Y, Callaghan W M, Kim S Y, *et al.* Maternal obesity and risk of gestational diabetes mellitus. *Diabetes Care* 2007;**30**(8):2070–6.

17. Yogev Y & Catalano P M. Pregnancy and obesity. *Obstet Gynecol Clin North Am* 2009;**36**(2):285–300.

18. National Institute for Health and Clinical Excellence (NICE). *Diabetes in Pregnancy. Management of Diabetes and its Complications from Pre-conception to the Postnatal Period.* NICE Clinical Guideline 63. 2008. www.nice.org.uk/nicemedia/pdf/CG063Guidance.pdf [Accessed January 4, 2012].

19. World Health Organization. *Definition, Diagnosis and Classification of Diabetes Mellitus and its Complications. Report of a WHO Consultation. Part 1: Diagnosis and Classification of Diabetes Mellitus.* 1999. www.staff.ncl.ac.uk/philip.home/who_dmg.pdf [Accessed January 4, 2012].

20. Metzger B E, Lowe L P, Dyer A R, *et al.* Hyperglycemia and adverse pregnancy outcomes. *N Engl J Med* 2008;**3358**(19):1991–2002.

21. Crowther C A, Hiller J E, Moss J R, *et al.* Effect of treatment of gestational diabetes mellitus on pregnancy outcomes. *N Engl J Med* 2005;**352**(24):2477–86.

22. Gillman M W, Oakey H, Baghurst P A, *et al.* Effect of treatment of gestational diabetes mellitus on obesity in the next generation. *Diabetes Care* 2010;**33**(5):964–8.

23. Yu C K, Teoh T G & Robinson S. Obesity in pregnancy. *BJOG* 2006;**113**(10):1117–25.

24. Bellamy L, Casas J P, Hingorani A D, *et al.* Type 2 diabetes mellitus after gestational diabetes: a systematic review and meta-analysis. *Lancet* 2009;**373**(9677):1773–9.

25. Poston L. Developmental programming and diabetes – the human experience and insight from animal models. *Best Pract Res Clin Endocrinol Metab* 2010;**24**(4):541–52.

26. Poston L, Harthoorn L F & Van Der Beek E M. Obesity in pregnancy: implications for the mother and lifelong health of the child. A consensus statement. *Pediatr Res* 2011;**69**(2):175–80.

27. Milne F, Redman C, Walker J, *et al.* Assessing the onset of pre-eclampsia in the hospital day unit: summary of the pre-eclampsia guideline (PRECOG II). *BMJ* 2009;**339**:b3129.

28. National Institute for Health and Clinical Excellence. *Hypertension in Pregnancy. The Management of Hypertensive Disorders During Pregnancy.* NICE Clinical Guideline 107. 2010. http://guidance.nice.org.uk/CG107 [Accessed January 4, 2012].

29. O'Brien T E, Ray J G & Chan W S. Maternal body mass index and the risk of preeclampsia: a systematic overview. *Epidemiology* 2003;**14**(3):368–74.

30. Cedergren M I. Maternal morbid obesity and the risk of adverse pregnancy outcome. *Obstet Gynecol* 2004;**103**(2):219–24.

31. Walsh S W. Obesity: a risk factor for preeclampsia. *Trends Endocrinol Metab* 2007;**18**(10):365–70.

32. Bhattacharya S, Campbell D M & Liston W A. Effect of body mass index on pregnancy outcomes in nulliparous women delivering singleton babies. *BMC Public Health* 2007;**7**:168.

33. Bhattacharya S. Higher BMI in pregnant women associated with a greater likelihood of pre-eclampsia, caesarian delivery and higher offspring birth weight and body fat. *Evid Based Med* 2010;**15**(5):152–3.

34. Rajasingam D, Seed P T, Briley A L, *et al.* A prospective study of pregnancy outcome and biomarkers of oxidative stress in nulliparous obese women. *Am J Obstet Gynecol* 2009;**200**(4):395e1–9.

35. Finucane M M, Stevens G A, Cowan M J, *et al.* National, regional, and global trends in body-mass index since 1980: systematic analysis of health examination surveys and epidemiological studies with 960 country-years and 9.1 million participants. *Lancet* 2011;**377**(9765):557–67.

36. Bellamy L, Casas J P, Hingorani A D, *et al.* Pre-eclampsia and risk of cardiovascular disease and cancer in later life: systematic review and meta-analysis. *BMJ* 2007;**335**(7627):974.

37. Bourjeily G, Paidas M, Khalil H, *et al.* Pulmonary embolism in pregnancy. *Lancet* 2010;**375**(9713):500–12.

38. Drife J. Thromboembolism. *Br Med Bull* 2003;**67**:177–90.

39. Larsen T B, Sorensen H T, Gislum M, *et al.* Maternal smoking, obesity, and risk of venous thromboembolism during pregnancy and the puerperium: a population-based nested case-control study. *Thromb Res* 2007;**120**(4):505–9.

40. Knight M. Antenatal pulmonary embolism: risk factors, management and outcomes. *BJOG* 2008;**115**(4):453–61.

41. Lippi G & Franchini M. Pathogenesis of venous thromboembolism: when the cup runneth over. *Semin Thromb Hemost* 2008;**34**(8):747–61.

42. Heslehurst N, Simpson H, Ells L J, *et al.* The impact of maternal BMI status on pregnancy outcomes with immediate short-term obstetric resource implications: a meta-analysis. *Obes Rev* 2008;**9**(6):635–83.

43. Zhang J, Bricker L, Wray S, *et al.* Poor uterine contractility in obese women. *BJOG* 2007;**114**(3):343–8.

44. Nuthalapaty F S & Rouse D J. The impact of obesity on obstetrical practice and outcome. *Clin Obstet Gynecol* 2004;**47**(4):898–913; discussion 80–1.

45. Sheiner E, Levy A, Menes T S, *et al.* Maternal obesity as an independent risk factor for caesarean delivery. *Paediatr Perinat Epidemiol* 2004;**18**(3):196–201.

46. Usha Kiran T S, Hemmadi S, Bethel J, *et al.* Outcome of pregnancy in a woman with an increased body mass index. *BJOG* 2005;**112**(6):768–72.

47. Poobalan A S, Aucott L S, Gurung T, *et al.* Obesity as an independent risk factor for elective and emergency caesarean delivery in nulliparous women – systematic review and meta-analysis of cohort studies. *Obes Rev* 2009;**10**(1):28–35.

48. Heslehurst N, Lang R, Rankin J, *et al.* Obesity in pregnancy: a study of the impact of maternal obesity on NHS maternity services. *BJOG* 2007;**114**(3):334–42.

49. Heslehurst N, Moore H, Rankin J, *et al.* How can maternity services be developed to effectively address maternal obesity? A qualitative study. *Midwifery* 2011;**27**(5):e170–7.

Potential mechanisms contributing to gestational diabetes and pre-eclampsia in the obese woman

Naveed Sattar and Dilys J. Freeman

Introduction

The previous chapter and prior reviews demonstrate clear associations between maternal obesity and a range of pregnancy complications. Chief among these are gestational diabetes mellitus (GDM) and pre-eclampsia (PE), but other complications are also overrepresented including greater miscarriage risk, more cesarean sections, and even a heightened risk for intrauterine growth restriction (IUGR). The present chapter will discuss potential mechanisms linking obesity to GDM and PE. It will discuss postulated pathways, particularly for the obesity–PE link, and will show that many of these causal inferences are generally unfounded or exaggerated. The chapter will also provide a framework for future studies and describe potential strategies whereby the causal pathways may be explored.

Obesity and GDM

The strong epidemiological association between obesity and type 2 diabetes mellitus (T2DM) is well described [1]. Similarly, as noted in the previous chapter, the same is also true for the obesity–GDM link. However, in recent years our understanding of the mechanisms linking obesity to diabetes in the non-pregnant arena has advanced considerably. A brief description of this highly relevant background is helpful for subsequent considerations of the pathways linking obesity to GDM.

Mechanisms linking obesity to diabetes in non-pregnant individuals

Surprisingly, this is an area that still attracts some debate. What is clear, however, is the emergence of one dominant hypothesis, specifically that of the role of ectopic fat leading to organ-specific insulin resistance via a process termed "lipotoxicity" [2]. It appears that individuals prone to diabetes show a greater propensity to accumulate visceral fat for a given weight; interestingly, this characteristic, in turn, may be a downstream consequence of an "impaired" subcutaneous fat storage capacity, mechanisms for which deserve far greater attention. An extreme example of this concept is lipodystrophy, a disorder where affected individuals have an impaired ability to store subcutaneous fat, and consequently accumulate fat in visceral and ectopic tissues and have marked insulin resistance [3]. At the other extreme, there are many people, particularly women, who despite attaining very high BMI, as great as 50 to 60 kg/m^2, remain insulin sensitive and normolipemic. Imaging studies have shown these individuals to have low levels of visceral and ectopic fat but a high subcutaneous fat content [4]. It also appears that certain ethnic groups at heightened diabetes risk may have a predisposition to store fat centrally, e.g., in South Asians fat accumulates at a lower average BMI and at an earlier age than in European Whites. Consequently type 2 diabetes develops as much as a decade earlier than in other ethnic groups [5]. In other words, the location of fat storage (subcutaneous vs. visceral/ectopic) appears critical to both the age and the BMI at which metabolic disorders develop. Figure 5.1 summarizes the concept of ectopic fat.

Chronologically, gain of liver fat appears to immediately precede development of diabetes in most individuals, whereas muscle insulin resistance appears to be a longer standing and earlier abnormality [6]. Considerable focus has been placed recently on the role of the liver in the development of diabetes. Associated

Maternal Obesity, ed. Matthew W. Gillman and Lucilla Poston. Published by Cambridge University Press. © Cambridge University Press 2012.

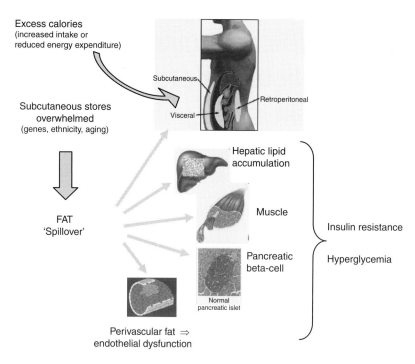

Excess calories
(increased intake or
reduced energy expenditure)

Subcutaneous

Retroperitoneal

Visceral

Subcutaneous stores
overwhelmed
(genes, ethnicity, aging)

FAT
'Spillover'

Hepatic lipid
accumulation

Muscle

Insulin resistance

Pancreatic
beta-cell

Hyperglycemia

Normal
pancreatic islet

Perivascular fat ⇒
endothelial dysfunction

Figure 5.1. Simple concept of ectopic fat and development of insulin resistance and frank diabetes in non-pregnant individuals. This figure provides a simple conceptual illustration of the development and location of ectopic fat in individuals once they have "overwhelmed" their ability to store safe subcutaneous fat. Certain factors such as gender (females with greater storage capacity), genetics (with family history of diabetes as a broad proxy measure), ethnicity (e.g., South Asians), and aging have relevance to an individual's ability to store fat subcutaneously. Other factors may also be relevant such as smoking but more data are needed to examine this. In temporal terms, liver fat accumulation may be closer to the time of development of diabetes whereas muscle insulin resistance is a more proximal development. Perivascular fat may contribute to vascular dysfunction via a process of adverse vasocrine signaling leading in turn to impaired nutrient blood flow – i.e., vascular insulin resistance. Finally, some recent evidence indicates excess fat may also accumulate in the pancreas to contribute to beta-cell dysfunction, and thus development of diabetes. (See figure in color plate section.)

with this, the condition of non-alcoholic fatty liver, attributed to hepatic insulin resistance [7], is very common (>50%) among subjects with T2DM.

The molecular mechanisms leading to excess hepatic fat accumulation remain elusive. Some suggest hyperinsulinemia drives hepatic *de novo* lipogenesis and hepatic fat excess [6] whereas others propose that continued excess caloric intake, particularly in the form of carbohydrate, is the principal factor responsible [8] although, of course, the two processes are interacting and often occur in parallel. Regardless of the exact process, excess hepatic fat is causally linked to hepatic insulin resistance via a number of potential cellular pathways including activation of inflammatory signaling pathways, endoplasmic reticulum stress, excess production of reactive oxygen species, mitochondrial dysfunction, accumulation of triglycerides and/or fatty acyl intermediates, and activation of serine-threonine kinases, as recently reviewed [9]. Individuals with excess hepatic fat are therefore unable to suppress hepatic gluconeogenesis normally in response to insulin and continued excessive hepatic glucose production contributes to diabetes development.

There is general agreement that in individuals destined to develop T2DM, as peripheral or hepatic insulin resistance increases, the pancreas's ability to hypersecrete insulin is eventually overwhelmed and frank diabetes ensues. Historically, most investigators considered predisposition to pancreatic failure to be largely genetically governed. However, a new concept that excess fat accumulating in the pancreas can impair pancreatic beta-cell function is also emerging [10]. This exciting development suggests that, at least in some patients, pancreatic function may be recoverable with substantial weight loss. The apparent "cure" or, better termed, "remission" from T2DM in patients following substantial weight loss from bariatric surgery, including some previously treated with insulin, would tend to support this possibility [11].

Other proposed mechanisms linking obesity to T2DM include release of systemic cytokines and a low-grade inflammatory state, as well as altered adipokine status, in particular lower adiponectin levels. However, these relationships may be overplayed as there is scant evidence for a causal role for C-reactive protein (CRP) in T2DM [12] and several anti-inflammatory interventions have not improved insulin resistance in man. Equally of interest, while adiponectin appears to have a clear role in animal models in mediating insulin sensitivity, there is strong evidence in humans to suggest that hyperinsulinemia lowers adiponectin levels rather than the reverse, as would be anticipated [13]. In other words, in humans higher adiponectin levels represent a "readout" of insulin sensitivity.

Obesity and risk for GDM

In simple terms, the association between insulin resistance and GDM makes clinical sense since late pregnancy is an insulin-resistant state. An early gestational (week 6–10) decrease in maternal fasting glucose of 2 mg/dl has been observed with little further decrease by the third trimester [14]. Since the decline occurs before a stage at which fetal utilization of glucose could make a significant contribution, this suggests that maternal metabolic and hormonal factors alter plasma glucose concentration independently of the conceptus. Late pregnancy is associated with a more than 50% decrease in peripheral insulin sensitivity assessed by euglycemic hyperinsulinemic clamp tests [15]. Data from euglycemic hyperinsulinemic clamp tests carried out prior to pregnancy and at around 13 and 35 weeks of gestation [16] demonstrate a 65% increase in both basal insulin and C-peptide (an indicator of insulin secretion) with advancing gestation and the metabolic clearance of insulin increases significantly. These changes in insulin kinetics may partly explain the hyperinsulinemia of pregnancy and almost certainly represent a physiological response to the insulin resistance of pregnancy. Changes in insulin sensitivity related to later pregnancy appear to be primarily at the peripheral level and secondarily at the hepatic level [17].

The elevated levels of non-esterified free fatty acids in later pregnancy, driven by pregnancy hormonal changes, may contribute to the peripheral insulin resistance [18,19]. The mechanism is likely to be accumulation of muscle cell diacylglycerol, which activates protein kinase C, leading to reduced tyrosine phosphorylation of IRS-1. In turn, this prevents phosphoinositol-3 kinase activation, a necessary step in insulin-stimulated glucose uptake.

The physiological decline in fasting glucose in early gestation is lower in mothers with greater BMI and there appears little reduction in severely obese women [14]. In the third trimester of pregnancy obese women demonstrate both peripheral and hepatic insulin resistance manifested as reduced insulin-mediated glucose disposal, a large reduction in insulin-stimulated carbohydrate oxidation, and a reduction in insulin suppression of endogenous glucose production, all of which is reversed in the postpartum period [20]. Obese women

show lower insulin sensitivity during pregnancy compared to control groups in both small longitudinal [21] and larger cross-sectional studies [22].

In pregnancy, maternal fat metabolism is of increasing importance as gestation advances in order to spare carbohydrate for the fetus. In keeping with this principle, the gestational hyperlipidemia is exaggerated in obese women so that triglyceride levels are higher than in leaner women [22]. Endothelial function is improved in pregnancy but to a lesser extent in obese mothers [22]. The reduced endothelial function in obese women may be linked to insulin resistance via inflammation and impaired nitric oxide production [23], but it may also be a contributory factor toward development of diabetes by contributing to a reduction in nutrient delivery to peripheral tissues.

As anticipated in obese pregnancy, women begin pregnancy with a "baseline" of greater insulin resistance and hypertriglyceridemia and both of these reach a peak in the second trimester rather than in the third as in lean women. In other words, obese women may be less flexible in their metabolic response to pregnancy and the total exposure to adverse metabolic conditions is greater (Figure 5.2). This aspect of metabolic change has attracted much less attention and is not yet fully described.

Summary of potential mechanisms linking obesity to GDM

In light of the above, several mechanisms may link obesity to heightened risk for GDM (Table 5.1). The higher insulin resistant state at pregnancy onset is certainly a major contributory factor, so that for an equivalent insulin-resistant effect of later pregnancy, obese women are much more likely to reach a threshold of insulin resistance beyond which the pancreas is unable to fully compensate. Additionally, obese women may experience greater fluxes of fatty acids, leading in turn to greater change in insulin resistance in pregnancy, or else they may experience greater accumulation of hepatic fat and thus greater hepatic insulin resistance. There is also the possibility that the normal enhancement of pancreatic beta-cell insulin release could be compromised in obese pregnancy by lipotoxic factors [24], but this is speculative and requires investigation. Others have shown associations between changes in systemic cytokines and insulin resistance in pregnancy [25], and although plasma cytokines are elevated in obese compared to lean pregnant women

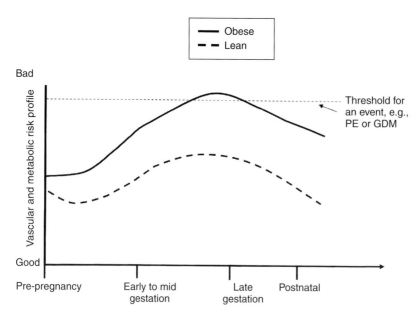

Figure 5.2. Proposed model of metabolic and vascular risk changes during pregnancy in lean and obese women. In lean women there is an initial general improvement in vascular risk profile as a response in early pregnancy (i.e., increased endothelium-dependent function, increased HDL-cholesterol, and reduction in blood pressure), with many changes driven by early pregnancy-related hormonal changes. However, as pregnancy proceeds toward the third trimester, metabolic and vascular stresses increase such that many of the early favorable changes start to reverse or attenuate back toward non-pregnant levels. In obese women, pre-pregnancy metabolic risk profile is less than optimal and obese women may show either an attenuated initial improvement in metabolic response to pregnancy and/or a lower maximal improvement, such that in some women the increasing metabolic and vascular stresses in the second half of pregnancy vastly exceed early benefits or acquired buffering capacity. As a result, more overweight or obese women are at increased risk of developing gestational diabetes mellitus (GDM) or pre-eclampsia (PE).

[22], causality has not been established. Despite there being little evidence in non-pregnant individuals for any benefit of anti-inflammatory therapies, it is plausible that the greater perivascular fat mass may perturb vascular function via locally released cytokines, which act to impede insulin-mediated NO production allowing insulin-mediated endothelin release to dominate [26]. There is some evidence that systemic inflammation is associated with microvascular dysfunction in pregnancy [23]. Given the demands of the peripheral circulation to accommodate greater blood flow in pregnant women, factors, such as excess perivascular fat, which can impair normal vasodilatation [27] may contribute to metabolic and vascular complications in obese pregnant women.

Do risk factors for GDM give mechanistic insight?

In support of a pivotal role for insulin resistance, numerous risk factors that predispose a woman to GDM are associated with greater whole-body insulin resistance and/or greater hepatic insulin resistance. In a recent study [28] we confirmed that women with a family history of diabetes, as well as those from South Asian communities, are at greater risk of GDM, independent of BMI. Such findings fit well with the

patterns of excess risk for T2DM in non-pregnant individuals. We also showed first trimester blood pressure as well as plasma tissue plasminogen activator antigen (t-PA) and low high-density lipoprotein (HDL)-cholesterol independently predicted GDM. Each of these three factors has been shown to predict diabetes in the non-pregnant population and all correlate with insulin resistance, albeit to differing extents. Interestingly, t-PA antigen while considered by many to reflect vascular dysfunction, also correlates very strongly with hepatic insulin resistance and degree of liver fat [29].

Clinical profile of women with GDM post-pregnancy

Further compounding the role of hepatic metabolism and insulin resistance in the origins of GDM, a recent study [30] has shown that women with a history of GDM, but glucose tolerant post-pregnancy, exhibit near double the liver fat content compared to women with a similar BMI but without previous GDM. Of equal interest, muscle insulin sensitivity was only slightly lower in women with prior GDM compared to the women with no history of GDM. Other groups have also observed a near doubling in the prevalence of fatty liver in women with prior GDM, suggesting

Table 5.1 Potential mechanisms contributing to greater GDM risk in obese women, the relative strength of evidence for their contributions, and suggestions for future areas of investigation

Pathway of interest	Level of evidence for causal role	Consequences/future ways forward
Greater baseline insulin resistance linked to family history of diabetes, ethnic origin, fat distribution (more central fat), and overall increased BMI	Robust	Effects of lifestyle intervention to lower pre-pregnancy insulin resistance via weight loss and activity Effects of lifestyle intervention in early pregnancy on changes in insulin sensitivity and pregnancy outcomes (work ongoing as described in later chapters)
Greater reduction in peripheral insulin resistance, ± lack of increase in early insulin sensitivity	Modest	Role of free fatty acids, and pregnancy hormonal changes
Greater hepatic fat accumulation	Modest	More studies required on hepatic fat accumulation in obese pregnancy, including identification of reliable surrogate markers of liver fat accumulation during pregnancy
Altered pancreatic function	Modest	Pancreatic beta-cell exhaustion must be a factor in GDM development but the relative importance of hereditary factors vs. fat accumulation is not clear More studies required on pancreatic beta-cell function in obese pregnancy – including use of urinary markers of beta-cell function (urinary C-peptide?)
Altered vascular function	Modest	More investigation required on a potential link between altered vascular function and impaired nutrient delivery in obese pregnancy
Greater systemic inflammatory status	Weak	Studies of anti-inflammatory intervention indicated but may be ethically questionable in pregnancy Studies of genetic variants related to pro-inflammatory state required but to date information on genes predictive of diabetes are generally lacking

excess liver fat to be a robust finding [31]. All of the above observations suggest the need for further studies to dissect the role of the liver, and its fat-handling capacity, in the development of GDM.

Lifestyle factors

A discussion on mechanisms for the development of GDM would be incomplete without addressing the role of lifestyle factors including excessive caloric intake or lower physical activity. By definition, women who are obese when pregnant have been on a greater life course trajectory of weight gain than their lean counterparts, so their net calorie excess has inevitably been much greater before pregnancy. However, obese women typically gain less weight than leaner women in pregnancy [32] so that their BMI or insulin resistance entering pregnancy appears the dominant factor driving their risk of diabetes [33]. Irrespective of this observation,

and as described in Chapter 15, several ongoing studies are testing the potential of lifestyle changes to prevent GDM or improve insulin sensitivity in obese pregnant women and the results of these are awaited with interest.

Obesity and PE

Pre-eclampsia is commonly described as the "disease of theories," a label that has remained unchanged for many years. Of interest, the heightened PE risk with greater BMI has only become apparent in the last two decades but, as yet and not unsurprisingly, the mechanisms for this relationship also remain unclear. Several of the postulated causal pathways are described below (see Table 5.2). Most theories stem from observational studies and inevitably suffer from the potential limitations of reverse causality, or residual confounding.

Table 5.2 Potential mechanisms contributing to greater PE risk in obese women, the relative strength of evidence for their contributions, and suggestions for future areas of investigation

Pathway of interest	Level of evidence for causal role	Consequences/future ways forward
Obesity links to hypertension and proteinuria	Modest	The stronger link between obesity and milder PE suggests the association may be partly accounted for by the general association of obesity with blood pressure and proteinuria risk
Insulin resistance	Modest	Insulin resistance linked to many implicated pathways
		Ongoing studies of effects of lifestyle and metformin in obese pregnancy will inform
		Larger studies required to address body-fat composition and risk for PE or to investigate phenotyping in women with prior PE
Dyslipidemia	Modest	Dyslipidemia could be secondary to disease process but altered lipid metabolism (including elevations in FFA) may be relevant to liver and kidney complications in PE
		Studies of genetic variants associated with dyslipidemia and PE risk required
		Effect of statins on PE – ongoing pilot study addressing surrogate endpoint should include long-term childhood follow-up
Inflammation	Weak	Studies of genetic variants associated with inflammation and PE risk required
		Anti-inflammatory therapies – much more robust evidence required before given serious consideration – potential adverse effects
Altered vascular function Altered ADMA	Weak	More work on a potential link between altered vascular function and impaired placental nutrient delivery in obese pregnancy
		Trials of arginine and other NO precursors in high-risk pregnancies but current results mixed
Lowered buffering capacity	Modest	Poorer nutrient status and so lower antioxidant buffering capacity to counter oxidative stress from poorly perfused placenta/other oxidative processes?
		Lower HDL-cholesterol to counteract pro-oxidative stress?
		Impaired vascular function to accommodate vascular blood flow demands

Obesity-related hypertension and proteinuria in non-pregnant subjects: a framework to anticipate more PE in obese women?

There is plentiful evidence that obesity is the major risk factor for essential hypertension in non-pregnant subjects. In addition, although less well appreciated, there is a clear link between obesity/metabolic syndrome and risk for proteinuria [34]. This relationship is likely causal since weight loss leads to a reduction in proteinuria in non-pregnant subjects [35]. Given that hypertension and proteinuria in combination define women with PE, we should not be surprised by an association between obesity and risk for PE. The observation that adiposity is more strongly associated with a rise in risk of mild PE, whereas associations with severe PE as defined by blood pressure >160/110 mmHg appear more modest [36], suggests that this simple explanation connecting obesity to PE is perhaps most pertinent to a subset of PE phenotypes. Further studies including the tracking of proteinuria changes in relation to baseline BMI in pregnancy would be helpful. A brief overview of the other relevant pathways postulated to link obesity to PE is given below.

Cardiovascular disease (CVD) risk factors and PE risk in obese women

There is a well-described association between PE and subsequent CVD risk [37], especially for those women with a history of early severe PE. Indeed, susceptibility for CVD risk may precede the development of PE and may be causative for the disease. Pregnancy may simply "unmask" an underlying propensity for CVD, which otherwise would only become manifest in later life. The reasons underpinning the association with cardiovascular risk and PE are not entirely clear; researchers have variably ascribed hypertension, lipid abnormalities, vascular dysfunction, pro-inflammatory and insulin resistance mechanisms as potential causal pathways [38]. Since obesity is linked to all these abnormalities, each requires attention in relation to the heightened risk of PE.

Obesity, lipids, and PE risk

Pre-eclampsia is characterized by dyslipidemia, predominantly hypertriglyceridemia. Women destined to develop PE demonstrate elevated triglyceride concentrations early in pregnancy and, linked to this, higher plasma free fatty acid (FFA) concentrations. The higher triglyceride levels are associated with an increase in smaller, denser low-density lipoprotein (LDL) particles, which are prone to oxidation [38]. Furthermore, the rise in FFA may facilitate exaggerated lipid accumulation in the liver and kidneys thus contributing to some of the complications of PE [38]. While these lipid changes are intriguing and also may have relevance to the appearance of foam cells in the spiral arteries in the placenta of women with PE, definitive evidence of causality cannot be inferred. Many women have significantly elevated triglyceride levels but do not develop PE; rather, lipid alterations in conjunction with other changes in PE may serve to accentuate the condition. Alternatively, there may be other as yet undefined disturbances in lipid metabolism that contribute. Some have postulated a lipolytic factor released by the placenta to be the main driver of elevations in FFA and triglycerides [39] but this remains to be characterized. Increased FFA flux may also drive ectopic fat accumulation in PE with similar downstream effects as described earlier for GDM [40].

The elevation of lipids in PE could also serve as a protective mechanism to improve placental nutrient transfer, thereby counteracting deficiencies arising from compromised placental blood flow. This is a common theme in PE, whereby the adverse maternal changes, including dyslipidemia and, more critically, elevated blood pressure, while potentially harmful to the mother, could maintain nourishment of the fetus. This raises an important issue since a randomized controlled trial to determine the potential benefit of treatment with lipid-lowering statins in women with

PE has recently commenced (www.controlled-trials.com/ISRCTN23410175). This pilot trial, the primary outcome of which is a change in surrogate markers of risk (soluble fms-like tyrosine kinase 1 (sFlt-1) at 48 hours post-randomization) will also address infant outcomes.

Obesity, inflammation, and PE risk

There remains considerable interest in the hypothesis that suggests PE arises from an inflammatory state. There is some evidence for heightened CRP and cytokine levels in women with PE [41] as well as changes in the circulating and placental inflammatory cell profile [42], with changes in the latter likely to be more significant than the subtle elevations in systemic cytokines. In light of these associations as well as the knowledge that obesity is linked to low-grade inflammatory response in pregnancy [22], many researchers have postulated that obesity heightens PE risk via this pathway. While a full discussion is beyond the scope of this chapter, these observational studies [22,42] do not prove causality. The magnitude of change in inflammatory cytokine concentration in isolation is too small to be considered causal. There are, as far as we are aware, no studies of anti-inflammatory interventions that have addressed the prevention or treatment of PE. Randomized controlled trials have shown that low-dose aspirin has a protective effect in the prevention of PE, reducing the incidence by 10% but, at the doses prescribed (approx. 60 mg), aspirin has negligible effect on inflammatory pathways in man. Whether there is a genuine potential to intervene to prevent or treat PE with novel anti-inflammatory treatments remains to be proven. This strategy could theoretically adversely influence the delicate and complex balance between pro- and anti-inflammatory pathways in normal pregnancy. Finally, at least some of the cellular inflammatory changes in PE may be secondary to the disease process – i.e., a result of aberrant vascular function.

Obesity, vascular dysfunction, and PE risk

Pre-eclampsia is characterized by impaired maternal vascular function. As noted above, obesity is linked to vascular dysfunction, which is proposed to occur via a process of vasocrine signaling [26]. In isolation this is unlikely to be causative but may potentiate the effect of other factors detrimental to vascular health.

Elevation in plasma concentrations of asymmetric dimethylarginine (ADMA), an inhibitor of nitric oxide synthesis, has been shown to predict coronary heart disease (CHD) and PE [43]. The ADMA concentration is influenced by several factors including obesity, inflammation, and dietary factors and it has been postulated that ADMA represents a unifying link between obesity and PE risk [43]. This is of some interest given the potential therapeutic role of enhanced dietary arginine to counter the effects of ADMA. Evidence from trials is mixed regarding the value of nitric oxide donors and precursors to prevent PE [44], although a more recent study was positive [45].

Obesity, lifestyle factors, insulin resistance, and PE risk

Given that insulin resistance is linked to inflammation, dyslipidemia, vascular dysfunction, and hypertension, and is most likely upstream of all of these abnormalities, it is clear that insulin resistance could be a major link between obesity and PE. Women with GDM have a heightened risk of PE as do women with T2DM. Women with PE have a higher risk of diabetes in later life [46], perhaps not unsurprisingly given the likely high prevalence of greater BMI. Reducing insulin resistance via either lifestyle changes or pharmacotherapy might therefore lessen PE risk, but here there is a lack of good data to inform. There is preliminary evidence from non-controlled studies of a potential reduction in PE and pregnancy-induced hypertension with metformin treatment in women with PCOS [47], but a recent randomized controlled trial from Norway of 257 women with PCOS did not find any reduction in PE risk (nor in the risk for GDM, or preterm delivery) with metformin vs. placebo given from the first trimester to delivery, although numbers of each of these outcomes were too small to draw firm conclusions [48]. Two ongoing randomized controlled trials of metformin in obese pregnant women in the UK (EMPOWaR, ISRCTN 51279843 and MOP, NCT01273584) are likely to provide valuable insight although the primary outcome in both trials is birthweight, not PE.

Lifestyle interventions in obese pregnant women may also prove effective. Observational studies suggest that physical activity seems to be associated with lower PE risk [49] but these studies are prone to residual confounding including by obesity – obese individuals being on average less physically active. In addition, the role of dietary composition vs. excess caloric intake in PE risk requires exploration. Despite the complexity of measuring dietary intake, the relationship between robust biomarkers of dietary intake and risk for PE would be of interest in order to establish the potential for dietary intervention for the treatment of PE. Unfortunately, there are few such robust markers and even measures such as blood vitamin concentrations are subject to considerable confounding, as we have recently demonstrated [50]. Thus the results of randomized trials of antioxidant vitamins are the most important pieces of evidence on which to base conclusions. Here, the current evidence does not favor use of antioxidant supplements to prevent PE [51,52].

Substantial weight loss via bariatric surgery can considerably lessen the risk of PE as demonstrated in a recent retrospective analysis in which risk for PE or eclampsia was 80% lower in the same women after surgery [53]. Thus, while obesity appears causally related to risk of PE, there appears to be no single mechanism that is able to explain this link.

Other pathways of interest

Successful placentation is essential for healthy pregnancy outcome, and in PE partial failure of trophoblast invasion is likely to play a major role in the disease process. Whether obesity can adversely influence placentation and placental function and thereby contribute to the primary pathology in PE is not well established. Equally, whether adipokine changes play a role is also speculative, and current data provide little evidence of causal links. Indeed, adiponectin levels are elevated in PE, perhaps as a salvage mechanism [54]. Finally, it may be the case that obese women (with the associated metabolic and vascular changes) are not only closer to the threshold required to 'express' PE but, in addition, they have a lower buffering capacity – associated with some of the pathways described above – to cope with the metabolic changes in pregnancy (see Table 5.2).

Conclusion

We have reviewed many of the mechanisms that may explain the relationship between obesity and GDM and with PE. With respect to GDM, we have focused attention on the role of total and ectopic fat deposition as key determinants of the level of insulin resistance with which women enter pregnancy (Figure 5.1). The baseline level of insulin resistance, perhaps more so than any other features (as reviewed in Table 5.1), appears critical to women's risk of developing GDM. Given the rising levels of obesity worldwide, ongoing studies as described in other chapters of this book are designed to determine whether beneficial lifestyle changes can be successfully initiated in obese pregnant women and, if so, whether such changes can attenuate risk for pregnancy complications including GDM.

With respect to the obesity–PE association, it appears that there is no single mechanistic explanation. We have reviewed the potential roles of many different pathways, expressing our views on the strength of evidence to support each pathway, and giving suggestions for future relevant studies (Table 5.2). However, it appears that, as with the obesity–CVD link in the general population [55], obesity likely enhances risk of PE through a combination of interlinked downstream mechanisms and that no one pathway is dominant. Whether lifestyle changes initiated in early pregnancy can lessen PE risk remains to be seen. In the meantime, the key public health message is to place additional emphasis and resources to help young women maintain a healthy body weight and thus minimize their chances of pregnancy complications.

References

1. Eckel R H, Kahn S E, Ferrannini E, *et al.* Obesity and type 2 diabetes: what can be unified and what needs to be individualized? *J Clin Endocrinol Metab* 2011;**96**:1654–63.

2. Cusi K. The role of adipose tissue and lipotoxicity in the pathogenesis of type 2 diabetes. *Curr Diab Rep* 2010;**10**:306–15.

3. Huang-Doran I, Sleigh A, Rochford J J, *et al.* Lipodystrophy: metabolic insights from a rare disorder. *J Endocrinol* 2011;**207**:245–55.

4. Stefan N, Kantartzis K, Machann J, *et al.* Identification and characterization of metabolically benign obesity in humans. *Arch Intern Med* 2008;**168**:1609–16.

5. Cleland S J & Sattar N. Impact of ethnicity on metabolic disturbance, vascular dysfunction and atherothrombotic cardiovascular disease. *Diabetes Obes Metab* 2005;**7**:463–70.

6. Taylor R. Pathogenesis of type 2 diabetes: tracing the reverse route from cure to cause. *Diabetologia* 2008;**51**:1781–9.

7. Preiss D & Sattar N. Non-alcoholic fatty liver disease: an overview of prevalence, diagnosis, pathogenesis and treatment considerations. *Clin Sci (Lond)* 2008;**115**:141–50.

8. Stefan N, Kantartzis K & Haring H U. Causes and metabolic consequences of fatty liver. *Endocr Rev* 2008;**29**:939–60.

9. Hotamisligil G S & Erbay E. Nutrient sensing and inflammation in metabolic diseases. *Nat Rev Immunol* 2008;**8**:923–34.

10. Lim E L, Hollingsworth K G, Aribisala B S, *et al.* Reversal of type 2 diabetes: normalisation of beta cell function in association with decreased pancreas and liver triacylglycerol. *Diabetologia* 2011;**54**:2506–14.

11. Sjostrom L, Lindroos A K, Peltonen M, *et al.* Lifestyle, diabetes, and cardiovascular risk factors 10 years after bariatric surgery. *N Engl J Med* 2004;**35**:2683–93.

12. Timpson N J, Lawlor D A, Harbord R M, *et al.* C-reactive protein and its role in metabolic syndrome: mendelian randomisation study. *Lancet* 2005;**366**:1954–9.

13. Cook J R & Semple R K. Hypoadiponectinemia – cause or consequence of human "insulin resistance"? *J Clin Endocrinol Metab* 2010;**95**:1544–54.

14. Mills J L, Jovanovic L, Knopp R, *et al.* Physiological reduction in fasting plasma glucose concentration in the first trimester of normal pregnancy: the diabetes in early pregnancy study. *Metabolism* 1998;**47**:1140–4.

15. Catalano P M, Tyzbir E D, Roman N M, *et al.* Longitudinal changes in insulin release and insulin resistance in nonobese pregnant women. *Am J Obstet Gynecol* 1991;**165**:1667–72.

16. Catalano P M, Drago N M, Amini S B. Longitudinal changes in pancreatic beta-cell function and metabolic clearance rate of insulin in pregnant women with normal and abnormal glucose tolerance. *Diabetes Care* 1998;**21**:403–8.

17. Catalano P M, Hoegh M, Minium J, *et al.* Adiponectin in human pregnancy: implications for regulation of glucose and lipid metabolism. *Diabetologia* 2006;**49**:1677–85.

18. Sivan E, Homko C J, Whittaker P G, *et al.* Free fatty acids and insulin resistance during pregnancy. *J Clin Endocrinol Metab* 1998;**83**:2338–42.

19. Sivan E & Boden G. Free fatty acids, insulin resistance, and pregnancy. *Curr Diab Rep* 2003;**3**:319–22.

20. Sivan E, Chen X, Homko C J, *et al.* Longitudinal study of carbohydrate metabolism in healthy obese pregnant women. *Diabetes Care* 1997;**20**:1470–5.

21. Catalano P M, Huston L, Amini S B, *et al.* Longitudinal changes in glucose metabolism during pregnancy in obese women with normal glucose tolerance and gestational diabetes mellitus. *Am J Obstet Gynecol* 1999;**180**:903–16.

22. Ramsay J E, Ferrell W R, Crawford L, *et al.* Maternal obesity is associated with dysregulation of metabolic, vascular, and inflammatory pathways. *J Clin Endocrinol Metab* 2002;**87**:4231–7.

23. Stewart F M, Freeman D J, Ramsay J E, *et al.* Longitudinal assessment of maternal endothelial function and markers of inflammation and placental function throughout pregnancy in lean and obese mothers. *J Clin Endocrinol Metab* 2007;**92**:969–75.

24. Giacca A, Xiao C, Oprescu A I, *et al.* Lipid-induced pancreatic beta-cell dysfunction: focus on in vivo studies. *Am J Physiol Endocrinol Metab* 2011;**300**:e255–62.

25. Kirwan J P, Hauguel-De Mouzon S, Lepercq J, *et al.* TNF-alpha is a predictor of insulin resistance in human pregnancy. *Diabetes* 2002;**51**:2207–13.

26. Yudkin J S, Eringa E & Stehouwer C D. "Vasocrine" signalling from perivascular fat: a mechanism linking insulin resistance to vascular disease. *Lancet* 2005;**365**:1817–20.

27. Aghamohammadzadeh R, Withers S B, Lynch F M, *et al.* Perivascular adipose tissue from human systemic and coronary vessels: The emergence of a new pharmacotherapeutic target. *Br J Pharmacol* 2011, doi: 10.1111/j.1476–5381.2011.01479.x.

28. Savvidou M, Nelson S M, Makgoba M, *et al.* First-trimester prediction of gestational diabetes mellitus: examining the potential of combining maternal characteristics and laboratory measures. *Diabetes* 2010;**59**:3017–22.

29. Sattar N, Wannamethee S G & Forouhi N G. Novel biochemical risk factors for type 2 diabetes: pathogenic insights or prediction possibilities? *Diabetologia* 2008;**51**:926–40.

30. Prikoszovich T, Winzer C, Schmid A I, *et al.* Body and liver fat mass rather than muscle mitochondrial function determine glucose metabolism in women with a history of gestational diabetes mellitus. *Diabetes Care* 2011;**34**:430–6.

31. Forbes S, Taylor-Robinson S D, Patel N, *et al.* Increased prevalence of non-alcoholic fatty liver disease in European women with a history of gestational diabetes. *Diabetologia* 2011;**54**:641–7.

32. Fraser A, Tilling K, MacDonald-Wallis C, *et al.* Associations of gestational weight gain with maternal body mass index, waist circumference, and blood pressure measured 16 y after pregnancy: the Avon Longitudinal Study of Parents and Children (ALSPAC). *Am J Clin Nutr* 2011;**93**:1285–92.

33. Herring S J, Oken E, Rifas-Shiman S L, *et al.* Weight gain in pregnancy and risk of maternal hyperglycemia. *Am J Obstet Gynecol* 2009;**201**:61e1–7.

34. Whaley-Connell A, Pavey B S, Afroze A, *et al.* Obesity and insulin resistance as risk factors for chronic kidney disease. *J Cardiometab Syndr* 2006;**1**:209–14.

35. Afshinnia F, Wilt T J, Duval S, *et al.* Weight loss and proteinuria: systematic review of clinical trials and comparative cohorts. *Nephrol Dial Transplant* 2010;**25**:1173–83.

36. Bodnar L M, Catov J M, Klebanoff M A, *et al.* Prepregnancy body mass index and the occurrence of severe hypertensive disorders of pregnancy. *Epidemiology* 2007;**18**:234–9.

37. Sattar N & Greer I A. Pregnancy complications and maternal cardiovascular risk: opportunities for intervention and screening? *BMJ* 2002;**325**:157–60.

38. Sattar N, Gaw A, Packard C J, *et al.* Potential pathogenic roles of aberrant lipoprotein and fatty acid metabolism in pre-eclampsia. *Br J Obstet Gynaecol* 1996;**103**:614–20.

39. Endresen M J, Lorentzen B & Henriksen T. Increased lipolytic activity and high ratio of free fatty acids to albumin in sera from women with preeclampsia leads to triglyceride accumulation in cultured endothelial cells. *Am J Obstet Gynecol* 1992;**167**:440–7.

40. Jarvie E, Hauguel-de-Mouzon S, Nelson S M, *et al.* Lipotoxicity in obese pregnancy and its potential role in adverse pregnancy outcome and obesity in the offspring. *Clin Sci (Lond)* 2010;**119**:123–9.

41. Freeman D J, McManus F, Brown E A, *et al.* Short- and long-term changes in plasma inflammatory markers associated with preeclampsia. *Hypertension* 2004;**44**:708–14.

42. Walsh S W. Obesity: a risk factor for preeclampsia. *Trends Endocrinol Metab* 2007;**18**:365–70.

43. Roberts J M, Bodnar L M, Patrick T E, *et al.* The role of obesity in preeclampsia. *Pregnancy Hypertens* 2011;**1**:6–16.

44. Meher S & Duley L. Nitric oxide for preventing pre-eclampsia and its complications. *Cochrane Database Syst Rev* 2007;CD006490.

45. Vadillo-Ortega F, Perichart-Perera O, Espino S, *et al.* Effect of supplementation during pregnancy with L-arginine and antioxidant vitamins in medical food on pre-eclampsia in high risk population: randomised controlled trial. *BMJ* 2011;**342**:d2901.

46. Libby G, Murphy D J, McEwan N F, *et al.* Pre-eclampsia and the later development of type 2 diabetes in mothers and their children: an intergenerational study from the Walker cohort. *Diabetologia* 2007;**50**:523–30.

47. De Leo V, Musacchio M C, Piomboni P, *et al.* The administration of metformin during pregnancy reduces polycystic ovary syndrome related gestational complications. *Eur J Obstet Gynecol Reprod Biol* 2011;**157**:63–6.

48. Vanky E, Stridsklev S, Heimstad R, *et al.* Metformin versus placebo from first trimester to delivery in polycystic ovary syndrome: a randomized, controlled multicenter study. *J Clin Endocrinol Metab* 2010;**95**:e448–55.

49. Sorensen T K, Williams M A, Lee I M, *et al.* Recreational physical activity during pregnancy

and risk of preeclampsia. *Hypertension* 2003;**41**:1273–80.

50. Talwar D, McConnachie A, Welsh P, *et al.* Which circulating antioxidant vitamins are confounded by socioeconomic deprivation? The MIDSPAN family study. *PLoS One* 2010;**5**:1024–31.

51. McCance D R, Holmes V A, Maresh M J, *et al.* Vitamins C and E for prevention of pre-eclampsia in women with type 1 diabetes (DAPIT): a randomised placebo-controlled trial. *Lancet* 2010;**376**:259–66.

52. Rumbold A, Duley L, Crowther C A, *et al.* Antioxidants for preventing pre-eclampsia. *Cochrane Database Syst Rev* 2008;CD004227.

53. Bennett W L, Gilson M M, Jamshidi R, *et al.* Impact of bariatric surgery on hypertensive disorders in pregnancy: retrospective analysis of insurance claims data. *BMJ* 2010;**340**:c1662.

54. Ramsay J E, Jamieson N, Greer I A, *et al.* Paradoxical elevation in adiponectin concentrations in women with preeclampsia. *Hypertension* 2003;**42**:891–4.

55. Wormser D, Kaptoge S, Di Angelantonio E, *et al.* Separate and combined associations of body-mass index and abdominal adiposity with cardiovascular disease: collaborative analysis of 58 prospective studies. *Lancet* 2011;**377**:1085–95.

Chapter

6

Fetal and infant outcomes in obese pregnant women

Ruth Bell, Peter W. G. Tennant, and Judith Rankin

Introduction

Fetal loss, stillbirth, infant death, and major structural congenital anomaly are among the most serious adverse outcomes that have been associated with maternal obesity. This chapter summarizes the available epidemiological evidence, and discusses potential explanations and public health implications.

Maternal obesity and the risk of fetal and infant death

Fetal death and maternal obesity

Fetal death is the delivery of a fetus or infant that shows no signs of life. Fetal deaths are categorized as stillbirths or miscarriages on the basis of gestational age at delivery. A stillbirth is the delivery of a baby at a gestational age beyond the accepted threshold for viability that shows no signs of life, and a miscarriage is a fetal loss at an earlier gestational age. The gestational age threshold defining stillbirth varies between countries, from 20 weeks in the United States [1], 24 weeks in the UK [2], and 28 weeks in other parts of Europe [3].

Around 1 in 200 births in developed countries ends in a stillbirth [4,5], with limited evidence of improvement in recent years [1,2]. Known maternal risk factors for stillbirth include advanced age, nulliparity, ethnic background, maternal diabetes, hypertension, obesity, and smoking [6–8]. The majority of stillbirths, around 85%, occur before the onset of labor (antepartum stillbirths) and the remainder occur during labor (intrapartum stillbirths) [2]. In epidemiological studies, a high proportion of stillbirths, 10% to 70% depending on cause of death classification, are described as "unexplained," with no apparent underlying cause [5,9]. While clinically many stillbirths occur unexpectedly in apparently uncomplicated pregnancies, if exhaustive post-mortem investigations are undertaken, an underlying cause can be identified in most cases [5]. However, in routine clinical practice, permission for autopsy is frequently either denied or not sought. The most frequent disorders include placental pathology, infection, umbilical cord abnormalities, congenital anomalies, and maternal medical disorders including diabetes and hypertension [9].

A number of epidemiologic studies have explored the relationship between maternal body mass index (BMI) in early pregnancy and the risk of stillbirth. Chu et al., in a meta-analysis of cohort and case-control studies, found the risk of stillbirth was doubled in obese women (BMI $\geq 30 \, kg/m^2$) compared with those of recommended BMI ($18.5–25 \, kg/m^2$) (summary odds ratio [OR] 2.07; 95% confidence interval [CI] 1.59–2.74). For overweight women there was also a significant increase in risk of stillbirth compared with those of recommended BMI (OR 1.47; 95% CI: 1.08–1.94) [10]. A recent meta-analysis of five cohort studies reported an increased risk of stillbirth in both obese (OR 1.63; 95% CI: 1.35–1.95) and overweight women (OR 1.23; 95% CI: 1.09–1.38) compared with recommended BMI [11–18]. Table 6.1 summarizes the cohort studies included in these meta-analyses, together with three further cohort studies [11–18]. Of the studies reporting more recent data (deliveries after 2002), one reported a doubling of risk, consistent with the earlier meta-analysis [17], while two found no significant association (OR 1.07; 95% CI: 0.74–1.56 and OR 1.04; CI: 0.79–1.37) [12,16]. A recent UK national study of births to women with a BMI $\geq 35 \, kg/m^2$ (morbid obese) reported a doubling of risk of stillbirth compared with the background population [19], consistent with

Maternal Obesity, ed. Matthew W. Gillman and Lucilla Poston. Published by Cambridge University Press. © Cambridge University Press 2012.

Table 6.1 Cohort studies of maternal body mass index and risk of stillbirth

Study	Setting and population	Definition of stillbirth	Definition of obesity/overweight (kg/m²)	Adjustment for covariates	OR for obesity	OR for overweight
Sebire et al. (2001)[a,b] [13]	UK 1989–1997 Regional multicenter study 287 213 singleton deliveries	Not stated (UK definition of stillbirth changed from 28 weeks to 24 weeks in 1992)	Obese 30+ Overweight 25–29.9 Reference 20.0–24.9 Early pregnancy	Maternal age, parity, ethnic group, smoking, history of hypertension or diabetes, gestational diabetes, pre-eclampsia	1.40 (1.14–1.71)	1.10 (0.94–1.28)
Cnattingius and Lambe (2002)[b] [14]	Sweden 1992–1997 National study 453 801 singleton deliveries	28 weeks	Obese 30+ Overweight 25–29.9 Reference 20.0–24.9 Early pregnancy	Maternal age, height, parity, cohabitation, education, country of birth	2.0 (1.7–2.4)	1.4 (1.2–1.5)
Cedergren (2004)[a] [28]	Sweden 1982–2001 National study 972 806 singleton deliveries	28 weeks (antepartum)	Obese 35–40 Overweight 29.1–35 Reference 19.8–26 Early pregnancy	Maternal age, parity, smoking, year of delivery	1.99 (1.57–2.51)	1.79 (1.59–2.01)
Kristensen et al. (2005)[a] [29]	Denmark 1989–1996 Single center 24 505 singleton deliveries	28 weeks	Obese 30+ Overweight 25–29.9 Reference 18.5–24.9 Self-reported recall pre-pregnancy	Maternal age, height, parity, smoking, education, employment, alcohol, caffeine, infant sex, lone parent status	3.1 (1.6–5.9)	1.2 (0.6–2.2)
Nohr et al. (2005)[a] [22]	Denmark 1998–2001 National study 54 505 singleton deliveries	28 weeks (antepartum)	Obese 30+ Overweight 25–29.9 Reference 18.5–24.9 Self-reported recall pre-pregnancy	Maternal age, height, parity, socio-occupational status, exercise, smoking, alcohol, coffee consumption	3.4 (2.1–5.5)	2.0 (1.4–3.0)
Getahun et al. (2007)[b] [11]	US 1989–1997 Regional multicenter study 626 883 singleton deliveries	20 weeks (antepartum)	Obese 30+ Overweight 25–29.9 Reference 18.5–24.9 Pre-pregnancy, not further specified	Maternal age, education, marital status, parity, late antenatal care, excess weight gain, smoking, fetal sex, previous preterm/SGA birth, SGA	White: hazard ratio (HR) 1.3 (1.1–1.6) African American: HR 1.2 (0.9–1.5)	White: HR 1.2 (1.1–1.4) African American: HR 1.2 (1.0–1.6)

Table 6.1 (cont.)

Study	Setting and population	Definition of stillbirth	Definition of obesity/overweight (kg/m²)	Adjustment for covariates	OR for obesity	OR for overweight
Salihu et al. (2007) [18]	US 1978–1997 Regional multicenter study 1 577 082 singleton deliveries	20 weeks	Obese 30+ Overweight 25–29.9 Reference 18.5–24.9 Measured height, self-reported pre-pregnancy weight	Maternal age, race, education, marital status, smoking, prenatal care, fetal sex, year of birth	1.5 (1.3–1.7)	n/a
Smith et al. (2007)[b] [15]	Scotland 1992–2001 Regional multicenter study 216 563 singleton deliveries	24 weeks (antepartum unrelated to congenital anomaly)	Obese 30+ Overweight 25–29 Reference 20–24 Weight recorded at 15–21 weeks gestation	Maternal age, deprivation category, height, smoking status, marital status, alpha-fetoprotein and hCG levels	1.96 (1.47–2.60)	1.44 (1.13–1.82)
Hauger et al. (2008) [16]	Argentina 2003–2006 Regional multicenter study 60 505 singleton deliveries (excluding anomalies)	22 weeks (or birthweight 500 g)	Obese 30+ Overweight 25–29.9 Reference 18.5–24.9 Measured height and self-reported pre-pregnancy weight	Not stated	1.07 (0.74–1.56)	1.07 (0.82–1.39)
Khashan and Kenny (2009)[b] [12]	UK 2004–2006 Regional multicenter study 99 403 singleton deliveries	24 weeks	Obese 30–39.9 Overweight 25–29.9 Reference 18.5–24.9 Early pregnancy height and weight	Maternal age, parity, deprivation, ethnicity, and infant sex	1.04 (0.79–1.37)	1.02 (0.82–1.28)
Tennant et al. (2011) [17]	UK 2003–2005 Regional multicenter study 40 932 singleton deliveries	20 weeks (antepartum)	Obese 30+ Overweight 25–29.9 Reference 18.5–24.9 Measured or self-reported in early pregnancy	Maternal age, ethnicity, smoking, deprivation. Pre-existing diabetes and major congenital anomaly excluded	2.3 (1.6–3.3)	1.3 (0.9–1.9)

[a] Included in meta-analysis by Chu et al. [10]
[b] Included in meta-analysis by Flenady et al. [8]

the earlier meta-analysis. Thus, the evidence overall suggests an increased risk of stillbirth of around two-fold in obese women compared with those with recommended BMI. For overweight women, most studies report an elevated odds ratio (Table 6.1), but lower than for obese women, suggesting a dose–response effect with increasing BMI.

Evidence concerning the relationship between maternal obesity and early fetal loss is limited, mainly because miscarriage, unlike stillbirth, is not routinely recorded at the time of the birth registration or in health care information systems. Published research is largely confined to studies of women receiving fertility treatment. These women may have an elevated risk of miscarriage due to their underlying fertility problems, and so the results may not be generalizable to all women. Metwally et al. included 16 such studies in a meta-analysis and reported an overall OR of 1.67 (95% CI: 1.25–2.25) for overweight or obese women compared to women with recommended BMI [20]. This is similar in magnitude to estimates of the effect of obesity on stillbirth, and raises the possibility that obesity may be associated with increased risk of fetal death throughout pregnancy, regardless of gestational age.

In the general population, fetal loss rates are highest at earlier gestations, and decline with gestation before increasing at and beyond term [21]. Only two studies have explored whether the risk of fetal death associated with maternal obesity varies with gestation. Nohr et al. examined the relationship between fetal loss and gestational age separately by BMI category, and found that the risk associated with maternal obesity increased with increasing gestational age, being greatest at term (37 or more completed weeks) [22]. In contrast, Tennant et al. found no evidence of interaction between maternal obesity and gestational age on fetal death from 20 weeks gestation; i.e., the elevated risk associated with obesity appeared consistent throughout the latter half of pregnancy [17].

Thus current data suggests that obesity increases the risk of fetal death from the second trimester onward, possibly with a greater effect on stillbirth at or beyond term. Evidence of increased risk of first trimester fetal loss is confined to women seeking fertility treatment, but is consistent with an effect of similar magnitude.

Infant death and maternal obesity

An infant death is the death of a live-born baby within the first year. Mortality rates are highest in the period immediately after birth and decline over the first year; thus around two thirds of infant deaths occur in the neonatal period (first 28 days of life) [23]. Many infant deaths, particularly those occurring in the neonatal period, are related to preterm delivery, either spontaneous or elective [23,24]. Post-neonatal deaths (during 28 to 365 days of life) are considerably less common, and often attributed to sudden infant death syndrome (SIDS) or infection. Congenital anomaly is an important cause of death throughout the first year of life. In most developed countries, infant mortality has fallen steadily over the past two decades; however, variations between regions and population subgroups persist [25]. Infant mortality is associated with maternal risk factors including parity, smoking, and ethnic background; however, the strongest association is with socioeconomic deprivation [26,27].

Five cohort studies have reported an increased risk of neonatal mortality in women with maternal obesity [17,28–31], with ORs ranging between 1.6 and 2.6. One recent report from North West England found no evidence of an association with neonatal mortality (RR for obese vs. recommended BMI 0.89; 95% CI: 0.61–1.30) [12]. This study, however, reported a particularly high neonatal mortality rate for infants of women of normal BMI, and the lowest mortality rate for overweight women, and was conducted in a population with a high proportion of non-White women.

Only two studies have reported on the association with post-neonatal mortality. Chen et al. reported a significant association (OR 1.28; 95% CI: 1.02–1.61) [30], while Tennant et al., in a smaller study, found no significant association, despite an apparently larger effect size (OR 1.80; 95% CI: 0.71–4.56) [17]. Within each of these studies, the OR for post-neonatal death was substantially smaller than for neonatal death.

The epidemiological evidence therefore indicates an association between maternal obesity and neonatal death of a similar magnitude to the association with stillbirth (around two-fold). There is very sparse evidence relating to an effect on mortality beyond the neonatal period, but available evidence is consistent with any effect being less than for neonatal mortality.

Interpretation

Causality

Establishing an epidemiological association between maternal obesity and mortality is insufficient by itself

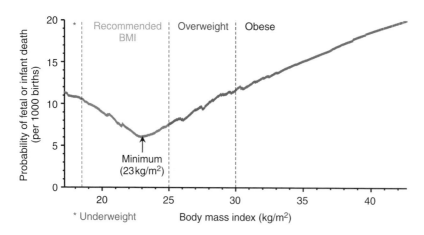

Figure 6.1. Probability of a fetal or infant death with increasing pre-pregnancy body mass index. Reproduced with permission from Tennant *et al.* [17], who constructed the figure using locally weighted scatter plot regression. (See figure in color plate section.)

to indicate a causal relationship. Other explanations, such as confounding factors (i.e., risk factors that are associated with both maternal obesity and mortality) should be considered. Most large-scale epidemiological studies adjust for available known confounding factors including maternal age, parity, ethnicity, and socioeconomic status, but many do not have access to detailed information on individual clinical and demographic risk factors.

Nearly all published studies of fetal and infant mortality report increased risk, albeit to a smaller and sometimes non-significant level, for overweight women compared to those of recommended BMI (Table 6.1). Only one has investigated mortality outcomes across the full BMI spectrum. This analysis demonstrated a V-shaped relationship with the combined outcome of late fetal and infant death. The lowest mortality rate was observed for a maternal BMI of around 23, with increases in risk for early pregnancy BMI above and below this (Figure 6.1) [17]. This suggests that the relationship with increasing BMI shows a "dose–response" effect, with no clear threshold indicating increased risk; this is often considered indicative of a causal relationship. It also suggests that there may be an optimal BMI, below which risks of adverse outcome increase.

Furthermore, changes in maternal BMI between pregnancies have been shown to change the risk of both stillbirth and some obesity-related pregnancy complications [32]. Women who gained more than three BMI units (kg/m^2) between pregnancies were at increased risk of stillbirth, while those who lost more than one BMI unit had reduced risks of related complications such as pre-eclampsia. This evidence, which links changes in BMI within the same individuals to their subsequent pregnancy outcomes, strongly suggests

the relationship between maternal BMI and fetal and infant mortality is causal, rather than resulting from correlation with other environmental influences.

Cause of death

Maternal obesity is associated with increased risk of specific pregnancy complications, which may lead to fetal or infant death. The best characterized associations are with pre-eclampsia and hypertensive disorders [33], and with diabetes, both pre-existing type 2 diabetes and gestational diabetes [34].

Analysis of cause of stillbirth in obese women suggests that some of the increased risk can be attributed to increases within specific cause of death categories, including pre-eclampsia [17], and fetoplacental dysfunction [22,29]. Congenital anomaly is a major cause of both stillbirth and infant death, and has been associated with maternal obesity (see below). However, the increased stillbirth risk associated with maternal obesity is not confined to specific causes, but is observed across all cause of death categories.

Studies of neonatal and post-neonatal death indicate an elevated risk across all causes of death [13,17,28,29]. In the general population, neonatal mortality rates are strongly associated with rates of preterm delivery. Studies investigating the effect of maternal BMI on gestational age at delivery have reported inconsistent results, due in part to the scarcity of large datasets that robustly distinguish spontaneous preterm labor from elective early delivery arising from concerns about fetal well-being. A recent systematic review reported a significant association between maternal obesity and overweight for induced preterm birth (RR 1.30; 95% CI: 1.23–1.37) but not for spontaneous preterm birth (RR 0.93; 95% CI: 0.85–1.01) [35].

While elective preterm delivery may increase the risk of neonatal death, and in some cases may result in a fetus dying after delivery rather than before, it is unlikely that an increased rate of induced preterm birth explains the association between maternal obesity and neonatal death. It may rather reflect the increased rate of underlying obesity-related complications such as pre-eclampsia and maternal diabetes, which are common medical indications for elective delivery.

Mechanisms

Underlying metabolic mechanisms between obesity and fetal or infant death have been reviewed by Nelson *et al.* [36] and are discussed in Chapters 5 and 15. In brief, excess maternal adiposity is correlated with metabolic risk factors including reduced insulin sensitivity, lipid disorders, and increased levels of inflammatory mediators. These are thought to directly contribute to the development of gestational hypertension, pre-eclampsia and other disturbances of placental function, and also to impaired glucose tolerance and gestational diabetes [37,38].

Other potential explanations have been put forward to explain the increased risk of fetal and infant mortality with increased maternal BMI. Increased maternal BMI is associated with increased birthweight via maternal hyperglycemia [39]. However, increased fetal fat mass may co-exist with disorders of placental vasculature in obese women, thus increasing the difficulty of identifying a compromised fetus from serial growth ultrasound scans using conventional growth standards [40]. Assessment of fetal size, both clinically and by ultrasound, may also be more difficult in women with high BMI [41]. Thus, some of the excess risk of stillbirth in obese pregnant women may be attributable to lower rates of recognition of poor fetal growth and fetal compromise.

More speculative potential explanations include sleep apnea [42], reduced ability to detect fetal movements [6], lower rates of antenatal diagnosis of congenital anomaly [41], and residual confounding, for example of poor socioeconomic conditions and dietary quality, which are rarely adjusted for in population-based studies. Such residual confounding may be a potentially important explanation for any association between maternal obesity and post-neonatal deaths, where there is less plausibility of a direct causal association.

Ethnicity

Most published work on maternal obesity and fetal and infant mortality has been conducted in North America and Europe, in populations of mainly White ethnicity. Some studies suggest that the effect of maternal obesity may differ in different ethnic groups. A stronger association with the risk of stillbirth and infant death has been reported for Black American women [18,43]. A study of Chinese women reported a stillbirth OR consistent with the findings in White populations [44]. However, other research has reported no differences between ethnic groups [45]. Further research is needed in different populations to explore these potential differences in more detail.

The relationship between adiposity and BMI varies between ethnic groups. Furthermore, Asian populations have an increased risk of general morbidity at lower BMI levels than among European populations. The World Health Organization (WHO) has therefore proposed lower BMI thresholds to define underweight, ideal weight, overweight, and obese among Asian populations [46]. Thus far, research investigating pregnancy outcomes in relation to maternal BMI has not used population-specific BMI categories. Recent work in England reported that the proportion of women of South Asian origin who were classified obese at the start of pregnancy doubled when using the WHO definition for Asian populations [47]. Given known differences in perinatal mortality rates within maternal ethnic groups, research is needed using the BMI categories for Asian populations to accurately estimate pregnancy risks associated with maternal BMI.

Maternal obesity and congenital anomaly

Congenital anomaly is a term that describes a diverse range of disorders of fetal development that result in structural or other abnormalities present at birth. Congenital anomalies affect around 2% to 4% of all deliveries [48] and are one of the major causes of stillbirths and infant deaths, accounting for 9% of stillbirths and 23% of neonatal deaths in the UK [2] and 20% of infant deaths in the USA [49]. Congenital anomalies are also a significant contributor to morbidity in childhood and beyond. Chromosomal (non-structural) anomalies account for about a quarter of all anomalies [48]. The most common structural anomalies reported in developed countries are cardiovascular, nervous system (predominantly neural tube defects), and urinary anomalies.

A number of epidemiological studies, primarily from North America and Northern Europe, have

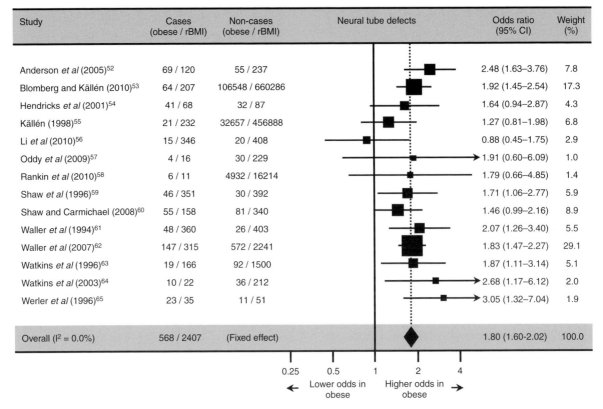

Figure 6.2. Association between maternal obesity (compared with recommended weight) and the risk of a pregnancy affected by a neural tube defect. The estimates from each study (box) are plotted together with the level of uncertainty (whiskers) and summarized by fixed effect meta-analysis (rhombus). The size of each data marker is proportional to the weight that each study was assigned toward the summary value.

investigated the association between congenital anomalies and pre-pregnancy or early pregnancy obesity, and their findings have been recently summarized in two systematic reviews [50,51]. The available evidence suggests a consistent association between maternal obesity and neural tube defects and cardiovascular anomalies. Updating these reviews to include recent studies, we calculated a pooled OR of 1.80 (95% CI: 1.60–2.02) for neural tube defects in obese women compared with those of recommended weight [52–65] (Figure 6.2) and 1.20 (95% CI: 1.15–1.25) for cardiovascular anomalies [53,57,58,61,62,64,66–70] (Figure 6.3).

The evidence for obesity contributing to other anomaly subtypes is sparser and less consistent, but positive associations have been reported for cleft palate, cleft lip and palate, anorectal atresia, and limb reduction anomalies [51] and, more recently, with bilateral renal agenesis [71], and microtia [72]. A small number of congenital anomalies are more common among

underweight women, including gastroschisis, genital anomalies, and atrial septal defects [51,73].

As the prevalence of individual congenital anomaly subtypes is low, and the effect size for many subtypes appears modest, most studies are underpowered to establish whether maternal overweight in addition to obesity is significantly associated with congenital anomaly. Thus evidence for a dose–response effect is sparse. The meta-analysis by Stothard et al. reported a significantly increased risk of neural tube defects in overweight women (OR 1.2; 95% CI: 1.04–1.38) [51]. However, no studies have been sufficiently powered to analyze BMI as a continuous variable and hence there is currently no data about the optimum BMI in relation to congenital anomaly occurrence.

Interpretation

Given the heterogeneity of the anomalies potentially associated with maternal obesity, it is likely that there

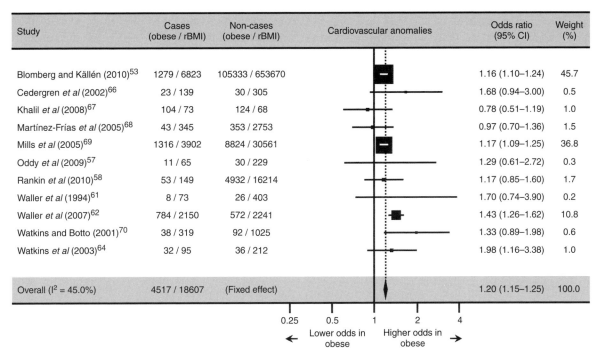

Study	Cases (obese / rBMI)	Non-cases (obese / rBMI)	Cardiovascular anomalies	Odds ratio (95% CI)	Weight (%)
Blomberg and Källén (2010)[53]	1279 / 6823	105333 / 653670		1.16 (1.10–1.24)	45.7
Cedergren et al (2002)[66]	23 / 139	30 / 305		1.68 (0.94–3.00)	0.5
Khalil et al (2008)[67]	104 / 73	124 / 68		0.78 (0.51–1.19)	1.0
Martínez-Frías et al (2005)[68]	43 / 345	353 / 2753		0.97 (0.70–1.36)	1.5
Mills et al (2005)[69]	1316 / 3902	8824 / 30561		1.17 (1.09–1.25)	36.8
Oddy et al (2009)[57]	11 / 65	30 / 229		1.29 (0.61–2.72)	0.3
Rankin et al (2010)[58]	53 / 149	4932 / 16214		1.17 (0.85–1.60)	1.7
Waller et al (1994)[61]	8 / 73	26 / 403		1.70 (0.74–3.90)	0.2
Waller et al (2007)[62]	784 / 2150	572 / 2241		1.43 (1.26–1.62)	10.8
Watkins and Botto (2001)[70]	38 / 319	92 / 1025		1.33 (0.89–1.98)	0.6
Watkins et al (2003)[64]	32 / 95	36 / 212		1.98 (1.16–3.38)	1.0
Overall (I² = 45.0%)	4517 / 18607	(Fixed effect)		1.20 (1.15–1.25)	100.0

0.25 0.5 1 2 4

← Lower odds in obese   Higher odds in obese →

Figure 6.3. Association between maternal obesity (compared with recommended weight) and the risk of a pregnancy affected by a cardiovascular anomaly. The estimates from each study (box) are plotted together with the level of uncertainty (whiskers) and summarized by fixed effect meta-analysis (rhombus). The size of each data marker is proportional to the weight that each study was assigned toward the summary value.

are a number of potential underlying mechanisms. These have been reviewed in detail by Carmichael et al. [74]. One likely pathway is maternal diabetes and early pregnancy hyperglycemia. Pre-existing diabetes is a well-established risk factor for congenital anomalies, particularly cardiovascular anomalies and neural tube defects [75], and the risk of type 2 diabetes, which is frequently undiagnosed, is strongly associated with BMI [76]. The causal mechanism is thought to involve a direct effect of hyperglycemia resulting in oxidative stress, which disrupts expression of critical genes controlling embryonic development [77]. This pathway has been elucidated in vitro and in animal studies in relation to diabetes and neural tube defects [78], but inducing oxidative stress in the absence of hyperglycemia has similar effects [79]. Moreover, epidemiological studies that have excluded women with known diabetes report little impact on the association between obesity and anomalies [51,58]. Thus other mechanisms are likely to be involved.

It is possible that undiagnosed diabetes, or hyperglycemia that does not meet the diagnostic criteria for diabetes, may be a factor in the increased risk of congenital anomalies in obese women. Gestational diabetes (diabetes first recognized during pregnancy) has been associated with an increased risk of congenital anomalies [80]. While gestational diabetes is not usually detected until later in pregnancy, when morphogenesis is complete, a diagnosis of gestational diabetes may be a marker of altered glucose levels early in pregnancy.

Nutrition-related mechanisms have been considered [74]. These include micronutrient defects, such as folate deficiency. Folate is known to be protective of neural tube defects and also possibly other congenital anomalies, including cardiovascular anomalies [81]. Women with high BMI have been shown to have lower serum folate levels [82], and the association of higher maternal weight with neural tube defects persists following flour fortification, suggesting that the protective effect of folate may be reduced in women with high BMI compared to leaner women (as assessed by highest vs. lowest quartiles of maternal weight) [83]. Thus differences in folic acid uptake and/or metabolism may explain some of the variation in risk of at least some congenital anomalies. This issue is discussed in Chapter 16.

Other micronutrient deficiencies are associated with a number of specific congenital anomalies [78,84]. For example, increasing BMI has been associated with lower levels of carotenoids, vitamin C, selenium, and vitamin D [85]. Alterations in micronutrient status between obese and recommended weight women may result from poorer diet quality, dieting, use of weight-loss products, and differences in metabolism.

Other authors have suggested that differential antenatal detection in women with high BMI may result in a higher birth prevalence of congenital anomalies, due to a lower rate of selective termination of affected pregnancies. Accurate ultrasound scanning is more difficult in obese women [41]. However, in a sensitivity analysis, Stothard et al. found no evidence that epidemiological studies of maternal BMI and congenital anomalies that included cases resulting in termination of pregnancy differed in their findings from those confined to live and stillbirths [51]. Furthermore, Rankin et al. did not find a significant difference in the proportion of termination of pregnancy between mothers who were underweight, of normal weight, overweight, or obese [58].

Further research involving larger sample sizes is needed to investigate whether there is an association with other congenital anomalies and to gain insight into the underlying mechanisms.

Population impact and public health implications

Population impact

The impact of maternal obesity on adverse fetal and infant outcomes depends on both rates of obesity, and of adverse pregnancy outcome, in the population in question. One study, in a UK population, estimated an obese woman's absolute risk of stillbirth or infant death to be 7.6 per 1000 births higher than in women of recommended BMI, compared with a rate in women of recommended BMI of 8.6 per 1000 [17]. In the USA, where the prevalence of obesity among women of childbearing age is 34% [86], and where there are around 4 million births a year [87], this would equate to an extra 10 000 stillbirths or infant deaths a year, or a fifth of such cases.

This demonstrates how an increase in the probability of a rare event, when considered on a population basis, can translate into a large absolute number of events. The impact of obesity on the absolute number of congenital anomalies is less than on stillbirth, due to smaller effect sizes and/or lower prevalences of the specific congenital anomaly subtypes that have been associated with maternal obesity (approximately 8 per 1000 births are affected by a cardiovascular anomaly and 0.5–1.0 per 1000 births are affected by a neural tube defect [88]). Assuming the absolute risks reported by Stothard et al., this suggests that maternal obesity may result in around 600 neural tube defects and 800 cardiovascular anomalies each year in the USA. However, the economic impact may be substantial, due to the specialist health care needs of many children and adults living with congenital anomalies [89].

Reducing the rate of infant and early childhood mortality remains an important public health goal both globally and for many national governments [27]. Reducing child mortality in the under-fives is one of the United Nations' Millennium Development Goals. Nearly two fifths of global deaths in the under-fives are estimated to occur in the neonatal period [90]. With the increasing global prevalence of obesity, this goal appears particularly challenging as, without effective interventions to reduce obesity-related mortality, or improvements in other areas, the neonatal mortality rate can be expected to increase. Rising maternal obesity is also likely to complicate efforts to reduce socio-economic inequalities in the rates of stillbirth and infant death. Obesity has a complex relationship with socio-economic status, with higher BMI in women typically correlating with deprivation in developed countries but with wealth in less developed countries [90,91]. In developed countries therefore, action to prevent and treat obesity in young women may represent a viable method to reduce inequalities in pregnancy outcomes. Indeed, the UK Department of Health has identified reducing obesity among poorer communities as a central action in its aim to reduce the socioeconomic gap in infant mortality [27].

Public health implications

This chapter has considered only the implications for fetal and infant outcomes of entering pregnancy with a high maternal BMI, and has not considered the potential impact of weight gain during pregnancy. For congenital anomaly, in particular, the maternal environment in the first weeks of pregnancy is the critical focus for prevention, since organogenesis is completed during this time (e.g., neural tube development is complete by day 56). For most women, the first antenatal appointment will take place after this window.

Thus prevention of obesity-related fetal loss, infant death, and congenital anomaly requires emphasis on the prevention of obesity among teenage and young women as part of a broad-based population-level obesity prevention strategy. For young women who are already at a high BMI, effective weight-loss interventions should be made available and targeted to this group. It has been suggested that weight-loss interventions be offered to overweight and obese women who are planning pregnancy as part of preconception care. However, evidence about the safety of rapid and/or substantial weight loss in the periconception period is currently lacking. Furthermore, a high proportion of pregnancies are unplanned. Thus while reducing the prevalence of obesity in women of reproductive age may be considered a high priority, this may be better achieved by approaches outside reproductive health care services.

In many health care systems, older adults or those with co-morbidities are commonly prioritized for weight-loss interventions. However, the adverse reproductive effects of obesity have generally not been taken into account when considering the relative cost-effectiveness of weight-loss interventions in different population subgroups. Similarly, it is important to evaluate the potential for screening for undiagnosed diabetes in young women, particularly those who are obese, using economic models that account for the reproductive risks of pre-gestational diabetes. Pre-existing but undiagnosed diabetes may be one potential explanation for the increased rates of adverse pregnancy outcome in obese women.

Ideally, women should be supported to optimize their weight prior to considering pregnancy. It is likely that underweight may also increase fetal and infant risks and that optimum BMI in relation to these outcomes is in the middle of the recommended BMI range [17]. However, any pre-pregnancy reduction in weight in women with a higher than recommended BMI is likely to reduce the risk of adverse fetal and infant outcome, as long as there are no adverse effects to peri-conception weight loss [32]. Nevertheless, engaging with women to address their weight prior to conception is likely to be challenging. Many pregnancies are unplanned, and many women, and health care professionals, may be unaware of the potential impact of obesity on pregnancy outcome. Experience

with women with diabetes suggests that even when there is widespread awareness of increased pregnancy risks, and preconception advice and support is available, many women do not engage with these services or prepare adequately for pregnancy. Thus primary care and community-based approaches to obesity prevention and treatment in young women, which are not specifically linked to pregnancy preparation, remain important. Further, women may be more receptive to weight-loss intervention after pregnancy, and successful intervention at this time is likely to have a positive effect on the outcome of any subsequent pregnancies. However, postnatal weight-loss interventions have generally reported high drop-out rates [92].

Although obesity appears to be associated with a non-specific increase in fetal and infant mortality, some serious but treatable pregnancy complications are more common in obese women. These include gestational diabetes and pre-eclampsia. Both of these conditions are amenable to early diagnosis and effective intervention. Hence it is important that the clinical management of these conditions is optimized, and that obese women are identified in early pregnancy and targeted for antenatal surveillance and intervention as recommended. Similarly, maternity services need to be aware of the potentially reduced sensitivity of ultrasound detection of congenital anomaly in obese women, and plan for longer appointment times and appropriate counseling of such women as necessary.

Research gaps

There are a number of gaps in the epidemiological literature. One important issue that has been insufficiently addressed is the need to better define and characterize the effect of increased maternal adiposity in non-White populations. This may require the use or development of adjusted BMI categories in different ethnic groups. Larger studies are required to enable exploration of the effect of BMI as a continuous variable and thus better characterize both the optimum BMI, and the effect of increasing and decreasing BMI. Larger studies would also permit further investigation of the association with less common outcomes, such as specific congenital anomaly subtypes and post-neonatal mortality.

Clinical studies are required to develop and evaluate effective behavioral interventions to reduce weight in women both pre- and post-pregnancy. These need to address important issues such as uptake and completion, as well as the effect on both weight and subsequent reproductive outcomes. Further research to elucidate underlying mechanisms is also needed, which could lead to the development of more specific therapeutic targets.

Conclusion

Maternal obesity has a significant impact on the risk of fetal and neonatal mortality, and on the development of congenital anomaly, at both individual and population level. This burden is likely to increase as a result of current global trends in obesity. Tackling this problem requires action on a number of levels, including the implementation of existing knowledge about effective public health and clinical interventions, as well as further research across relevant public health, clinical, and scientific disciplines to advance understanding and discovery of novel preventive and therapeutic approaches.

References

1. MacDorman M & Kirmeyer S. Fetal and perinatal mortality, United States, 2005. *Natl Vital Stat Rep* 2009;**57**:1–19.

2. Centre for Maternal and Child Enquiries (CMACE). *Perinatal Mortality 2008: United Kingdom.* (London; 2010).

3. Gissler M, Mohangoo A D, Blondel B, *et al.* Perinatal health monitoring in Europe: results from the EURO-PERISTAT project. *Inform Health Soc Care* 2010;**35**:64–79.

4. Stanton C, Lawn J E, Rahman H, Wilczynska-Ketende K & Hill K. Stillbirth rates: delivering estimates in 190 countries. *Lancet* 2006;**367**:1487–94.

5. Flenady V, Middleton P, Smith G, *et al.* Stillbirths: the way forward in high-income countries. *Lancet* 2011;**377**:1703–17.

6. Fretts R C. Etiology and prevention of stillbirth. *Am J Obstet Gynecol* 2005;**193**:1923–35.

7. Reddy U, Laughon S, Sun L, *et al.* Prepregnancy risk factors for antepartum stillbirth in the United States. *Obstet Gynecol* 2010;**116**:1119–26.

8. Flenady V, Koopmans L, Middleton P, *et al.* Major risk factors for stillbirth in high-income countries: a systematic review and meta-analysis. *Lancet* 2011;**377**:1331–40.

9. Smith G C S & Fretts R C. Stillbirth. *Lancet* 2007;**370**:1715–25.

10. Chu S Y, Kim S Y, Lau J, *et al.* Maternal obesity and risk of stillbirth: a metaanalysis. *Am J Obstet Gynecol* 2007;**197**:223–8.

11. Getahun D, Ananth C & Kinzler W. Risk factors for antepartum and intrapartum stillbirth: a population-based study. *Am J Obstet Gynecol* 2007;**196**:499–507.

12. Khashan A & Kenny L. The effects of maternal body mass index on pregnancy outcome. *Eur J Epidemiology* 2009;**24**:697–705.

13. Sebire N J, Jolly M, Harris J P, *et al.* Maternal obesity and pregnancy outcome: a study of 287,213 pregnancies in London. *Int J Obesity Related Metabol Disord* 2001;**25**:1175.

14. Cnattingius S & Lambe M. Trends in smoking and overweight during pregnancy: prevalence, risks of pregnancy complications, and adverse pregnancy outcomes. *Seminars Perinatology* 2002;**26**:286–95.

15. Smith G, Shah I, White I, *et al.* Maternal and biochemical predictors of antepartum stillbirth among nulliparous women in relation to gestational age of fetal death. *BJOG* 2007;;**114**(6):705–14.

16. Hauger M S, Gibbons L, Vik T & Belizán J M. Prepregnancy weight status and the risk of adverse pregnancy outcome. *Acta Obstet Gynecol Scand* 2008;**87**(9):953–9.

17. Tennant P W G, Rankin J & Bell R. Maternal body mass index and the risk of fetal and infant death: a cohort study from the North of England. *Human Reprod* 2011;**26**:1501–11.

18. Salihu H, Dunlop A, Hedayatzadeh M, *et al.* Extreme obesity and risk of stillbirth among black and white gravidas. *Obstet Gynecol* 2007;**110**:552–7.

19. Centre for Maternal and Child Enquiries. *Maternal Obesity in the UK: Findings from a National Project.* (London: CMACE, 2010).

20. Metwally M, Ong K J, Ledger W L & Li T C. Does high body mass index increase the risk of miscarriage after spontaneous and assisted conception? A meta-analysis of the evidence. *Fertil Steril* 2008;**90**:714–26.

21. Kramer M S, Liu S, Luo Z C, *et al.* Analysis of perinatal mortality and its components: time for a change? *Am J Epidemiol* 2002;**156**:493–7.

22. Nohr E A, Bech B H, Davies M J, *et al.* Prepregnancy obesity and fetal death: a study within the Danish National Birth Cohort. *Obstet Gynecol* 2005;**106**:250–9.

23. Mathews T & MacDorman M F. Infant mortality statistics from the 2006 period linked birth/infant death data set. *Natl Vital Stat Rep* 2010;**58**:1–31.

24. Smith L K, Manktelow B N, Draper E S, Springett A & Field D J. Nature of socioeconomic inequalities in neonatal mortality: population based study. *BMJ* 2010;**341**:c6654.

25. UN Inter-agency Group for Child Mortality Estimation. *Levels and Trends in Child Mortality.* (United Nations Childrens Fund; 2010).

26. Kramer M S. The epidemiology of adverse pregnancy outcomes: an overview. *J Nutr* 2003;**133**(5 Suppl 2):1592S–6S.

27. D H Health Inequalities Unit. *Review of the Health Inequalities Infant Mortality PSA Target.* (London: Department of Health, 2007).

28. Cedergren M I. Maternal morbid obesity and the risk of adverse pregnancy outcome. *Obstet Gynecol* 2004;**103**:219–24.

29. Kristensen J, Vestergaard M, Wisborg K, Kesmodel U & Secher N J. Pre-pregnancy weight and the risk of stillbirth and neonatal death. *BJOG* 2005;**112**:403–8.

30. Chen A, Feresu S A, Fernandez C & Rogan W J. Maternal obesity and the risk of infant death in the United States. *Epidemiology* 2009;**20**:74–81.

31. Nohr E, Vaeth M, Bech B, *et al.* Maternal obesity and neonatal mortality according to subtypes of preterm birth. *Obstet Gynecol* 2007;**110**:1083–90.

32. Villamor E & Cnattingius S. Interpregnancy weight change and risk of adverse pregnancy outcomes: a population-based study. *Lancet* 2006;**368**:1164–70.

33. Bodnar L M, Ness R B, Markovic N & Roberts J M. The risk of preeclampsia rises with increasing prepregnancy body mass index. *Ann Epidemiol* 2005;**15**:475–82.

34. Chu S Y, Callaghan W M, Kim SY, *et al.* Maternal obesity and risk of gestational diabetes mellitus. *Diabetes Care* 2007;**30**:2070–6.

35. McDonald S, Han Z, Mulla S & Beyene J. Overweight and obesity in mothers and risk of preterm birth and low birth weight infants: systematic review and meta-analyses. *BMJ* 2010;**341**:c3428.

36. Nelson S M, Matthews P & Poston L. Maternal metabolism and obesity: modifiable determinants of pregnancy outcome. *Hum Reprod Update* 2010;**16**:255–75.

37. Sattar N, Ramsay J, Crawford L, Cheyne H & Greer I. Classic and novel risk factor parameters in women with a history of preeclampsia. *Hypertension* 2003;**42**:39–42.

38. Wolf M, Kettyle E, Sandler L, *et al.* Obesity and pre-eclampsia: the potential role of inflammation. *Obstet Gynecol* 2001;**98**:757–62.

39. Nohr E A, Vaeth M, Baker J L, *et al.* Combined associations of prepregnancy body mass index and gestational weight gain with the outcome of pregnancy. *Am J Clin Nutr* 2008;**87**:1750–9.

40. Gardosi J, Clausson B & Francis A. Maternal obesity and the risk of stillbirth in small-for-gestational-age babies identified by customised birthweight centiles. *Arch Dis Child (Fetal Neonatal Ed)* 2008;**93**(Suppl 1):Fa5.

41. Phatak M & Ramsay J. Impact of maternal obesity on procedure of mid-trimester anomaly scan. *J Obstet Gynaecol* 2010;**30**:447–50.

42. Franklin K, Holmgren P, Jonsson F, *et al.* Snoring, pregnancy-induced hypertension, and growth retardation of the fetus. *Chest* 2000, **117**:137–41.

43. Thompson D R, Clark C L, Wood B & Zeni M B. Maternal obesity and risk of infant death based on Florida birth records for 2004. *Pub Health Rep* 2008;**123**:487–93.

44. Leung T Y, Leung T N, Sahota D S, *et al.* Trends in maternal obesity and associated risks of adverse pregnancy outcomes in a population of Chinese women. *BJOG* 2008;**115**:1529–37.

45. Baeten J M, Bukusi E A & Lambe M. Pregnancy complications and outcomes among overweight and obese nulliparous women. *Am J Public Health* 2001;**91**:436–40.

46. WHO Expert Consultation. Appropriate body-mass index for Asian populations and its implications for policy and intervention strategies. *Lancet* 2004;**363**:157–63.

47. Heslehurst N, Sattar N, Rajasingham D, *et al.* Maternal obesity and ethnic groups: trends in 552,303 births over thirteen years in England, UK. *Arch Dis Child (Fetal Neonatal Ed)* 2010;**95**:Fa33–4.

48. Rankin J, Pattenden S, Abramsky L, *et al.* Prevalence of congenital anomalies in five British regions, 1991–1999. *Arch Dis Child (Fetal Neonatal Ed)* 2005;**90**:Fa374–9.

49. Heron M, Hoyert D, Murphy S, *et al.* Deaths: final data for 2006. *Natl Vital Stat Rep* 2009;**57**(14):1–134.

50. Rasmussen S A, Chu S Y, Kim S Y, Schmid C H & Lau J. Maternal obesity and risk of neural tube defects: a metaanalysis. *Am J Obstet Gynecol* 2008;**198**:611–19.

51. Stothard K J, Tennant P W G, Bell R & Rankin J. Maternal overweight and obesity and the risk of congenital anomalies. *JAMA* 2009;**301**:636–50.

52. Anderson J L, Waller D K, Canfield M A, *et al.* Maternal obesity, gestational diabetes, and central nervous system birth defects. *Epidemiology* 2005;**16**:87–92.

53. Blomberg M I & Källén B. Maternal obesity and morbid obesity: the risk for birth defects in the offspring. *Birth Defects Res A Clin Mol Teratol* 2010;**88**:35–40.

54. Hendricks K A, Nuno O M, Suarez L, Larsen R. Effects of hyperinsulinemia and obesity on risk of neural tube defects among Mexican Americans. *Epidemiology* 2001;**12**:630–5.

55. Källén K. Maternal smoking, body mass index, and neural tube defects. *Am J Epidemiol* 1998;**147**:1103–11.

56. Li Z, Liu J, Ye R, *et al.* Maternal prepregnancy body mass index and risk of neural tube defects: a population-based case-control study in Shanxi

province, China. *Birth Defects Res A Clin Mol Teratol* 2010;**88**:570–4.

57. Oddy W H, De Klerk N H, Miller M, Payne J & Bower C. Association of maternal pre-pregnancy weight with birth defects: evidence from a case-control study in Western Australia. *Aust N Z J Obstet Gynaecol* 2009;**49**:11–15.

58. Rankin J, Tennant P W G, Stothard K J, *et al.* Maternal body mass index and congenital anomaly risk: a cohort study. *Int J Obesity* 2010;**34**:1371–80.

59. Shaw G M, Velie E M & Schaffer D. Risk of neural tube defect-affected pregnancies among obese women. *JAMA* 1996;**275**:1093–6.

60. Shaw G M & Carmichael S L. Prepregnant obesity and risks of selected birth defects in offspring. *Epidemiology* 2008;**19**:616–20.

61. Waller D K, Mills J L, Simpson J L, *et al.* Are obese women at higher risk for producing malformed offspring? *Am J Obstet Gynecol* 1994;**170**:541–8.

62. Waller D K, Shaw G M, Rasmussen S A, *et al.* Prepregnancy obesity as a risk factor for structural birth defects. *Arch Pediat Adol Med* 2007;**161**:745–50.

63. Watkins M L, Scanlon K S, Mulinare J & Khoury M J. Is maternal obesity a risk factor for anencephaly and spina bifida? *Epidemiology* 1996;**7**:507–12.

64. Watkins M L, Rasmussen S A, Honein M A, Botto L D & Moore C A. Maternal obesity and risk for birth defects. *Pediatrics* 2003;**111**:1152–8.

65. Werler M M, Louik C, Shapiro S & Mitchell A A. Prepregnant weight in relation to risk of neural tube defects. *JAMA* 1996;**275**:1089–92.

66. Cedergren M I, Selbing A J & Källén B A J. Risk factors for cardiovascular malformation – a study based on prospectively collected data. *Scand J Work Environ Health* 2002;**28**:12–17.

67. Khalil H S, Saleh A M & Subhani S N. Maternal obesity and neonatal congenital cardiovascular defects. *Int J Gynaecol Obstet* 2008;**102**:232–6.

68. Martínez-Frías M L, Frías J P, Bermejo E, *et al.* Pre-gestational maternal body mass index predicts an increased risk of congenital malformations in infants of mothers with gestational diabetes. *Diabet Med* 2005;**22**:775–81.

69. Mills J L, Troendle J, Conley M R, Carter T & Druschel C M. Maternal obesity and congenital heart defects: a population-based study. *Am J Clin Nutr* 2010;**91**:1543–9.

70. Watkins M L & Botto L D. Maternal prepregnancy weight and congenital heart defects in offspring. *Epidemiology* 2001;**11**:439–46.

71. Slickers J E, Olshan A F, Siega-Riz A M, Honein M A & Aylsworth A S. Maternal body mass index and lifestyle exposures and the risk of bilateral renal agenesis or hypoplasia. *Am J Epidemiology* 2008;**168**:1259–67.

72. Ma C, Carmichael S L, Scheuerle A E, Canfield M A & Shaw G M. Association of microtia with maternal obesity and periconceptional folic acid use. *Am J Med Genet A*, 2010;**152**:2756–61.

73. Draper E, Rankin J, Tonks A, *et al.* Recreational drug use – a major risk factor for gastroschisis? *Am J Epidemiology* 2008;**167**:485–91.

74. Carmichael S L, Rasmussen S A & Shaw G M. Prepregnancy obesity: a complex risk factor for selected birth defects. *Birth Defects Res A Clin Mol Teratol* 2010;**88**:804–10.

75. Balsells M, Garcia-Patterson A, Gich I & Corcoy R. Maternal and fetal outcome in women with type 2 versus type 1 diabetes mellitus: a systematic review and metaanalysis. *J Clin Endocrinol Metab* 2009;**94**:4284–91.

76. Wee C C, Hamel M B, Huang A, *et al.* Obesity and undiagnosed diabetes in the U.S. *Diabetes Care* 2008,**31**:1813–15.

77. Zabihi S & Loeken M R. Understanding diabetic teratogenesis: where are we now and where are we going? *Birth Defects Res A Clin Mol Teratol* 2010;**88**:779–90.

78. Wentzel P. Can we prevent diabetic birth defects with micronutrients? *Diabetes Obes Metab* 2009;**11**:770–8.

79. Loeken M R. Free radicals and birth defects. *J Matern Fetal Neonatal Med* 2004;**15**:6–14.

80. Correa A, Gilboa S M, Besser L M, *et al.* Diabetes mellitus and birth defects. *Am J Obstet Gynecol* 2008;**199**:237e1–9.

81. Czeizel A. Periconceptual folic acid and multivitamin supplementation for the prevention of neural tube defects and other congenital abnormalities. *Birth Defects Res A Clin Mol Teratol* 2009;**85**:260–8.

82. Mojtabai R. Body mass index and serum folate in childbearing age women. *Eur J Epidemiology* 2004;**19**:1029–36.

83. Ray J G, Wyatt P R, Vermeulen M J, Meier C & Cole D E C. Greater maternal weight and the ongoing risk of neural tube defects after folic acid flour fortification. *Obstet Gynecol* 2005;**105**:261–5.

84. Keen C, Clegg M, Hannah L, *et al.* The plausibility of micronutrient deficiency being a significant contributing factor to the occurrence of pregnancy complications. *J Nutrition* 2003;**133**:1597S–1605S.

85. Kimmons J, Blanck H, Tohill B, Zhang J & Khan L. Associations between body mass index and the prevalence of low micronutrient levels among US adults. *MedGenMed* 2006;**8**:59.

86. Flegal K, Carroll M, Ogden C & Curtin L. Prevalence and trends in obesity among US adults, 1999–2008. *JAMA* 2010;**303**:235–41.

87. Martin J, Hamilton B, Sutton P, *et al.* Births: final data for 2007. *Natl Vit Stat Rep* 2010;**58**:1–85.

88. Cragan J & Gilboa S. Including prenatal diagnoses in birth defects monitoring: experience of the Metropolitan Atlanta Congenital Defects Program. *Birth Defects Res A Clin Mol Teratol* 2009;**85**:20–9.

89. Waitzman N, Romano P & Scheffler R. Estimates of the economic costs of birth defects. *Inquiry* 1994;**31**:188–205.

90. Jamison D, Shahid-Salles S, Jamison J, Lawn J & Zupan J. Stillbirths and neonatal mortality in the context of the global burden of disease. In Lopez A, Mathers C, Ezzati M, Jamison D & Murray C. (eds.) *Global Burden of Disease and Risk Factors.* (Washington, DC: The World Bank, 2006).

91. McLaren L. Socioeconomc status and obesity. *Epidemiol Rev* 2007;**29**:29–48.

92. Kulhmann A, Dietz P, Galavotti C & England L. Weight management interventions for pregnant or postpartum women. *Am J Prev Med* 2008;**34**:523–8.

Chapter

7

Obesity in pregnancy and mental health

Louise M. Howard and Helen Croker

Introduction

There is increasing recognition internationally that the physical health of people is only possible if they are also mentally healthy [1]; this is even more pertinent in pregnancy where a mother's mental health can impact not only on her physical health but also the health of her baby in utero [2]. Obesity and mental health problems are both important causes of maternal deaths in the UK and other industrialized countries [3–5]. This chapter therefore aims to review the evidence on how obesity in pregnancy is related to mental disorders and the implications of this for the management of obesity in pregnancy.

The mental disorders we will focus on are often grouped together as severe mental illness, common mental disorders, and binge eating disorder (other eating disorders and learning difficulties are beyond the scope of this chapter). The main international classifications of mental disorders are the World Health Organization (WHO) ICD classification [6] and the American Diagnostic and Statistical Manual of Mental Disorders (DSM-IV) [7], both of which are currently being revised and updated (ICD-11 and DSM-V will be appearing in the next few years). We will use the current definitions in ICD-10 predominantly, other than for binge eating disorder, which is only included in the DSM classification currently (see also below).

Definition of mental disorders

Severe mental illness can be defined in a number of ways, either by diagnosis (usually the psychotic disorders, schizophrenia [and related disorders such as schizo-affective disorder], bipolar disorder, and psychotic depression) or by severity of disorder. For the purpose of this chapter we will use the term severe mental

illness to include psychotic disorders, i.e., schizophrenia (and other related psychotic disorders), bipolar disorder, and depressive psychosis.

Schizophrenia is characterized by fundamental and characteristic distortions of thinking and perception, and an inappropriate or lack of emotional responsiveness. Clear consciousness and intellectual capacity are usually maintained, although certain cognitive deficits can develop over time. Delusions and hallucinatory voices discussing the patient, disorganized speech, and negative symptoms (marked apathy, paucity of speech, and blunting or incongruity of emotional responses, usually resulting in social withdrawal and lowering of social performance) can occur.

Bipolar disorder is characterized by two or more episodes where the patient's mood and activity are substantially disturbed, on some occasions mood is elevated, and energy and activity increased (hypomania or mania) and on others mood is lowered, and energy and activity decreased (depression). Repeated episodes of hypomania or mania only (i.e., without depressive episodes) are classified as bipolar disorder (see ICD-10) [6]. Depressive psychosis is a severe depressive disorder with mood congruent delusions and/or hallucinations.

Common mental disorders include depressive disorders and anxiety disorders. Depressive symptoms have to be present for at least two weeks to fulfil criteria for a depressive disorder, and symptoms may include feeling sad or irritable most of the time, loss of pleasure or interest in things that used to be enjoyed, significant weight loss or gain unrelated to pregnancy, difficulty sleeping or oversleeping, feeling restless or slowed down, fatigue, feelings of worthlessness or excessive guilt, and difficulties concentrating, remembering, or making decisions. There may also be thoughts of

Maternal Obesity, ed. Matthew W. Gillman and Lucilla Poston. Published by Cambridge University Press. © Cambridge University Press 2012.

self-harm or suicide. Depressive disorders can also often have prominent anxiety symptoms.

Anxiety disorders include specific phobias, agoraphobia (fear and avoidance of crowds, public places, or traveling away from home), social phobia (marked fear of being the focus of attention, or fear of behaving in a way that will be embarrassing, and marked avoidance of situations in which there is fear of behaving in an embarrassing way), panic disorder (recurrent panic attacks), and generalized anxiety disorder (at least six months of prominent tension, worry, and feelings of apprehension about everyday events and problems, with anxiety symptoms). Anxiety symptoms include autonomic arousal symptoms (e.g., palpitations, sweating, trembling, dry mouth), difficulty in breathing, fears of dying or losing control (see ICD-10 for more details) [6].

Binge eating disorder was included in DSM-IV in 1994 as a provisional eating disorder. It is likely that it will be included in both ICD-11 and DSM-V as there is growing recognition of this disorder as a specific entity [8]. Binge eating disorder is characterized by frequent and persistent episodes of binge eating accompanied by feelings of loss of control and marked distress in the absence of regular compensatory behaviors. The disorder is associated with specific eating disorder psychopathology (e.g., dysfunctional body shape and weight concerns). Binge eating disorder is often associated with overweight and obesity, and psychiatric co-morbidity.

Prevalence of mental health problems in pregnancy

Mental disorders are common during pregnancy [9]; pregnancy is not, as is sometimes portrayed, a time of "blooming mental health" for all women. The commonest mental disorder in pregnancy is depression, and a meta-analysis of studies on the prevalence of depressive disorders in pregnancy found a point prevalence of up to 5.6% and an incidence of 7.5% for major depression at different times during pregnancy – rates not significantly different for women of similar age who are not pregnant or in the immediate postpartum [10]. Higher rates were found for minor depression (i.e., persistent depressive symptoms but not with many of the associated symptoms found in major depressive disorder such as sleep disturbance or loss of appetite). This relatively high prevalence has led to some countries advocating routine screening for depression

in pregnancy and postpartum [11]. The Edinburgh Postnatal Depression Scale [12] can be used during pregnancy for the detection of depressive symptoms, as it does not include the somatic symptoms of depression (e.g., fatigue) used by other depression scales, and which are likely to be present in pregnant women but do not indicate depression in pregnancy. A cut-off score of >12 indicates a probable depressive disorder in the third trimester (validation of cut-offs indicating probable clinical depression has not yet been carried out for first and second trimesters [13]). There remains some controversy internationally on the best way for maternity services to detect depression and UK NICE guidelines currently suggest using two Whooley questions [14], though there have been no validation studies of these in the perinatal period to date. It is important that depression is distinguished from depressive symptoms by clinical interview, as depressive symptoms can be short-lived and mild, with a good short-term and long-term prognosis, and therefore do not need treatment. Major depressive disorders by comparison are associated with considerable maternal and fetal/infant morbidity. They can be treated effectively by psychological interventions or antidepressants, with psychological interventions usually being first-line treatment for mild or moderate depression in pregnancy, though antidepressants will be needed for severe illnesses or milder disorders that do not respond to psychological treatments.

There has been less research on anxiety disorders in pregnancy so it is not clear whether the prevalence of anxiety disorders in pregnancy is different to that of non-pregnant women. However, symptoms of anxiety are found to be common [15]. One study of anxiety disorders reported a prevalence of the different types of anxiety disorders of 24% in the third trimester [16]. There is also evidence that both anxiety and depressive disorders are more likely in pregnancy if a woman has a past history of mental disorders, and a woman is at particularly high risk of relapse if she stops antidepressants as a result of the pregnancy [17].

Binge eating disorder has been researched less extensively than other mental disorders in pregnancy, but in a recent large cohort study, a prevalence of nearly 5% was found [18], with a surprisingly high proportion (49%) of the women who fulfilled criteria for binge eating disorder in pregnancy being incident cases (i.e., with onset after becoming pregnant).

Pregnancy is similarly not protective against relapse of bipolar disorder; in a prospective observational clinical cohort study, the risk of at least one recurrence of an affective (mood) episode in pregnancy was 71% in 89 pregnant women with DSM-IV bipolar disorder, with the risk highest in those women who stopped prophylactic mood stabilizers [19]. (However, of note, it is the postpartum period that is associated with the highest risk of relapse of a psychotic episode [20].) Bipolar disorder has a prevalence of 0.74% [21] and is therefore a rare condition in pregnancy.

Schizophrenia is also a rare disorder with a lifetime prevalence of 0.4% [22]. Women with schizophrenia have a considerably lower fertility than women with the disorders discussed above, which appears to be partly due to the prolactin-raising effect of some antipsychotics and partly due to their difficulty in sustaining relationships [23]. However, with the increasing use of atypical antipsychotics, many of which are not associated with hyperprolactinemia, it is likely that more women with schizophrenia will have children, though maternity services will still see only one case in every 1000 to 2000 women. There is some evidence that women with schizophrenia are less likely to engage with antenatal services [2], often due to a fear of involvement of child protection services.

Obstetric outcomes in women with mental disorders

There is a growing literature documenting the increased risk of adverse obstetric outcomes in women with mental disorders. Psychotic disorders (bipolar disorder and schizophrenia and related disorders) are associated with prematurity and small for gestational age babies [15], stillbirths [24], and neonatal deaths [25]. A recent meta-analysis reported that depression in pregnancy is associated with low birthweight and prematurity [26] and we have found that antenatal depression increases the risk of subsequent sudden infant death syndrome [27]. Antenatal anxiety is also associated with poorer obstetric outcomes [28] though there is less research on this. In addition there is some preliminary evidence that suggests binge eating disorder increases the risk for large for gestational age babies and the need for cesarean section [29].

It may not be the disorders themselves that are causing these adverse outcomes, but rather the socio-economic deprivation and lifestyle factors associated with the disorders, such as smoking and poor nutrition. There is evidence that some pregnant women with mental disorders are more likely to smoke [25,29,30],

abuse alcohol and other substances, and if acutely ill, have poor self-care including poor nutrition and poor engagement with antenatal care [2]. Finally, the treatment for the disorder may also contribute to adverse outcome – in utero exposure to atypical antipsychotic drugs may increase infant birthweight and risk of macrosomia [31] and antipsychotics in general may be associated with an increased risk of gestational diabetes [32] though olanzapine and clozapine are most likely to cause gestational diabetes.

It is not clear whether obesity is a causal or moderating factor explaining the relationship between mental disorders and poor obstetric outcomes, as body mass index (BMI) has rarely been included as a covariate in the studies examining the association between mental disorders and obstetric outcomes. With the increasing recognition of the importance of the impact of obesity on adverse outcomes, future research will clearly need to disentangle the effect of obesity from other potential risk factors, such as smoking, on fetal and maternal outcomes.

Prevalence of mental disorders in obese women during pregnancy

There are very limited data on the relationship between obesity and mental health during pregnancy, but there is growing evidence that obese pregnant women have poorer mental health than those not obese. There have only been a few studies looking at specific mental disorders and obesity in pregnancy, and those published have focused on depression. A recent review of the association between ante- and postnatal depressive symptoms and maternal obesity found that of eight studies that investigated maternal ante- and postnatal depressive symptoms and maternal obesity, only three reported a positive association and the association found was stronger for postnatal than antenatal depressive symptoms and BMI [33]. However, many of the studies included relied on self-reported depressive symptoms (rather than diagnoses of depression) and self-reported BMI.

The current evidence, though limited, therefore suggests that obesity may be associated with poorer mental health in pregnancy or the postpartum period. Weight gain, as well as pre-pregnancy weight, seem important in increasing the risk for mental disorders [34]. However, the direction of causality is not clear and there are no data to our knowledge on obesity and mental disorders other than depression in pregnancy.

The relationship between obesity and mental disorders in non-pregnant women

Since the data in pregnancy are currently so limited, the evidence in the broader literature on obesity and mental disorders in women is briefly reviewed here, using studies that have reported results for non-pregnant women. Most studies have been cross-sectional surveys but there are some recent longitudinal cohort studies, which we focus on below where they are available. The majority of studies have focused on anxiety and mood disorders, with fewer studies investigating severe mental disorders. However, there is a growing literature on this latter group, particularly since the advent of atypical antipsychotic medications which have a more pronounced impact on weight gain than older antipsychotics (see below).

Severe mental illness

Most of the research literature in this area has reported on psychotic disorders together with fewer studies investigating obesity in specific disorders such as schizophrenia. The research on psychotic disorders in general will therefore first be reviewed and then the available studies on specific disorders discussed.

Obesity and its co-morbidities are commonly cited as being higher in those with severe mental disorders compared to the general population, and to be particularly pronounced in women, with obesity rates of around 40% to 60% [35–37]. People with severe mental disorders are not only more likely to be overweight, but they are also more likely to smoke, have hyperglycemia and/or diabetes, hypertension, and dyslipidemia [38], all of which could potentially impact on adverse obstetric outcomes. Individuals with severe mental disorders consume a diet that is rich in total and saturated fats and refined carbohydrates while containing less fiber, fruit, and vegetables than the general population [39], possibly due to effects of medication on carbohydrate craving. Those taking clozapine, for example, have a significantly higher intake of sugar and total and saturated fat than those not taking this medication.

A meta-analysis of weight gain with different antipsychotics illustrated that there is considerable variation in risk between antipsychotics [40] – after ten weeks of treatment, weight gain was greatest with clozapine followed by olanzapine; quetiapine and risperidone have an intermediate risk while aripiprazole and ziprasidone have little effect on weight. Clozapine (the most effective antipsychotic drug available), olanzapine (a related compound), and some other atypical antipsychotics are also linked to diabetes and increases in plasma lipids [41], and antipsychotics in general have been associated with gestational diabetes [32]. The older "typical" antipsychotics, while probably less related to severe weight gain, currently tend not to be prescribed as much as the newer atypical antipsychotic drugs as they are associated with other adverse side effects including motor disorders (parkinsonian-like symptoms and tardive dyskinesia).

Lower levels of physical activity and greater social deprivation experienced by those with severe mental disorders may contribute further to increased obesity rates [39] – this may be particularly important for inpatients, where opportunities for physical activity are limited. These lifestyle behaviors and associated risk factors contribute to the two to three times increased risk of premature death (mean standardized mortality ratio 2.6) in those with schizophrenia compared with the general population [22]. These risk factors are also found in pregnant women with severe mental disorders [2].

Clinicians treating patients with severe mental disorders inevitably focus on treatment of the mental illness, which can lead to suboptimal care of associated obesity and other metabolic problems in both primary care [42] and secondary medical [43], psychiatric [44], and maternity [25] care. Access to treatment for physical problems, including obesity and associated metabolic disorders, is also often lower among psychiatric patients [45]. Such disparities in access may be partly due to delays in help-seeking, low motivation and apathy (symptoms of schizophrenia), or structural discrimination [46].

There is clear evidence that overweight and obesity are particularly problematic in individuals with schizophrenia. For patients with schizophrenia, the reported prevalence of obesity varies considerably, with rates twice as high as the general population in the USA reported [36], with some studies finding rates in women as high as 40% to >60%, with a much higher prevalence of abdominal obesity in women with schizophrenia compared to control groups [47]. Medication use is typically associated with having a higher weight. Other important factors increasing obesity risk include concurrent antidepressant or mood stabilizer use, and illness severity, presence of chronic disease, physical inactivity, and high alcohol consumption [37]. International guidelines therefore now highlight the importance of weight monitoring in patients with schizophrenia, advising patients on their diet and exercise, provision of lifestyle/weight management interventions, and training mental health professionals in this area [48].

North American studies have reported that approximately 30% to 45% of women with bipolar disorder are obese, significantly more than the general population [49]. However, as with studies of schizophrenia, many have not compared patients with control subjects or controlled for important variables such as age and gender. Many of the drugs prescribed for bipolar disorder contribute to weight gain, particularly atypical antipsychotics, lithium, certain antidepressants, and sodium valproate [50].

Clinical studies have found that women being treated for bipolar disorder are at increased risk of eating disorders [51], the majority of which are binge eating disorder. Overall, obesity appears to be more prevalent in individuals with bipolar disorder than the general population, and to be particularly pronounced in women with concurrent depression, medication use, and binge eating.

Common mental disorders

The prevalence of depressive and anxiety disorders in obese populations varies between studies, and rates are often not given separately for men and women. However, studies have tended to find that depression and anxiety are associated with obesity, although these are not consistent findings. The most recent systematic review of longitudinal studies reported a reciprocal relationship between depression and obesity, with depressive symptoms increasing future obesity risk and obesity increasing risk of future depression [52]. However, some recent longitudinal studies have had contradictory results – in longer follow-up studies (periods of ten to twelve years), obesity in women did not predict major depression [53] and depression did not predict obesity [54].

The links between obesity and depression are therefore complex and not fully understood. Hypothesized mechanisms include biological, psychological, and behavioral pathways [52]. Biological pathways may include inflammatory, metabolic, and endocrine systems, while shared psychological pathways include body dissatisfaction, lowered self-esteem, and distress,

and these are likely to be linked to sociocultural factors including demographic characteristics and societal weight discrimination. Behavioral pathways include unhealthy eating and inadequate physical activity.

The effect of antidepressant treatment on depression in obese women has only recently been investigated with reports that higher relative body weight or obesity predicts poor response to antidepressants, particularly in women [55]. Medications such as tricyclic antidepressants stimulate appetite, specifically carbohydrate craving [50], and lack of exercise during a depressive illness may also contribute. Some depressive disorders are associated with overeating rather than anorexia so the psychopathology of a depressive episode is also likely to play a part.

There have also been increasing numbers of studies published in recent years reporting higher rates of anxiety disorders in obese women compared with non-obese women. A recent systematic review of (predominantly cross-sectional) population studies found a significant pooled odds ratio of 1.4 (95%CI: 1.1–1.7) for anxiety disorders in obese compared to non-obese women, with a stronger relationship found with more severe obesity [56]; the two included longitudinal studies had contradictory findings. There are a number of anxiety subtypes and it is possible that these have different relationships with obesity; results were mixed in the seven studies in this review where analyses by subgroup were done, though specific phobias (specifically social phobia and agoraphobia) were consistently associated with obesity in women. As for depression, studies vary as to the extent of adjustment made in analyses for potential confounding factors. Given the small number of studies and differences in analyses used, potential mediating factors are unclear but it appears that obesity may have some independent effects on anxiety. It is also unclear from this evidence whether obesity increases the risk of anxiety or vice versa, or indeed whether there is a reciprocal relationship as has been hypothesized for depression. The proposed mediators between obesity and anxiety are far from understood but have been proposed to be related to obese individuals experiencing weight stigma, lower social support, and being of lower socioeconomic status [56].

Few studies have been carried out concerning common mental disorders in clinical groups of patients attending obesity services, but there is some evidence that those attending specialist obesity services have high rates of mental disorders. A survey of patients attending UK specialist obesity services found that approximately 37% of women had "probable" or severe depression and 22% had anxiety disorders [57].

Binge eating disorder

Of women seeking obesity treatment, 12% to 29% meet diagnostic criteria for binge eating disorder [58–60]. Rates of binge eating disorder in population samples of women are lower and have been reported to be 0.2% to 3.3% [61]. Data regarding prevalence in obese women are limited; in a general population sample, 5.2% of women reported experiencing binge eating disorder in the past six months and binge eating disorder was associated with higher weight, with 12.3% of women with binge eating disorder being obese compared to 2.9% in those without binge eating disorder [62].

Individuals with binge eating disorder are more likely to experience psychiatric co-morbidity than those without binge eating disorder. Mood disorders are particularly common; 46% of women with binge eating disorder in a community sample had experienced lifetime depressive episodes [62]. Rates of mood disorders in those reporting binge eating disorder tend to be higher in clinical samples than community samples; in women seeking treatment for binge eating disorder, 67% reported a lifetime history of mood disorder and 33% had a current mood disorder [63]. Data are lacking regarding the presence of anxiety disorders in women with binge eating disorder. As mentioned earlier, there is also some evidence of an increased risk of binge eating disorder in women with bipolar disorder. Moreover those with bipolar disorder are at greater risk of obesity if they experience co-morbid binge eating disorder [64].

Management of obesity in women with mental disorders

In view of the relatively common occurrence of mental health problems in obese women and the serious implications of both obesity and mental disorders on health and pregnancy outcome, pregnant women with both obesity and mental disorders clearly need help with both problems. However, there is a paucity of evidence for effective intervention approaches. We were unable to identify any studies evaluating the impact of interventions for obese pregnant women with mental disorders.

However, there are some encouraging intervention studies targeting (non-pregnant) obese individuals with a range of mental disorders, especially those targeting weight management. Randomized controlled trials (RCTs) using non-pharmacological interventions such as cognitive behavioral therapy or nutrition counseling to reduce weight in patients with schizophrenia found statistically significant reductions in weight compared with usual care [65]. There were no significant differences in outcomes between approaches, nor clear differences between group and individual programs [65]. Other recent studies have also had positive results for obese patients with schizophrenia; an intervention targeting physical activity by increasing motivation and skills for walking significantly increased time spent walking [66] and a combined nutritional, exercise, and behavioral group intervention produced significant reductions in weight [67]. Although the recent Cochrane review for weight-loss treatments in individuals with schizophrenia found limited research for non-pharmacological interventions, they made some tentative recommendations regarding treatment modalities that may be applicable in pregnant obese women with schizophrenia [65]. These were that interventions are likely to need to be highly structured and offer intensive support in the early stages, although this could be reduced over time. They also recommended that interventions focus on realistic goals including simple changes to reduce calorie intake (e.g., changing the types of food eaten and reducing portion sizes) and gradual increases in moderate intensity activity, and that behavior change should be supported with cognitive behavioral therapy strategies. In line with this, it appears likely that increases in physical activity would be best achieved by increasing walking [68]. Programs for those with severe mental illness who are obese typically use the same techniques as standard lifestyle modification programs (e.g., self-monitoring), but are adapted to take into account levels of cognitive impairment [35]. Behavioral components include monitoring of weight, diet and activity, goal setting, and overcoming barriers to change.

Structured cognitive behavioral therapy programs are well-established treatments for binge eating disorder [69], but while these typically reduce bingeing behavior, they appear less effective at reducing weight [70]. Major depressive disorder and binge eating disorder have both been independently associated with worse outcomes in obesity treatment programs [71]. More research is therefore generally needed to find optimally effective treatments for obesity in patients with mental disorders and more specifically for pregnant women. However, there is some evidence that moderate physical activity improves depressive symptoms [72] and may be of help in the perinatal period [73]. Moderate physical activity and nutritional advice are recommended for pregnant obese women and could therefore indirectly improve mental health as well as physical health. The challenge is to ensure that obese pregnant women with mental disorders are referred to appropriate specialist clinics and that they are helped to engage with obesity interventions.

Management of mental disorders in obese pregnant women

There is a very limited evidence base on treatment of mental disorders in pregnancy [14]. However, where possible (i.e., in mild or moderate common mental disorders such as depression or anxiety, or binge eating disorder) non-pharmacological interventions are first-line treatment. These include moderate exercise for mild depression (see above), and cognitive behavioral therapy or interpersonal therapy for mild or moderate depressive or anxiety disorders, and binge eating disorders. More severe disorders will usually need psychotropic medication, and a careful individualized risk–benefit analysis is needed, taking into account the risk of medication on the fetus and the risk of untreated illness [14]. The ethical and practical difficulties in carrying out RCTs of psychotropic medication in pregnancy has meant that risks and benefits of these medications have not been adequately investigated [74] and a discussion of the literature to date is beyond the scope of this chapter. However, general principles include using medication that has already been found to be effective in an individual woman and to avoid switching medication during pregnancy as this could lead to relapse [75]. Where treatment is to be initiated for the first time in an obese pregnant woman, it would be advisable to avoid medication that is particularly likely to lead to weight gain, e.g., olanzapine. However, weight-neutral psychotropic drugs are not always effective in severe disorders (e.g., treatment-resistant schizophrenia) and it may be necessary to use drugs that are known to cause weight gain, with appropriate advice on diet and exercise. Advice from perinatal psychiatrists who can make an individualized risk–benefit analysis in collaboration with the woman and her family is therefore advisable [14].

Implications

Pregnant women with mental disorders are more likely to be obese than pregnant women without mental disorders. Pregnant women with mental disorders are also at increased risk of adverse obstetric and fetal outcomes and this may be partly due to obesity and/or may be worsened by obesity. Mental disorders therefore need to be identified in obese pregnant women and both the mental disorder and the obesity need to be treated. There has been a tendency for health professionals and researchers to focus on postpartum mental disorders, but there is growing recognition now that the potential for antenatal disorders to lead to adverse outcomes for both mother and infant means that identification of mental disorders during pregnancy is essential [11].

This review has demonstrated that that there is a very limited evidence base on obesity and mental disorders in pregnancy, and virtually no evidence on which to base treatment decisions. More research is urgently needed on the prevalence of mental disorders in obese pregnant women, the mechanisms by which mental disorders are associated with obesity, and effective interventions for pregnant women with both mental disorders and obesity.

References

1. Prince M, Patel V, Saxena S, *et al.* No health without mental health. *Lancet* 2007;**370**:859–77.

2. Howard L M. Fertility and pregnancy in women with psychotic disorders. *Eur J Obstet Gynecol Reprod Biol* 2005;**119**(1):3–10.

3. Kildea S, Pollock W E & Barclay L. Making pregnancy safer in Australia: the importance of maternal death review. *Aust N Z J Obstet Gynaecol* 2008;**48**:130–6.

4. Schutte J M, Hink E, Heres M H B, *et al.* Maternal mortality due to psychiatric disorders in the Netherlands. *J Psychosom Obstet Gynaecol* 2008;**29**(3):150–2.

5. Cantwell R, Clutton-Brock T, Cooper G, *et al.* Saving Mothers' Lives: reviewing maternal deaths to make motherhood safer: 2006–2008. The eight report of the Confidential Enquiries into Maternal Deaths in the United Kingdom. *BJOG* 2011;**118**(Suppl 1):1–203.

6. WHO. *International Classification of Diseases and Related Health Problems, 10th Revision* (ICD-10): 2010. http://apps.who.int/classifications/apps/icd/icd10online/ [Accessed January 4, 2012].

7. American Psychiatric Association. *Diagnostic and Statistical Manual of Mental Disorders, Fourth Edition* (DSM-IV). (American Psychiatric Association, 2000).

8. Treasure J, Claudino A M, Zucker N. Eating disorders. *Lancet* 2010;**375**(9714):583–93.

9. Vesga-Lopez O, Bianco C, Keyes K, *et al.* Psychiatric disorders in pregnant and postpartum women in the United States. *Arch Gen Psychiatry* 2008;**65**(7):805–15.

10. Gavin N I, Gaynes B N, Lohr K N, *et al.* Perinatal depression: a systematic review of prevalence and incidence. *Obstet Gynecol* 2005;**106**(5 Pt 1):1071–83.

11. Bick D & Howard L M. When should women be screened for postnatal depression? *Expert Rev Neurother* 2010;**10**(2):151–4.

12. Cox J L, Holden J M & Sagovsky R. Detection of postnatal depression. Development of the 10-item Edinburgh Postnatal Depression Scale. *Br J Psychiatry* 1987;**150**:782–6.

13. Gibson J, McKenzie-McHarg K, Shakespeare J, *et al.* A systematic review of studies validating the Edinburgh Postnatal Depression Scale in antepartum and postpartum women. *Acta Psychiatr Scand* 2009;**119**(5):350–64.

14. National Institute for Health and Clinical Excellence. Antenatal and postnatal mental health. Clinical management and service guidance. NICE Clinical Guideline 45. Developed by the National Collaborating Centre for Mental Health. (NICE, 2007).

15. Leight K L, Fitelson E M, Weston C A, *et al.* Childbirth and mental disorders. *Int Rev Psychiatry* 2010;**22**(5):453–71.

16. Sutter Dallay A L, Giaconne-Marcesche V, Glatigny-Dallay E, *et al.* Women with anxiety disorders during pregnancy are at increased risk of intense postnatal depressive symptoms: a prospective survey of the MATQUID cohort. *Eur Psychiatry* 2004;**19**(8):459–63.

17. Cohen L S, Altshuler L L, Harlow B L, *et al.* Relapse of major depression during pregnancy in women who maintain or discontinue antidepressant treatment. *JAMA* 2006;**295**(5):499–507.

18. Bulik C M, Von Holle A, Hamer R, *et al.* Patterns of remission, continuation and incidence of broadly defined eating disorders during early pregnancy in the Norwegian Mother and Child Cohort Study (MoBa). *Psychol Med* 2007;**37**:1109–18.

19. Viguera A C, Whitfield T, Baldessarini R J, *et al.* Risk of recurrence in women with bipolar disorder during pregnancy: prospective study of mood stabilizer discontinuation. *Am J Psychiatry* 2007;**164**(12):1817–24.

20. Munk-Olsen T, Laursen T M, Pedersen C B, *et al.* New parents and mental disorders: a population-based register study. *JAMA* 2006;**296**(21):2582–9.

21. Ferrari A J, Baxter A J & Whiteford H A. A systematic review of the global distribution and availability of prevalence data for bipolar disorder. *J Affect Disord* 2011;**134**:1–13.

22. McGrath J, Saha S, Chant D, *et al.* Schizophrenia: a concise overview of incidence, prevalence, and mortality. *Epidemiol Rev* 2008;**30**:67–76.

23. Howard L M, Kumar C, Leese M, *et al.* The general fertility rate in women with psychotic disorders. *Am J Psychiatry* 2002;**159**(6):991–7.

24. Webb R, Abel K, Pickles A, *et al.* Mortality in offspring of parents with psychotic disorders: a critical review and meta-analysis. *Am J Psychiatry* 2005;**162**(6):1045–56.

25. Howard L M, Goss C, Leese M, *et al.* Medical outcome of pregnancy in women with psychotic disorders and their infants in the first year after birth. *Br J Psychiatry* 2003;**182**:63–7.

26. Grote N K, Bridge J A, Gavin A R, *et al.* A meta-analysis of depression during pregnancy and the risk of preterm birth, low birth weight and intrauterine growth restriction. *Arch Gen Psychiatry* 2010;**67**(10):1012–24.

27. Howard L M, Kirkwood D & Latinovic R. Sudden infant death syndrome and maternal depression. *J Clin Psychiatry* 2007;**68**(8):1279–83.

28. Alder J, Fink N, Bitzer J, *et al.* Depression and anxiety during pregnancy: a risk factor for obstetric, fetal and neonatal outcome? A critical review of the literature. *J Matern Fetal Neonatal Med* 2007;**20**(3):189–209.

29. Bulik C M, Von Holle A, Siega-Riz A M, *et al.* Birth outcomes in women with eating disorders in the Norwegian Mother and Child Cohort Study. *Int J Eat Disord* 2009;**42**(1):9–18.

30. Goodwin R D, Keyes K & Simuro N. Mental disorders and nicotine dependence among pregnant women in the United States. *Obstet Gynecol* 2007;**109**(4):875–83.

31. Newham J J, Thomas S H, MacRitchie K, *et al.* Birth weight of infants after maternal exposure to typical and atypical antipsychotics: prospective comparison study. *Br J Psychiatry* 2008;**192**(5):333–7.

32. Reis M & Källén B. Maternal use of antipsychotics in early pregnancy and delivery outcome. *J Clin Psychopharmacol* 2008;**28**(3):279–88.

33. Milgrom J, Skouteris H, Worotniuk T, *et al.* The association between ante- and postnatal depressive symptoms and obesity in both mother and child: a systematic review of the literature. *Women's Health Issues* 2012; e1–e10.

34. Bodnar L M, Wisner K L, Moses-Kolko E, *et al.* Prepregnancy body mass index, gestational weight gain and the likelihood of major depression during pregnancy. *J Clin Psychol* 2009;**70**(9):1290–6.

35. Allison D B, Newcomer J W, Dunn A L, *et al.* Obesity among those with mental disorders. A National Institute of Mental Health Meeting Report. *Am J Prev Med* 2009;**36**(4):341–50.

36. Dickerson F B, Brown C H, Kreyenbuhl J A, *et al.* Obesity among individuals with serious mental illness. *Acta Psychiatr Scand* 2006;**113**:306–13.

37. Hakko H, Komulainen M T, Koponen H, *et al.* Are females at special risk of obesity if they become psychotic? The Longitudinal Northern Finland 1966 Birth Cohort Study. *Schizophr Res* 2006;**84**:15–19.

38. De Hert M, Dekker J M, Wood D, *et al.* Cardiovascular disease and diabetes in people with severe mental illness position statement from the European Psychiatric Association (EPA), supported by the European Association for the Study of Diabetes (EASD) and the European Society of Cardiology (ESC). *Eur Psychiatry* 2009;**24**(6):412–24.

39. Holt R I G & Peveler R C. Obesity, serious mental illness and antipsychotic drugs. *Diabetes Obes Metab* 2009;**11**(7):665–79.

40. Allison D B, Mentore J L, Heo M, *et al.* Antipsychotic-induced weight gain: a comprehensive research synthesis. *Am J Psychiatry* 1999;**156**(11):1686–96.

41. De Hert M A, van Winkel R, Van Eyck D, *et al.* Prevalence of the metabolic syndrome in patients with schizophrenia treated with antipsychotic medication. *Schizophr Res* 2006;**83**(1):87–93.

42. Hippisley-Cox J, Parker C, Coupland C, *et al.* Inequalities in the primary care of patients with coronary heart disease and serious mental health problems: a cross-sectional study. *Heart* 2007;**93**:1256–62.

43. Druss B G, Bradford W D, Rosenheck R A, *et al.* Quality of medical care and excess mortality in older patients with mental disorders. *Arch Gen Psychiatry* 2001;**58**:565–72.

44. Mackin P, Bishop D R & Watkinson H M. A prospective study of monitoring practices for metabolic disease in antipsychotic-treated community psychiatric patients. *BMC Psychiatry* 2007;**7**:28.

45. Osborn D P, King M B & Nazareth I. Participation in screening for cardiovascular risk by people with schizophrenia or similar mental illnesses: cross sectional study in general practice. *BMJ* 2003;**326**:1122–3.

46. Howard L M, Barley E, Rigg A, *et al.* A diagnosis of cancer in people with severe mental illness: practical and ethical issues raised. *Lancet Oncol* 2010;**11**(8):797–804.

47. McEvoy J P, Meyer J M, Goff D C, *et al.* Prevalence of the metabolic syndrome in patients with schizophrenia: baseline results from the Clinical Antipsychotic Trials of Intervention Effectiveness (CATIE) schizophrenia trial and comparison with national estimates from NHANES III. *Schizophr Res* 2005;**80**:19–32.

48. National Institute for Health and Clinical Excellence. Core interventions in the treatment and management of schizophrenia in primary and secondary care. NICE Clinical Guideline 82. Developed by the National Collaborating Centre for Mental Health. (NICE, 2009).

49. Fagiolini A, Kupter D J, Houck PR, *et al.* Obesity as a correlate of outcome in patients with bipolar I disorder. *Am J Psychiatry* 2003;**160**:112–17.

50. Torrent C, Amann B, Sánchez-Moreno J, *et al.* Weight gain in bipolar disorder: pharmacological treatment as a contributing factor. *Acta Psychiatr Scand* 2008;**118**:4–18.

51. Diflorio A & Jones I. Is sex important? Gender differences in bipolar disorder. *Int Rev Psychiatry* 2010;**22**(5):437–52.

52. Luppino F S, de Wit L M, Bouvy P F, *et al.* Overweight, obesity, and depression. A systematic review and meta-analysis of longitudinal studies. *Arch Gen Psychiatry* 2010;**67**(3):220–9.

53. Gariepy G, Wang J L, Lesage A D, *et al.* The longitudinal association from obesity to depression: results from the 12-year National Population Health Survey. *Obesity* 2010;**18**:1033–8.

54. Patten S B, Williams J V A, Lavorato D H, *et al.* Major depression, antidepressant medication and the risk of obesity. *Psychother Psychosom* 2009;**78**:182–6.

55. Uher R, Mors O, Hauser J, *et al.* Body weight as a predictor of antidepressant efficacy in the GENDEP project. *J Affect Disord* 2009;**118**(1–3):147–54.

56. Gariepy G, Nitka D & Schmitz N. The association between obesity and anxiety disorders in the population: a systematic review and meta-analysis. *Int J Obes* 2010;**34**:407–19.

57. Tuthill A, Slawik H, O'Rahilly S, *et al.* Psychiatric co-morbidities in patients attending specialist obesity services in the UK. *Q J Med* 2006;**99**:317–25.

58. Azarbad L, Corsica J, Hall B, *et al.* Psychosocial correlates of Binge Eating Disorder in Hispanic, African American, and Caucasian women presenting for bariatric surgery. *Eat Behav* 2010;**11**:79–84.

59. Fandiño J, Moreira R O, Preissler C, *et al.* Impact of Binge Eating Disorder in the psychopathological profile of obese women. *Compr Psychiatry* 2010;**51**:110–14.

60. Riener R, Schindler K & Ludvik B. Psychosocial variables, eating behaviour, depression, and binge eating in morbidly obese subjects. *Eat Behav* 2006;**7**(4):309–14.

61. Dingemans A E, Bruna M J & van Furth E F. Binge Eating Disorder: a review. *Int J Obes* 2002;**26**:299–307.

62. Reichborn-Kjennerud T, Bulik C M, Sullivan P F, *et al.* Psychiatric and medical symptoms in binge eating in the absence of compensatory behaviours. *Obes Res* 2004;**12**(9):1445–54.

63. Grenon R, Tasca G A, Cwinn E, *et al.* Depressive symptoms are associated with medication use and lower health-related quality of life in overweight women with Binge Eating Disorder. *Womens Health Issues* 2010;**20**(6):435–40.

64. Keck P E & McElroy S L. Bipolar disorder, obesity, and pharmacotherapy-associated weight gain. *J Clin Psychiatry* 2003;**64**(12):1426–35.

65. Faulkner G, Cohn T & Remington G. Interventions to reduce weight gain in schizophrenia. *Cochrane Database Syst Rev* 2007;**1**:CD005148.

66. Beebe L H, Smith K, Burk R, *et al.* Effect of a motivational intervention on exercise behaviour in persons with schizophrenia spectrum disorders. *Community Ment Health J* 2011;**47**(6):628–36.

67. Chen C K, Chen Y C & Huang Y S. Effects of a 10-week weight control program on obese patients with schizophrenia or schizoaffective disorder: a 12-month follow up. *Psychiatry Clin Neurosci* 2009;**63**(1):17–22.

68. Ussher M, Stanbury L, Cheeseman V, *et al.* Physical activity preferences and perceived barriers to activity among persons with severe mental illness in the United Kingdom. *Psychiatr Serv* 2007;**58**(3):405–8.

69. Wilfley D E, Welch R R, Stein R I, *et al.* A randomized comparison of group cognitive-behavioral therapy and group interpersonal psychotherapy for the treatment of overweight individuals with binge-eating disorder. *Arch Gen Psychiatry* 2002;**59**(8):713–21.

70. Bulik C M, Brownley K A & Shapiro J R. Diagnosis and management of Binge Eating Disorder. *World Psychiatry* 2007;**6**(3):142–8.

71. Pagoto S, Bodenlos J S, Kantor L, *et al.* Association of major depression and Binge Eating Disorder with weight loss in a clinical setting. *Obesity* 2007;**15**(11):2557–9.

72. Krogh J, Nordentoft M, Sterne J A, *et al.* The effect of exercise in clinically depressed adults: systematic review and meta-analysis of randomized controlled trials. *J Clin Psychiatry* 2011;**72**(4):529–38.

73. Daley A, Jolly K & MacArthur C. The effectiveness of exercise in the management of post-natal depression: systematic review and meta-analysis. *Fam Pract* 2009;**26**(2):154–62.

74. Howard L M, Webb R & Abel K. Antipsychotic drugs for pregnant and breastfeeding women with non-affective psychosis. Editorial. *BMJ* 2004;**329**:933–4.

75. Taylor D, Paton C & Kapur S. *The Maudsley Prescribing Guidelines*, 10th edn. (London: Informa Healthcare, 2009).

Long-term consequences of obesity in pregnancy for the mother

Andrea Deierlein and Anna Maria Siega-Riz

Introduction

Current knowledge argues that pregnancy serves as a preview of a woman's long-term health. The numerous physiological changes during pregnancy, which stress the metabolic system [1], can reveal subclinical disease states as well as identify new ones [2,3]. Evidence for this assertion exists in studies that have examined the association between gestational diabetes mellitus (GDM) and subsequent type 2 diabetes mellitus (T2DM) [4], as well as hypertensive disorders during pregnancy and subsequent cardiovascular disease risk factors [5]. Whether pregnancy is on the causal pathway or simply a time period that allows these chronic diseases to be unmasked remains yet to be determined. Obese women are more likely to be at higher risk of developing complications such as GDM, hypertensive disorders, and pre-eclampsia during pregnancy [6–9]. In this chapter we will focus on the evidence for the association between gestational weight gain and postpartum weight retention among obese women, as well as the association between obesity and lack of breast-feeding, and how these associations are potentially interrelated to cause further disease in obese women.

Postpartum weight retention

Pregnancy and its associated weight gain may be potential "triggers" for the development of obesity in women [10,11]. Pooled estimates of average absolute postpartum weight retention in units of body mass index (BMI) (kg/m^2) are 2.42 (95% CI: 2.32–2.52) at six weeks, 1.14 (95% CI: 1.04–1.25) at six months, and 0.46 (95% CI: 0.38–0.54) at twelve months postpartum [12]. These estimates suggest that most women will lose the majority of weight that is associated with pregnancy within one year postpartum. However, many

studies have observed a wide range of variation in postpartum weight retention [13,14], with as many as 20% of women having substantial postpartum weight retention ranging over 5 kg (11 lbs) [13].

Gestational weight gain is the most important predictor of postpartum weight retention [15] and a contributor to the obesity epidemic among women of reproductive ages [16]. Compared to women with gestational weight gains within the recommended range, women with gains in excess of the range are at greater risk of not returning to their pre-pregnancy weight status and becoming overweight or obese [17,18]; at 21 years postpartum it is estimated that women with excessive gains are approximately 2 and 4.5 times more likely to be overweight and obese, respectively [17]. The recommended amount of weight gain during pregnancy varied over the twentieth century, culminating with the 1990 Institute of Medicine (IOM) gestational weight gain guidelines, which provided recommended weight gain ranges specific for pre-pregnancy BMI status [19]. These guidelines were revised in 2009 to adopt the International Obesity Task Force BMI categories [20] and set an upper limit of weight gain for obese women. The 2009 IOM recommendations for gestational weight gain are: underweight (BMI <18.5), 28–40 lbs (12.7–18.1 kg); normal weight (BMI 18.5–24.9), 25–35 lbs (11.3–15.9 kg); overweight (BMI 25.0–29.9), 15–25 lbs (6.8–11.3 kg); and obese (BMI ≥30), 11–20 lbs (5.0–9.1 kg) [21]. Currently, there are insufficient data to provide recommendations specific for women in an obesity class higher than class I (BMI 30–35). Although obese women have the lowest recommended weight gain range and tend to gain less weight during pregnancy than women in lower BMI groups, nearly half of obese women gain weight in excess of their specific recommendations (based on the

Maternal Obesity, ed. Matthew W. Gillman and Lucilla Poston. Published by Cambridge University Press. © Cambridge University Press 2012.

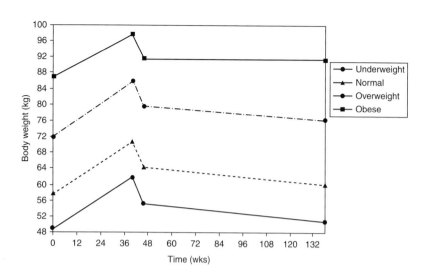

Figure 8.1. Patterns of maternal weight changes from preconception through gestation and early and late postpartum periods according to pregravid BMI group. Reproduced from reference [32] with permission from Macmillan Publishers Ltd.

1990 recommendations) [21]. Among obese women, it is estimated that each pound (0.5 kg) of gestational weight gain is associated with a 0.4 lb (0.2 kg) increase above pre-pregnancy weight at one year postpartum [22]. Additionally, the odds of retaining at least 10 lbs (4.5 kg) at one year postpartum are approximately 2 and 7.5 times higher in obese women who gain more than 15 lbs (6.8 kg) during pregnancy compared to those who gain 0–15 lbs (0–6.8 kg) [22].

Independent of gestational weight gain, there is some evidence to suggest that pre-pregnancy BMI contributes to postpartum weight retention [23–25]; each one unit increase in pre-pregnancy BMI is associated with a 0.10 kg (0.22 lbs) increase in weight retention from the start of a first pregnancy to the beginning of a second pregnancy [26]. Maternal obesity and increases in BMI between pregnancies are associated with adverse pregnancy complications, including gestational hypertension and diabetes [27,28], and decreased success of vaginal birth after cesarean delivery [29,30]. It is not clear, however, whether obese women are more likely to retain weight or to gain weight in the postpartum period [31]. There are a limited number of long-term observational studies that followed women beyond 12 months postpartum but there is some evidence that despite having similar (or even greater) postpartum weight losses during the early postpartum period (within approximately one year postpartum) [15,16,32,33], obese women have smaller postpartum weight losses and greater weight gains during later postpartum periods (>1 year postpartum) compared to women in lower pre-pregnancy BMI categories [11,32]. Among a large

urban population of women, early postpartum weight losses during the first six weeks post-delivery were similar across pre-pregnancy BMI categories (1990 categories: underweight, <19.8; normal weight, 19.8–26.0; overweight, >26.0–29.0; and obese, >29.0) but differed from late postpartum losses between six weeks and a median two years postpartum. Underweight and normal weight women continued to lose weight during this time while weight loss diminished among obese women (Figure 8.1). The adjusted postpartum weight changes as a percentage of gestational weight were 33.1%, 32.3%, 24.3%, and 2.8% for underweight, normal weight, overweight, and obese women, respectively [32].

Similar divergent postpartum weight changes in obese women are also observed for longer follow-up periods. In a population of White, predominantly middle-class women with singleton pregnancies, obese (BMI >29.9) women had a mean weight gain of 7.8 kg (17.2 lbs) compared to 7.1, 5.9, and 6.1 kg (15.6, 13.0, and 13.4 lbs) among underweight (BMI <19.8), normal weight (BMI 19.8–26.0), and overweight (BMI >26.0–29.0) women, respectively, at an approximate ten-year follow-up (mean 8.5 years) [35]. At the 15-year follow-up, obese women were an average of 15.5 kg (34.2 lbs) heavier than their pre-pregnancy weights, corresponding to a yearly weight gain of 2.3 lbs (1.0 kg). This exceeded yearly weight gains of 1.7, 1.2, and 1.0 lb(s) (0.77, 0.55, and 0.45 kg) in overweight, normal weight, and underweight women, respectively [23]. Among Black and White women in the Coronary Artery Risk Development in Young Adults (CARDIA) study, greater mean weight changes were observed at ten-year follow-up for women with BMI $\geq 25 \, kg/m^2$ with one or more "short" pregnancies (miscarriages and/or abortions) or one or more births compared to those who remained nulliparous. Weight changes ranged from 5 to 6 kg (11 to 13.2 lbs) and 3 to 5 kg (6.6 to 11 lbs) in White and Black women with BMI $\geq 25 \, kg/m^2$, respectively, while changes ranged from 0 to 1 kg (0 to 2.2 lbs) and 0 to 2 kg (0 to 4.4 lbs) in White and Black women with BMI $<25 \, kg/m^2$, respectively [34].

Few studies include anthropometric measurements other than weight and height as a means to estimate body fat and fat patterns of women during the perinatal period. In the few that did include these measurements, there is inconsistent evidence regarding the fat gains during pregnancy and fat losses during the postpartum period in obese women compared to their lower weight counterparts [36,37]. Regardless of the amount of fat gain during pregnancy, there may be important regional differences in fat accumulation during the postpartum in non-obese vs. obese women, such that obese women accumulate more fat in central locations (as determined by waist circumference and skinfold measurements of the suprailiac and subscapular regions), while non-obese women accumulate more fat in peripheral locations (as determined by skinfold measurements in the arms and costal regions) [34,38]. These differences in sites of fat accumulation are apparent in the postpartum and likely have important implications for later disease development since there is evidence that visceral fat thickness is more strongly associated with insulin resistance [39], diastolic blood pressure, glycemia, insulinemia, triglycerides, HDL-C, and total cholesterol/HDL-C ratio [40] than body fat in other locations.

In a small study of pregnant women, body weight and skinfold thicknesses (triceps, biceps, subscapular, suprailiac, and mid-thigh) were measured at 13 and 36 weeks gestation and six months postpartum and used to estimate body density and body fat mass [38]. All women gained weight between 13 and 36 weeks gestation and had substantial weight loss at six weeks postpartum followed by slight or no reductions in weight through six months postpartum. Despite no differences in weight change across BMI groups (underweight, BMI <19.8; normal weight, BMI 19.8–26.0; overweight, BMI >26.0–29.0; obese, BMI >29.0), statistically significant differences were found for changes in measurements of fat mass, total and suprailiac skinfold thicknesses, and waist-to-hip ratio among obese women during the postpartum period. Compared to normal weight women, obese women had less fat mass loss and gains in total skinfold thicknesses between 36 weeks gestation and six months postpartum and gains in waist-to-hip ratio between six weeks and six months postpartum [38].

Maternal obesity and infant feeding

Overweight and obese women are less likely to initiate breastfeeding and more likely to prematurely stop breastfeeding compared to their normal weight counterparts [41,42]. Possible reasons for a reduced likelihood of breastfeeding among overweight/obese women include physiological, medical, psychological, practical/mechanical, and sociocultural factors [41,43]. This is important because breastfeeding may have a protective effect against later adverse health outcomes that are associated with obesity, including some cancers, T2DM [44,45], metabolic syndrome [46,47], and cardiovascular diseases [48,49]. It is also hypothesized that breastfeeding plays a role in the "resetting" of maternal metabolism following pregnancy [50]; it is associated with favorable postpartum hormonal and metabolic changes that re-establish glucose homeostasis and increase lipid metabolism, and has been shown to reduce postpartum weight retention in some [50,51] but not all studies [15,52]. Exclusive or prolonged breastfeeding may also improve offspring outcomes including allergy, infection, cognitive ability, and perhaps obesity [53–55].

Summary

It is well established that obesity, independent of pregnancy, is associated with long-term metabolic consequences and chronic disease development, such as metabolic syndrome, T2DM, and cardiovascular diseases. It is less certain what role, if any, pregnancy may play in influencing the relationship between obesity and these later health outcomes in women. As discussed in Chapters 5 and 15, pregnancy results in states of hyperlipidemia and insulin resistance, which are amplified in obese women and also thought to have important implications for the development of GDM and hypertensive disorders [3,9].

There is currently little investigation of the interrelationships between obesity, pregnancy, and chronic disease. An increase in BMI of $\geq 3 \, kg/m^2$ between consecutive pregnancies is associated with an increased risk of GDM and hypertensive disorders in the second pregnancy [27]. Risks of hypertensive disorders are highest among obese women who maintained or increased their BMI between pregnancies [28]. Maternal obesity (BMI >29.0) is also associated with later development of T2DM/pre-T2DM and heart disease (CHD)/pre-CHD, where T2DM/pre-T2DM was defined as a diagnosis of T2DM, metabolic syndrome, or at least three risk factors for metabolic syndrome, and CHD/pre-CHD was defined as a diagnosis of CHD, hypertension, or dyslipidemia. At 15 years postpartum, obese women were nine times more likely to have pre-DM/DM and five times more likely to have pre-CHD/CHD compared to women who were underweight (BMI <19.8) and normal weight (BMI 19.8–26.0) prior to pregnancy [23]. Thus, among obese women, pregnancy is less likely to be playing a causal role but rather may be unmasking chronic diseases that will develop in the future.

Limitations of studies and gaps in our understanding

The current literature suggests that maternal obesity has many long-term health consequences for the mother; however, the degree to which pregnancy contributes to these outcomes is uncertain. It remains to be determined whether adverse health outcomes, such as postpartum weight retention and chronic disease development, vary not just by pre-pregnancy BMI status but by other social and behavioral factors as well. Body mass index is a crude measurement of body fat and does not provide information regarding body fat patterning, which may be more influential for chronic disease development. Much of the current evidence is based on studies with older cohorts or small sample sizes, which may lack adequate numbers of obese women. This was reflected in several studies that used cut-off points within the overweight range (BMI ≥25) rather than estimating effects within maternal overweight and obese categories. Associations of maternal obesity and adverse health outcomes may be missed when these categories are collapsed due to inadequate numbers of obese women. Long-term studies also often overlook adjustment for weight gain associated with aging, which may have important implications for estimating the effect of pregnancy and parity on weight development.

It is not certain whether the observed postpartum weight changes and chronic disease development are primarily due to pregnancy-related metabolic changes and weight retention or lifestyle behaviors related to

having a child, such as infant feeding practices and changes in physical activity and dietary habits. Overall, there is a need for prospective studies that follow women from preconception through menopause. It is important to document women's behaviors, anthropometric and body composition measures, and hormonal and endocrine markers prior to, during, and after pregnancy for many years to understand the interrelationships between pregnancy, weight development, and long-term health consequences.

References

1. Kaaja R J & Greer I A. Manifestations of chronic disease during pregnancy. *JAMA* 2005;**294**:2751–7.

2. Rich-Edwards J W, McElrath T F, Karumanchi S A & Seely E W. Breathing life into the lifecourse approach: pregnancy history and cardiovascular disease in women. *Hypertension* 2010;**56**:331–4

3. Sattar N & Greer I A. Pregnancy complications and maternal cardiovascular risk: opportunities for intervention and screening? *BMJ* 2002;**325**:157–60.

4. Bellamy L, Casas J P, Hingorani A D & Williams D. Type 2 diabetes mellitus after gestational diabetes: a systematic review and meta-analysis. *Lancet* 2009;**373**:1773–9.

5. Bellamy L, Casas J P, Hingorani A D & Williams D J. Pre-eclampsia and risk of cardiovascular disease and cancer in later life: systematic review and meta-analysis. *BMJ* 2007;**335**:974.

6. Saldana T M, Siega-Riz A M, Adair L S & Suchindran C. The relationship between pregnancy weight gain and glucose tolerance status among black and white women in central North Carolina. *Am J Obstet Gynecol* 2006;**195**:1629–35.

7. Thadhani R, Stampfer M J, Hunter D J, *et al.* High body mass index and hypercholesterolemia: risk of hypertensive disorders of pregnancy. *Obstet Gynecol* 1999;**94**:543–50.

8. Chu S Y, Callaghan W M, Kim S Y, *et al.* Maternal obesity and risk of gestational diabetes mellitus. *Diabetes Care* 2007;**30**:2070–6.

9. Bodnar L M, Catov J M, Klebanoff M A, Ness R B & Roberts J M. Prepregnancy body mass index and the occurrence of severe hypertensive disorders of pregnancy. *Epidemiology* 2007;**18**:234–9.

10. Linne Y, Barkeling B & Rossner S. Long-term weight development after pregnancy. *Obes Rev* 2002;**3**:75–83.

11. Hunt S C, Daines M M, Adams T D, Heath E M & Williams R R. Pregnancy weight retention in morbid obesity. *Obes Res* 1995;**3**:121–30.

12. Schmitt N M, Nicholson W K & Schmitt J. The association of pregnancy and the development of obesity – results of a systematic review and meta-analysis on the natural history of postpartum weight retention. *Int J Obes* 2007;**31**:1642–51.

13. Gunderson E P & Abrams B. Epidemiology of gestational weight gain and body weight changes after pregnancy. *Epidemiol Rev* 2000;**22**:261–74.

14. Nohr E A, Vaeth M, Baker J L, *et al.* Combined associations of prepregnancy body mass index and gestational weight gain with the outcome of pregnancy. *Am J Clin Nutr* 2008;**88**:1705.

15. Siega-Riz A M, Herring A H, Carrier K, *et al.* Sociodemographic, perinatal, behavioral, and psychosocial predictors of weight retention at 3 and 12 months postpartum. *Obesity (Silver Spring)* 2010;**18**:1996–2003.

16. Rasmussen K M, Abrams B, Bodnar L M, *et al.* Recommendations for weight gain during pregnancy in the context of the obesity epidemic. *Obstet Gynecol* 2010;**116**:1191–5.

17. Mamun A A, Kinarivala M, O'Callaghan M J, *et al.* Associations of excess weight gain during pregnancy with long-term maternal overweight and obesity: evidence from 21y postpartum follow-up. *Am J Clin Nutr* 2010;**91**:1336–41.

18. Amorim A R, Rossner S, Neovius M, Lourenco P M & Linne Y. Does excess pregnancy weight gain constitute a major risk for increasing long-term BMI? *Obesity (Silver Spring)* 2007;**15**:1287–86.

19. Institute of Medicine, Subcommittee on Nutrition Status and Weight Gain during Pregnancy. *Nutrition during Pregnancy.* (Washington, DC: National Academy of Sciences, 1990).

20. International Obesity Task Force: World Health Organization. *Obesity: Preventing and Managing the Global Epidemic.* Report of a WHO Consultation. WHO Technical Report Series 894. (Geneva, Switzerland: WHO, 1998).

21. Institute of Medicine. *Weight Gain During Pregnancy: Reexamining the Guidelines.* (Washington, DC: National Academies Press, 2009).

22. Vesco K K, Dietz P M, Rizzo J, *et al.* Excessive gestational weight gain and postpartum weight retention among obese women. *Obstet Gynecol* 2009;**114**:1069–75.

23. Rooney B L, Schauberger C W & Mathiason M A. Impact of perinatal weight change on long-term obesity and obesity-related illnesses. *Obstet Gynecol* 2005;**106**:1349–56.

24. Boardley D J, Sargent R G, Coker A L, Hussey J R & Sharpe P A. The relationship between diet, activity, and other factors, and postpartum weight change by race. *Obstet Gynecol* 1995;**86**:834–8.

25. Joseph N P, Hunkali K B, Wilson B, *et al.* Pre-pregnancy body mass index among pregnant adolescents: gestational weight gain and long-term postpartum weight retention. *J Pediatr Adolesc Gynecol* 2008;**21**:195–200.

26. Ostbye T, Krause K M, Swamy G K & Lovelady C A. Effect of breastfeeding on weight retention from one pregnancy to the next: results from the North Carolina WIC program. *Prev Med* 2010;**51**:368–72.

27. Villamor E & Cnattingius S. Interpregnancy weight change and risk of adverse pregnancy outcomes: a population-based study. *Lancet* 2006;**368**:1164–70.

28. Mostello D, Chang J J, Allen J, *et al.* Recurrent preeclampsia: the effect of weight change between pregnancies. *Obstet Gynecol* 2010;**116**:667–72.

29. Durnwald C P, Ehrenberg H M & Mercer B M. The impact of maternal obesity and weight gain on vaginal birth after cesarean section success. *Obstet Gynecol* 2004;**191**:954–7.

30. Juhasz G, Gyamfi C, Gyamfi P, Tocce K & Stone J L. Effect of body mass index and excessive weight gain on success of vaginal birth after cesarean delivery. *Obstet Gynecol* 2005;**106**:741–6.

31. Harris H E & Ellison G T H. Do the changes in energy balance that occur during pregnancy predispose parous women to obesity? *Nutr Res Rev* 1997;**10**:57–81.

32. Gunderson E P, Abrams B & Selvin S. Does the pattern of postpartum weight change differ according to pregravid body size? *Int J Obes* 2001;**25**:853–62.

33. Walker L O, Sterling B S & Timmerman G M. Retention of pregnancy-related weight in the early postpartum period: implications for women's health services. *JOGNN* 2005;**34**:418–27.

34. Gunderson E P, Murtaugh M A, Lewis C E, *et al.* Excess gains in weight and waist circumference associated with childbearing: the Coronary Artery Risk Development in Young Adults Study (CARDIA). *Int J Obes* 2004;**28**:525–35.

35. Rooney B L & Schauberger C W. Excess pregnancy weight gain and long term obesity: one decade later. *Obstet Gynecol* 2002;**100**:245–52.

36. Lederman S A, Paxton A, Heymsfield S B, *et al.* Body fat and water changes during pregnancy in women with different body weight and weight gain. *Obstet Gynecol* 1997;**90**:483–8.

37. Butte N F, Ellis K J, Wong W W, Hopkinson J M & Smith E O. Composition of gestational weight gain impacts maternal fat retention and infant birth weight. *Am J Obstet Gynecol* 2003;**189**:1423–32.

38. Soltani H & Fraser R B. A longitudinal study of maternal anthropometric changes in normal weight,

overweight, and obese women during pregnancy and postpartum. *Br J Nutr* 2000;**84**:95–101.

39. Berg A H & Scherer P E. Adipose tissue, inflammation, and cardiovascular disease. *Circ Res* 2005;**96**:939–49.

40. Bartha J L, Marin-Segura P, Gonzalez-Gonzalez N L, *et al.* Ultrasound evaluation of visceral fat and metabolic risk factors during early pregnancy. *Obesity* 2007;**15**:2233–39.

41. Amir L H & Donath S. A systematic review of maternal obesity and breastfeeding intention, initiation, and duration. *BMC Pregnancy Childbirth* 2007;**7**:9.

42. Baker J L, Michaelsen K F, Thorkild I A S & Rasmussen K M. High prepregnant body mass index is associated with early termination of full and any breastfeeding in Danish women. *Am J Clin Nutr* 2007;**86**:404–11.

43. Mehta U J, Siega-Riz A M & Herring A H. Effect of body image on pregnancy weight gain. *Matern Child Health J* 2011;**15**:324–32.

44. Stuebe A M, Rich-Edwards J W, Willett W C, Manson J E & Michels K B. Duration of lactation and incidence of type 2 diabetes. *JAMA* 2005;**294**:2601–10.

45. Schwarz E B, Brown J S, Creasman J M, *et al.* Lactation and maternal risk of type 2 diabetes: a population-based study. *Am J Med* 2010;**123**:863.e1–6.

46. Ram K T, Bobby P, Hailpern S M, *et al.* Duration of lactation is associated with lower prevalence of the metabolic syndrome in midlife – SWAN, the Study of Women's Health Across the Nation. *Am J Obstet Gynecol* 2008;**198**:268.e1–6.

47. Gunderson E P, Jacobs D R Jr., Chiang V, *et al.* Duration of lactation and incidence of the metabolic syndrome in women of reproductive age according to gestational diabetes mellitus status: a 20-Year prospective study in CARDIA (Coronary Artery Risk Development in Young Adults). *Diabetes* 2010;**59**:495–504.

48. Stuebe A M, Michels K B, Willett W C, *et al.* Duration of lactation and incidence of myocardial infarction in middle to late adulthood. *Am J Obstet Gynecol* 2009;**200**:138.e1–8.

49. Schwarz E B, Ray R M, Stuebe A M, *et al.* Duration of lactation and risk factors for maternal cardiovascular disease. *Obstet Gynecol* 2009;**113**:974–82.

50. Stuebe A M & Rich-Edwards J W. The reset hypothesis: lactation and maternal metabolism. *Am J Perinatol* 2009;**26**:81–8.

51. Kac G, Benicio M, Velasquez-Melendez G, Valente J G & Struchiner C. Breastfeeding and postpartum weight retention in a cohort of Brazilian women. *Am J Clin Nutr* 2004;**79**:487–93.

52. Janney C A, Zhang D & Sowers M. Lactation and weight retention. *Am J Clin Nutr* 1997;**66**:1116–24.

53. Kramer M S & Kakuma R. Optimal duration of exclusive breastfeeding. *Cochrane Database Syst Rev* 2002;**1**:CD003517.

54. Fewtrell M, Wilson D C, Booth I & Lucas A. Six months of exclusive breast feeding: how good is the evidence? *BMJ* 2010;**342**:c5955.

55. Cope M B & Allison D B. Critical review of the World Health Organization's (WHO) 2007 report on "evidence of the long-term effects of breastfeeding: systematic reviews and meta-analysis" with respect to obesity. *Obes Rev* 2008;**9**:594–605.

Long-term consequences of maternal obesity and gestational weight gain for offspring obesity and cardiovascular risk: intrauterine or shared familial mechanisms?

Abigail Fraser and Debbie A. Lawlor

Introduction

Cardiovascular disease (CVD) is a leading cause of death in low-, middle-, and high-income countries, accounting for a quarter of deaths globally in 2001 [1]. Until recently most of our knowledge concerning etiological risk factors for CVD focused on adulthood. Indeed, there is good evidence that major adult risk factors such as smoking, diet, physical activity, hypertension, and obesity explain much of the variation in geographical and secular trends of CVD incidence and it has been suggested that there is no need to investigate further [2]. However, it has also been known for decades that the pathophysiological process of atherosclerosis begins in childhood and young adulthood [3,4]. Obesity and other cardiovascular risk factors such as hyperlipidemia, high blood pressure, and insulin resistance are present in childhood and track into adulthood [5–8], and a growing body of evidence has consistently shown associations of obesity in childhood and adolescence with mortality and cardiovascular morbidity later in life [9]. The adverse consequences of childhood obesity are not limited to the cardiovascular system, indeed it can affect almost every organ system and has other serious complications such as diabetes, fatty liver, asthma, and may have psychosocial complications as well [10].

In both the USA and in England approximately one in five women of reproductive age is now obese [11,12]. This increasing prevalence of overweight and obesity among women of childbearing age is a growing concern, since, as reviewed in Chapters 5, 8, and 16, obesity in pregnancy is associated with increased risk of most pregnancy complications, such as gestational diabetes mellitus (GDM), hypertensive disorders of pregnancy (HDP), delivery of a large for gestational age baby, and congenital defects [13]. The prevalence of childhood overweight and obesity has also increased worldwide in recent decades, though with some possibility that this increase is now leveling [10].

It has been suggested that long-term implications of maternal pre- or early pregnancy obesity and greater gestational weight gain (GWG) for offspring health are the driving force behind the current obesity epidemic [14]. If greater maternal adiposity results in in utero programming of the developing fetus to later overweight/obesity, the public health consequences would be extreme, as this could drive the obesity epidemic through subsequent generations irrespective of any improvements in key risk factors for obesity [14]. This is because women going into their pregnancy with greater adiposity would program their offspring to greater adiposity and their daughters would go into their pregnancies with greater adiposity and so on.

In this chapter we examine what is currently known about maternal adiposity and GWG and their associations with long-term offspring health, focusing on obesity and cardiovascular risk factors in offspring. We pay particular attention to study designs that might shed light on whether or not associations are causal, and if causal what the likely underlying mechanisms might be.

Consistent evidence demonstrates that pre-pregnancy body mass index (BMI) is inversely associated with GWG, although more overweight and obese women exceed the range of Institute of Medicine

Maternal Obesity, ed. Matthew W. Gillman and Lucilla Poston. Published by Cambridge University Press. © Cambridge University Press 2012.

(IOM)-recommended GWG compared with underweight and normal weight women [15]. We will therefore address pre-/early pregnancy adiposity and GWG separately. We begin by summarizing the potential mechanisms that could explain the influence of maternal adiposity and GWG on offspring health. We then critically examine the evidence of associations of maternal adiposity and GWG with offspring adiposity and cardiovascular risk factors and discuss whether it is likely that associations are causal or not. Throughout the chapter we address adiposity across the whole distribution as well as extremes of overweight/obesity since, for the large part, adiposity is linearly associated with cardiovascular risk factors and events in both adults [16] and children [17]. It is also important in terms of public health impact and for the development of interventions, to establish whether any associations of maternal pre-/early pregnancy adiposity with offspring outcomes are continuous across the distribution or threshold effects occur at the extreme only.

Mechanisms

Maternal pre-/early pregnancy adiposity

The main question with regard to potential underlying mechanisms of the association between maternal and offspring adiposity is whether it is due to intrauterine effects, extrauterine effects, or both.

The developmental overnutrition hypothesis

The fetal overnutrition hypothesis (also known as fetal teratogenesis) was first proposed in the 1950s by Pederson to explain the association between maternal diabetes in pregnancy and excessive growth in the developing fetus [18]. According to this hypothesis the greater delivery of glucose to the fetus in the diabetic pregnancy results in fetal hyperinsulinemia (a necessary response to prevent fetal hyperglycemia) and as a consequence increased insulin-mediated fetal growth. In the 1980s this hypothesis was broadened to include the possibility that other fuels, in addition to glucose, such as free fatty acids, ketone bodies, and amino acids also contributed to fetal hyperinsulinemia and increased fetal growth [19], and in the 1990s to include non-diabetic but overweight/obese pregnancies as a key modifiable exposure [20]. It was postulated that diabetes, obesity, and greater GWG independently affect the transfer of metabolic substrates to the fetus, which in turn influence secretion of insulin and growth of the

fetus [20]. Further, there has been speculation that this overnutrition may lead to permanent changes in appetite control, metabolism, and neuroendocrine function resulting in long-term increased risk of obesity, and vascular and metabolic disorders in the offspring [21]. This extended version of the original fetal overnutrition/fetal teratogenesis hypothesis is also referred to as the developmental overnutrition hypothesis.

In support of the developmental overnutrition hypothesis, high concentrations of maternal glucose among those with gestational diabetes have been shown to increase nutrient (glucose, amino acids, free fatty acids) transfer to the fetus and result in fetal hyperinsulinemia and increased fetal growth [18,19]. In studies of humans, fetal hyperinsulinemia has been detected in the offspring of diabetic mothers both in utero (assessed in samples of amniotic fluid) [22–24] and immediately after birth (assessed in samples of cord blood) and is associated with greater fetal growth [25]. The Hyperglycemia and Adverse Pregnancy Outcome (HAPO) study showed a positive linear relationship between maternal glucose and birthweight [26]. In vitro animal and human studies have also demonstrated that fetal pancreatic development and fat stores are influenced by the availability of fetal fuels – in particular glucose, lipids, and amino acids – which are in turn determined by maternal adiposity, insulin secretion and responsiveness, plasma levels of glucose, free fatty acids, and inflammatory signals [19,27].

Epigenetics

Animal studies have shown that maternal diet can induce epigenetic changes in offspring and cause long-term alterations in the expression of genes involved in obesity and energy metabolism [28]. In humans, maternal hyperglycemia has been found to correlate with placental leptin gene DNA methylation levels (fetal side: r = –0.44; maternal side: r = 0.53) [29]. These studies suggest that epigenetic changes may explain the association between maternal obesity and long-term offspring health, but replication of these initial findings is required before we can assume they are robust. These epigenetic processes may be part of the mechanisms underlying developmental overnutrition. See Chapter 13 for more discussion of the epigenetics of maternal obesity.

Shared familial genetics or environmental exposures

Offspring will inherit approximately half of their genes from their mother. Hence it is possible that greater maternal adiposity, GWG, and greater off-spring adiposity result from common genetic make up. Environmental exposures and behaviors (such as dietary patterns and levels of physical activity) also cluster within families. Therefore another possible explanation is that these behaviors explain the relationship between maternal and offspring obesity.

Gestational weight gain

Of total weight gain in healthy women approximately 55% is related to fat deposition, blood volume expansion, and increases in breast and uterine tissue, a further 15% to 20% is due to the placenta and amniotic fluid, and 25% to 30% fetal tissue [15]. Rates of deposition of maternal fat parallel GWG with women gaining between 2 and 6 kg of fat during pregnancy [30]. Pregnancy is associated with maternal deposition of both subcutaneous and visceral fat, with most subcutaneous deposition being centrally located [30,31]. Maternal pregnancy-related fat accumulation is relatively constant from the start of pregnancy to the middle of the second trimester when the rate of accumulation flattens [30,32]. In general this fat accumulation is a normal physiological response to pregnancy and together with women becoming temporarily more insulin resistant during pregnancy is important for providing the developing fetus with essential nutrients for normal growth and development.

Mechanisms underlying the potential associations of GWG with offspring adiposity and cardiovascular risk include the following:

Tracking of body size or composition. Intrauterine fetal growth clearly contributes to GWG and determines birthweight. Size at birth is positively associated with later size – including BMI, fat, and lean mass [33]. Hence any associations of GWG with offspring adiposity later in life could partially reflect tracking of offspring body composition.

Complications of pregnancy. There is some evidence that greater GWG is associated with a greater risk of gestational diabetes [34,35], and pre-eclampsia is associated with edema and related maternal GWG [36]. Maternal diabetes is associated with greater adiposity and diabetes risk in offspring (see below) and pre-eclampsia is consistently associated with higher offspring blood pressure [37,38]. Hence the association of GWG with cardiovascular risk factors could be mediated by complications of pregnancy.

Developmental overnutrition resulting from greater maternal deposition of fat early in pregnancy, as described in detail above.

Shared familial genetics or environmental exposure. Characteristics associated with greater weight gain at different stages across the offspring's life course (genetic, shared familial behaviors) could result in greater maternal GWG as well as greater weight gain in offspring and hence greater adiposity later in their life. However, arguments against this assertion are that more adipose mothers gain *less* weight in pregnancy [15], and a recent study found no evidence of association of established adiposity-related genetic variants with GWG [39].

Evidence of association of prenatal exposure to diabetes with offspring adiposity and cardiovascular risk factors

Although the focus of this chapter is on maternal pre-/early pregnancy adiposity and offspring outcomes, a key mechanism proposed for this association is via maternal diabetes and glucose metabolism and developmental overnutrition. It has been estimated that up to half of the cases of gestational diabetes can be attributed to pre-pregnancy obesity [40], and the risk of gestational diabetes increases by 0.92% (95% CI: 0.73–1.10) for every unit increase in BMI [41]. There is also some evidence that GWG preceding a diagnosis of gestational diabetes is associated with an increased risk of GDM [34,35].

In studies of the Pima Indians of Arizona (a population with very high prevalences of obesity and type 2 diabetes), mean BMI, fasting glucose and insulin, and type 2 diabetes are greater in offspring (during childhood, adolescence, and early adulthood) born to mothers who had diabetes during their pregnancy compared to either the offspring of mothers who developed diabetes later in their lives or those who never developed diabetes [42]. In a sibling study (182 individuals from 52 families), also conducted in the Pimas, risk of obesity and type 2 diabetes was greater among offspring born after the mother had been diagnosed with diabetes than in their siblings born before their mother's diagnosis [43]. Sibling studies are a powerful approach for determining causality as they inherently control for maternal genetic variation and any environmental exposures that have remained constant or very similar across pregnancies. Hence, in this context, a difference in the risk of obesity and type 2 diabetes between siblings is likely due, at least in part, to discordant exposure to maternal diabetes in utero.

The same study also found that within siblings there was no association of paternal diabetes around the time of pregnancy with these offspring outcomes [43]. Comparing the association of paternal and maternal diabetes with offspring outcomes is another way of exploring whether exposure to diabetes in utero is causally associated with offspring outcomes. If exposure to diabetes in utero directly affects the offspring, the maternal–offspring association will be much stronger than the paternal–offspring association. However, associations driven by shared familial, social, genetic, and environmental factors are likely to produce similar maternal–paternal associations. Therefore findings from the Pima sibling study suggest that, at least in a population at high risk for obesity and diabetes, intrauterine mechanisms make an important contribution to the link between gestational diabetes and offspring greater adiposity, insulin resistance, and type 2 diabetes.

More recently the association of diabetes (type 1, type 2, or gestational) or hyperglycemia during pregnancy with offspring obesity and cardiovascular risk has been examined in European and North American populations, with the majority of such studies finding that the offspring of mothers with gestational diabetes or hyperglycemia have greater BMI and fasting glucose and insulin (see [44–46] and citations therein). Some of these suggest that this association is confounded by maternal pre-pregnancy BMI since the association attenuates towards the null with adjustment for maternal BMI. However, given the graded association of BMI (both in and outside pregnancy) with fasting or postload glucose and the evidence that glucose freely crosses the placenta and results in increases in fetal insulin secretion in a graded manner, under the developmental overnutrition hypothesis, maternal BMI and gestational diabetes/ hyperglycemia may be part of the same causal exposure. Adjustment of one for the other may therefore represent overadjustment. A recent large study of Swedish men that included a within-sibling analysis (280 866 men from 248 293 families) found that the BMI of men whose mothers had diabetes during their pregnancy was on average 0.94 kg/m^2 greater (95% CI: 0.35–1.52) than in their brothers born before their mother was diagnosed with diabetes [45]. There was no within-sibling association

of maternal early pregnancy BMI in that study and adjustment for it did not alter the diabetes–offspring BMI association. These findings suggest that, as in the Pima Indians, intrauterine mechanisms contribute importantly to the link between maternal diabetes in pregnancy and later offspring adiposity in a relatively lean European population and that this association is not strongly confounded by early pregnancy BMI.

Association of maternal adiposity with offspring adiposity and cardiovascular risk factors

A number of studies have demonstrated that maternal pre- or early pregnancy BMI is positively associated with offspring BMI in later life (for example [47,48] and recently reviewed in [30] and [49]). However, there is little evidence that intrauterine mechanisms play a substantial role in this association.

Evidence from studies comparing associations of maternal and paternal BMI with offspring adiposity is conflicting. Some studies have found stronger associations of maternal BMI with offspring adiposity than of paternal BMI (e.g., [50]), including studies that measured parental BMI pre-pregnancy [51,52]. However, the differences between the maternal and paternal associations in these studies are small and unlikely to be important drivers of the obesity epidemic [53]. Furthermore, in the larger studies, the magnitudes of associations of maternal BMI with offspring adiposity are similar to those of paternal BMI with offspring adiposity [54–56], suggesting that these associations are driven by shared familial genetic or lifestyle characteristics. Furthermore, a large sibling study found that maternal early pregnancy BMI was positively associated with offspring BMI in the whole cohort and between non-siblings, but not within siblings (Figure 9.1) [45]. These results also suggest that the association observed in the cohort as a whole and in other studies might be explained by confounding due to characteristics that are identical or very similar in siblings such as maternal genotype, socioeconomic position, diet, and patterns of physical activity. Finally, a Mendelian randomization study in which maternal genetic variation in the fat mass and obesity-associated (*FTO*) gene, conditional upon offspring *FTO*, was used as an instrumental variable to estimate the causal effect of exposure to greater maternal adiposity in utero also did not support a strong effect [53].

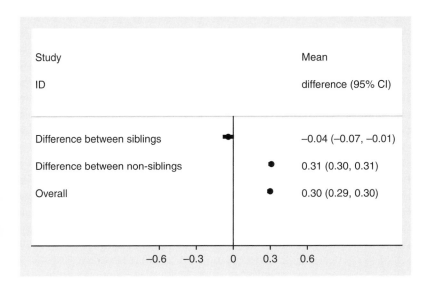

Figure 9.1. Associations of maternal early pregnancy BMI with offspring BMI. Reproduced with permission from [45].

The one exception to these general findings is with extreme maternal obesity in pregnancy. In an elegant sibling study, adiposity was lower and insulin sensitivity and lipid profile were improved in the offspring of mothers with extreme obesity (BMI >40) born after their mother had undergone bariatric surgery and subsequent weight loss, than in those born before she had received this surgery [57].

Summary of the evidence regarding the effect of pre-/early pregnancy BMI (and gestational diabetes) on offspring adiposity and related outcomes

Taken together these studies suggest that maternal obesity results in long-term effects on offspring adiposity and associated metabolic disturbance via intrauterine mechanisms in the extremes of clinical obesity or where there exists metabolic disturbance such as diabetes in pregnancy. Variation across most of the distribution of maternal pre-/early pregnancy BMI (below extreme obesity levels of $40 \, \text{kg/m}^2$), and without diabetes, may not have long-term effects on offspring risk. The public health implications of this are that maternal obesity per se is unlikely, so far, to have made a major contribution to the obesity epidemic. Furthermore, if the aim is to prevent long-term offspring overweight/obesity and cardiovascular risk via intrauterine mechanisms related to maternal overweight/obesity then it may make most sense to focus interventions on those with impaired glucose–insulin homeostasis or with

morbid obesity. From a public health perspective more may be gained, in terms of obesity and cardiovascular disease prevention, from interventions that prevent overweight/obesity in all family members and across the life course rather than focusing specifically on women of reproductive age.

Association of GWG with offspring adiposity and cardiovascular risk factors

Several studies have examined associations of GWG with offspring adiposity and a large majority have reported positive associations with measures of offspring adiposity in childhood [48,58–60], adolescence [61], and adulthood (Table 9.1) [62]. Other studies have examined the association with cardiovascular risk factors, most commonly offspring blood pressure, with conflicting results (Table 9.1) [58,62–66]. In ALSPAC, a UK-based prospective pregnancy cohort (http://www.bristol.ac.uk/alspac/), repeat measures of weight in pregnancy (median: 10; interquartile range: 8–11) are available for ~12 500 women. These women had a due date between April 1991 and December 1992, and in the early 1990s weight was still measured routinely in antenatal clinics in the UK. These repeat measures were modeled using a linear spline multilevel model with two levels: woman and measurement occasion, relating weight (outcome) to gestational age (exposure). Knots (points where the slope, i.e., the rate of GWG, changes) were placed at 18 and 28 weeks of gestation

Table 9.1 Studies assessing the association of GWG with offspring adiposity and cardiovascular risk factors later in life

Study	Sample size	Assessment of GWG	Relevant outcomes	Age (years) at outcome assessment	Main findings	Confounders controlled for
Southampton Women's Survey, UK [72]	948	Difference between weight measured at 34 weeks gestation and before pregnancy.	Fat mass, fat-free mass.	0, 4, 6	GWG was positively associated with fat mass at six and with fat-free mass at four when adjusting for potential confounders.	Sex, age at measurement, childhood height, pre-maternal pregnancy BMI, maternal smoking in pregnancy, age, height, parity, educational attainment, breastfeeding duration, birthweight.
Avon Longitudinal Study of Parents and Children, UK [38]	5154 for adiposity and blood pressure. 3457 for blood assays.	Repeat measures (median: 10; range: 1–17) abstracted from medical records.	BMI, waist circumference, fat mass, blood pressure, lipids, apolipoproteins, adiponectin, leptin, C-reactive protein, interleukin-6.	9	Greater recommended GWG by 2009 IOM guidelines was associated with greater offspring BMI, waist, fat mass, leptin, systolic blood pressure, C-reactive protein, and interleukin-6 and lower HDL-cholesterol and apolipoprotein-A1. Greater recommended GWG associated with reduced adiposity but similar otherwise to offspring of women who gained as recommended. Early pregnancy GWG associated with offspring adiposity but GWG in mid-pregnancy was associated with adiposity only in GWG >500 g. GWG in mid-pregnancy was associated with adverse lipid and inflammatory profiles, largely mediated by adiposity.	Age, gender, pre-pregnancy weight and GWG in previous weeks, parity, social class, smoking in pregnancy, age at birth, and mode of delivery.
Australia [62]	2432	Difference between maximum weight in pregnancy abstracted from	BMI, blood pressure.	21	Offspring BMI was on average 0.3 kg/m² (95% CI: 0.1–0.4) higher for each 0.1 kg/wk greater GWG after adjustment for potential	Age, sex, maternal age, education, parity, cigarette smoking, and pre-pregnancy BMI.

92

Study	N	Measurement	Outcomes	Age (years)	Results	Confounders adjusted
		medical records and self-reported pre-pregnancy weight.			confounding factors. Mean change in systolic and diastolic blood pressure per 0.1 kg GWG: 0.2 (95% CI: −0.2–0.6) and 0.0 (−0.3–0.3) respectively. Adjusting for current BMI attenuated blood pressure associations further.	
Portugal [59]	4845	Self-reported.	Overweight.	6–12	Odds of overweight increased across the distribution of GWG. ≥16 kg weight compared to ≤9 kg: multivariable OR = 1.27 (95% CI: 1.01–1.61).	Gender, age, birthweight, order of birth, breastfeeding, smoking during pregnancy, physical activity, parental BMI, parental education, calcium-to-protein ratio intake, and energy intake.
Bassett Mothers Health Project, USA [73]	208	Weight and height measured at antenatal visits and abstracted from medical records.	Overweight.	3	Net GWG (total GWG minus birthweight) was not associated with risk of overweight, but the risk of overweight associated with net GWG increased with increasing pre-pregnancy BMI.	Gestational age, pre-pregnancy BMI, income, maternal smoking in pregnancy, breastfeeding, birthweight.
Project Viva, USA [58]	1044	Difference between the last weight recorded before delivery and self-reported pre-pregnancy weight.	BMI, overweight, subscapular and triceps skinfold thicknesses, blood pressure.	3	Greater GWG was associated with greater BMI, sum of subscapular and triceps skinfold thickness, odds of overweight, and systolic blood pressure.	Maternal prenatal smoking, race/ethnicity, household income, marital status, glucose tolerance, gestation length, breastfeeding duration, sex, birthweight.
Growing Up Today Study cohort and their mothers, members of the Nurses' Health Study II, USA [61]	11 994	Self-reported.	BMI, overweight, obesity.	9–14	For each 5 lbs (2.3 kg) of GWG gain child BMI z-score increased by 0.03 units (95% CI: 0.02–0.04), equivalent to 1.3 lbs (0.6 kg) for an average 14-year-old boy or girl. The OR for obesity was 1.08 (1.05–1.13) when adjusting for all potential confounders and mediators.	Maternal age and smoking, household income and paternal education, child race/ethnicity, gestational age, sex, age in 1996, Tanner stage, pre-pregnancy BMI, gestational diabetes, breastfeeding duration, child behaviors including weekly hours of television and videos, physical activity, daily sugar-sweetened beverage intake, daily fried food, birthweight.

Table 9.1 (cont.)

Study	Sample size	Assessment of GWG	Relevant outcomes	Age (years) at outcome assessment	Main findings	Confounders controlled for
Motherwell birth cohort study, Scotland [74]	276	Difference between weight at last and first antenatal booking, abstracted from medical records.	Four-site skinfold thicknesses, waist circumference, BMI, percentage body fat, and fat mass.	27–30	GWG was positively associated with all outcomes.	Age, sex, smoking status, social class, activity level, birthweight.
Nurses' Health Study II and the Nurses' Mothers' Cohort, USA [75]	26 506	Retrospective self-reported.	Overweight, obesity.	18, 35–36	A U-shaped association between GWG and offspring obesity was found for obesity at 18 and at 35–36.	Maternal BMI, maternal smoking during pregnancy, nausea during pregnancy, maternal age at time of daughter's birth, birth order, parental history of diabetes, paternal BMI, mother living with father at time of child's birth, paternal level of education, birthweight.
Special Supplemental Nutrition Program for Women, Infants, and Children (WIC), USA [47]	8494	Self-reported. Net GWG (kg/wk) defined as self GWG minus birthweight/ length of gestation.	Obesity.	2–4	No association between net GWG and the odds of obesity at two, three, and four years of age.	Birthweight, birth year, sex, mother's age, race/ethnicity, education level, marital status, parity, pre-pregnancy BMI, and smoking during pregnancy.
Collaborative Perinatal Project, USA [60]	10 226	Difference between weight measured at delivery and self-reported pre-pregnancy weight.	Overweight.	7	GWG was positively associated with the risk of offspring overweight. Multivariable OR per 1 kg = 1.03 (95% CI: 1.01–1.05).	Maternal race, age, pre-pregnancy BMI, number of cigarettes smoked per day, gestational age, child sex, age, first-born status, study site, birthweight.
German Health Interview and Examination Survey for Children and Adolescents (KiGGS), Germany [76]	10 784	Self-reported based on medical certificate.	Overweight.	3–17	GWG was positively associated with the risk of offspring overweight. OR per kg = 1.01 (95% CI: 1.00–1.02) when adjusting for potential confounders including birthweight.	Sex, age, social status, pregnancy smoking, breastfeeding, birthweight, child's TV watching, physical activity.

Cohort	n	Weight measure	Outcome	Age	Results	Adjustments
The Copenhagen Perinatal Cohort, Denmark [77]	4234	Probably from medical records.	BMI, overweight, obesity.	1–42	At 42, there was a small effect of GWG on BMI (0.10 kg/m² per kg GWG; 95% CI: 0.04–0.17), and an increased risk of obesity (8% per kg GWG; 3, 13%).	Sex, maternal age, maternal pre-pregnancy BMI, parental social status, breadwinner's education, single-mother status, prematurity, birthweight, edema, and smoking during pregnancy.
Sweden [78]	1657	Medical records.	BMI.	18	No association. Results not shown.	Age, mother's age, parity, mother's education, smoking, pre-pregnancy BMI, birthweight for gestational age at birth.
Gambia [65]	675	Weight gain in the last three months of gestation calculated from weight measured at six months gestation and weight measured 30 days before birth.	Blood pressure.	1–9	In children one to seven years old there was no association of GWG with systolic blood pressure. Among children eight to nine years old there was an inverse relationship.	Weight at 7.5 months, maternal height, and blood pressure.
UK [63]	296	Difference in weight measured at 18 and 28 weeks gestation.	Blood pressure.	11	Overall, GWG was weakly inversely related to blood pressure. However, among women with triceps skinfold thickness at 18 weeks below the group median, GWG was inversely associated with offspring blood pressure; systolic blood pressure increased by 11.3 mmHg (95% CI: 2.2–20.4) and diastolic blood pressure by 10.1 mmHg (95% CI: 3.2–17.1) per kg/wk decrease.	Weight, cuff size, time of day, sex, ethnic group.
Jamaica [64]	77	Difference in weight measured at 15 and 35 weeks gestation.	Blood pressure.	10–12	GWG was inversely associated with blood pressure. Systolic blood pressure rose by 0.6 mmHg (95% CI: 0.1–1.0) for each 1 kg decrease in GWG.	Offspring sex, weight at 11, maternal hemoglobin, and triceps thickness at 15 weeks gestation.
Israel [66]	10883	Not reported.	Blood pressure.	17	No strong evidence of associations of GWG with blood pressure. In women the mean difference in systolic blood pressure per 1 kg GWG was 0.02 (95% CI: –0.06–0.11) and in men –0.3 (95% CI: –0.09–0.04).	Birthweight corrected for gestational age, birth order, ethnic origin, social status, height and BMI at 17, mother's educational attainment, and pre-pregnancy BMI.

to best fit the data. This method enables us to examine the timing of GWG in relation to outcomes and could potentially provide insight into underlying mechanisms, since weight gain at the beginning of pregnancy closely reflects maternal fat gain while weight gain later on in pregnancy reflects fetal components. Using these data, we found that GWG in early pregnancy was linearly associated with greater offspring adiposity, while GWG in mid-pregnancy was associated with offspring adiposity and blood pressure only in women who gained >500 g per week. This suggests that maternal fat accretion early in pregnancy may be driving associations. Gestational weight gain was also associated with adverse lipid and inflammatory profiles, with these associations largely mediated via associations with offspring adiposity [48].

Despite the consistency of studies, it remains difficult to determine whether associations of GWG with offspring adiposity are causal, that is act via intrauterine mechanisms. The associations are independent of maternal pre- or early pregnancy BMI, which suggests that they are unlikely to be solely driven by genetic and lifestyle characteristics related to greater adiposity in general. Moreover, genetic variants associated with adiposity outside pregnancy are not associated with GWG in the ALSPAC cohort [39].

A recent sibling comparison found that GWG within siblings was positively associated with birthweight and the authors concluded that this suggested the association was unlikely to be confounded by background family socioeconomic position [67]. They also implied that these findings provided indirect evidence that the association of GWG with later offspring adiposity was unlikely to be confounded by fixed family characteristics. However, in general, studies examining the associations of GWG with later offspring adiposity have found that birthweight does not mediate this association [48,58,59,62,]. This would suggest that associations of GWG with later adiposity are not a simple reflection of body size tracking throughout life. A large sibling study that examined the association of maternal GWG with offspring BMI at age 18 found no evidence of an association within siblings (mean difference in offspring BMI = 0.00; 95% CI: –0.02–0.02 kg/m^2 per 1 kg difference in maternal GWG) in mothers with a normal pre-pregnancy weight. In contrast, among overweight and obese mothers, greater GWG was associated with greater offspring BMI at 18 (mean difference in offspring BMI = 0.06; 95% CI: 0.01–0.12). These findings raise the possibility that among normal weight women the positive association of GWG with later offspring BMI is driven largely by shared familial (genetic and/or environment) risk factors, whereas in women who are overweight or obese in early pregnancy greater GWG appears to be associated with later greater offspring BMI via intrauterine mechanisms in addition to shared familial characteristics [68]. Alternatively, this may reflect deposition and persistence of differential fat depots between normal and overweight women, as analyses of skinfold thicknesses show that obese women put on more fat in the upper body compartment but that lean women put on more fat in the lower body compartment [69–71].

Summary of the evidence regarding the effect of GWG on offspring adiposity and related outcomes

Gestational weight gain is positively associated with offspring obesity and other cardiovascular risk factors in later life. It is, however, unclear whether these associations are due to causal intrauterine mechanisms. Results of a single sibling study suggest that intrauterine mechanisms may explain associations of GWG with offspring adiposity in early adulthood, only in overweight/obese women but not in normal weight women. Gestational weight gain is a multifaceted risk factor and reflects a number of different maternal and fetal components. It would be useful to see if these findings are replicated in other studies with relevant sibling data. However, unless we can identify the contributions of different components (maternal fat accretion, amniotic fluid, fetal weight, placenta, etc.) to the overall GWG, it is hard to interpret findings in a causal framework. One way of identifying these separate contributions would be by serial imaging measurements throughout pregnancy.

Summary

Existing evidence suggests that intrauterine mechanisms are likely to result in long-term effects on offspring adiposity and cardiovascular risk factors among the extremely obese, in those with diabetes, and in association with greater amounts of GWG. However, given that evidence is not so compelling among women with less severe obesity, maternal adiposity is probably not a main driver of the obesity epidemic currently. That said, if women of reproductive health continue to become more and more obese and the prevalence of type 2 diabetes and gestational diabetes continues to increase, it is possible that maternal adiposity will become a bigger contributor to any ongoing epidemic as more women of reproductive age would fall into the extreme phenotypes of clinical obesity or diabetes during pregnancy. Furthermore, promoting a healthy weight in women of reproductive age is sensible not only with regard to reproductive health but also for a wide range of other health outcomes in both the women themselves and their offspring. There is also still a need to better understand the short- and long-term effects of different patterns of GWG for both mother and off-spring. In particular a more nuanced decomposition of this into maternal fat deposition (which in terms of amount and location may be detrimental to health) and healthy growth of the fetus and vascular response of the mother (which are unlikely to be detrimental to health) is required.

References

1. Lopez A D, Mathers C D, Ezzati M, Jamison D T & Murray C J L (eds.) *Global Burden of Disease and Risk Factors.* (Washington, DC: World Bank, 2006).

2. Magnus P & Beaglehole R. The real contribution of the major risk factors to the coronary epidemics: time to end the "only-50%" myth. *Arch Intern Med* 2001;**161**(22):2657–60.

3. Enos M W, Holmes L C R & Beyer C J. Coronary disease among United States soldiers killed in action in Korea. *JAMA* 1953;**152**:1090–3.

4. Newman W P, Freedman D S, Voors A W, *et al.* Relation of serum lipoprotein levels and systolic blood pressure to early atherosclerosis. *N Engl J Med* 1986;**314**(3):138–44.

5. McCarthy H D, Ellis S M & Cole T J. Central overweight and obesity in British youth aged 11–16 years: cross sectional surveys of waist circumference. *BMJ* 2003;**326**(7390):624.

6. Freedman D S, Dietz W H, Srinivasan S R, *et al.* The relation of overweight to cardiovascular risk factors among children and adolescents: the Bogalusa Heart Study. *Pediatrics* 1999;**103**(6 Pt 1):1175–82.

7. Tounian P, Aggoun Y, Dubern B, *et al.* Presence of increased stiffness of the common carotid artery and endothelial dysfunction in severely obese children: a prospective study. *Lancet* 2001;**358**(9291):1400–4.

8. Fagot-Campagna A, Pettitt D J, Engelgau M M, *et al.* Type 2 diabetes among North American children and adolescents: an epidemiologic review and a public health perspective. *J Pediatr* 2000;**136**(5):664–72.

9. Reilly J J & Kelly J. Long-term impact of overweight and obesity in childhood and adolescence on morbidity and premature mortality in adulthood: systematic review. *Int J Obes* 2011;**35**(7):891–8.

10. Han J C, Lawlor D A & Kimm S Y. Childhood obesity. *Lancet* 2010;**375**(9727):1737–48.

11. Chu S, Kim S & Bish C. Prepregnancy obesity prevalence in the United States, 2004–2005. *Mat Child Health J* 2009;**13**(5):614–20.

12. NHS Information Centre. Lifestyle statistics. Statistics on obesity, physical activity and diet, England, February 2009. www.ic.nhs.uk/webfiles/publications/opan09/OPAD_Feb_2009_final_revised_Aug11.pdf [Accessed January 27, 2012].

13. Catalano P M & Ehrenberg H M. Review article: the short- and long-term implications of maternal obesity on the mother and her offspring. *BJOG* 2006;**113**(10):1126–33.

14. Ebbeling C B, Pawlak D B & Ludwig D S. Childhood obesity: public-health crisis, common sense cure. *Lancet* 2002;**360**(9331):473–82.

15. Institute of Medicine and National Research Council. *Weight Gain During Pregnancy: Reexamining the Guidelines.* (Washington DC: National Academies Press, 2009).

16. Whitlock G, Lewington S, Sherliker P, *et al.* Body-mass index and cause-specific mortality in 900 000 adults: collaborative analyses of 57 prospective studies. *Lancet* 2009;**373**(9669):1083–96.

17. Lawlor D A, Benfield L, Logue J, *et al.* Association between general and central adiposity in childhood, and change in these, with cardiovascular risk factors in adolescence: prospective cohort study. *BMJ* 2010;**341**:c6224.

18. Pederson J. Weight and length at birth of infants of diabetic mothers. *Acta Endocrinol (Copenh)* 1954;**16**:330–42.

19. Freinkel N. Banting Lecture 1980. Of pregnancy and progeny. *Diabetes* 1980;**29**(12):1023–35.

20. Whitaker R C & Dietz W H. Role of the prenatal environment in the development of obesity. *J Pediatr* 1998;**132**(5):768–76.

21. Oken E & Gillman M W. Fetal origins of obesity. *Obes Res* 2003;**11**(4):496–506.

22. Persson B, Heding L G, Lunell N O, *et al.* Fetal beta cell function in diabetic pregnancy. Amniotic fluid concentrations of proinsulin, insulin, and C-peptide during the last trimester of pregnancy. *Am J Obstet Gynecol* 1982;**144**(4):455–9.

23. Silverman B L, Metzger B E, Cho N H, *et al.* Impaired glucose tolerance in adolescent offspring of diabetic

mothers. Relationship to fetal hyperinsulinism. *Diabetes Care* 1995;**18**(5):611–7.

24. Silverman B L, Landsberg L & Metzger B E. Fetal hyperinsulinism in offspring of diabetic mothers. Association with the subsequent development of childhood obesity. *Ann N Y Acad Sci* 1993;**699**:36–45.

25. Dornhorst A, Nicholls J S, Ali K, *et al.* Fetal proinsulin and birth weight. *Diabet Med* 1994;**11**(2):177–81.

26. The HAPO Study Cooperative Research Group. Hyperglycemia and adverse pregnancy outcomes. *N Engl J Med* 2008;**358**(19):1991–2002.

27. Ramsay J E, Ferrell W R, Crawford L, *et al.* Maternal obesity is associated with dysregulation of metabolic, vascular, and inflammatory pathways. *J Clin Endocrinol Metab* 2002;**87**(9):4231–7.

28. Freeman D J. Effects of maternal obesity on fetal growth and body composition: implications for programming and future health. *Semin Fetal Neonatal Med* 2010;**15**(2):113–18.

29. Bouchard L, Thibault S, Guay S P, *et al.* Leptin gene epigenetic adaptation to impaired glucose metabolism during pregnancy. *Diabetes Care* 2010;**33**(11):2436–41.

30. Nelson S M, Matthews P, Poston L. Maternal metabolism and obesity: modifiable determinants of pregnancy outcome. *Hum Reprod Update* 2010;**16**(3):255–75.

31. Sohlstrom A & Forsum E. Changes in adipose tissue volume and distribution during reproduction in Swedish women as assessed by magnetic resonance imaging. *Am J Clin Nutr* 1995;**61**(2):287–95.

32. Pitkin R M. Nutritional support in obstetrics and gynecology. *Clin Obstet Gynecol* 1976;**19**(3):489–513.

33. Rogers I S, Ness A R, Steer C D, *et al.* Associations of size at birth and dual-energy X-ray absorptiometry measures of lean and fat mass at 9 to 10 y of age. *Am J Clin Nutr* 2006;**84**(4):739–47.

34. Herring S J, Oken E, Rifas-Shiman S L, *et al.* Weight gain in pregnancy and risk of maternal hyperglycemia. *Am J Obstet Gynecol* 2009;**201**(1):61–7.

35. Hedderson M M, Gunderson E P & Ferrara A. Gestational weight gain and risk of gestational diabetes mellitus. *Obstet Gynecol* 2010;**115**(3):597–604.

36. Steegers E A, von Dadelszen P, Duvekot J J, *et al.* Pre-eclampsia. *Lancet* 2010;**376**(9741):631–44.

37. Ferreira I, Peeters L L & Stehouwer C D. Preeclampsia and increased blood pressure in the offspring: meta-analysis and critical review of the evidence. *J Hypertens* 2009;**27**(10):1955–9.

38. Geelhoed J J, Fraser A, Tilling K, *et al.* Preeclampsia and gestational hypertension are associated with childhood blood pressure independently of family adiposity measures: the Avon Longitudinal Study of Parents and Children. *Circulation* 2010;**122**(12):1192–9.

39. Lawlor D, Fraser A, MacDonald-Wallis C, *et al.* Maternal and offspring adiposity related genetic variants and gestational weight gain. *Am J Clin Nutr* 2011;**94**(1):149–55.

40. Kim S Y, England L, Wilson H G, *et al.* Percentage of gestational diabetes mellitus attributable to overweight and obesity. *Am J Public Health* 2010;**100**(6):1047–52.

41. Torloni M R, Betrán A P, Horta B L, *et al.* Prepregnancy BMI and the risk of gestational diabetes: a systematic review of the literature with meta-analysis. *Obes Rev* 2009;**10**(2):194–203.

42. Pettitt D J, Nelson R G, Saad M F, *et al.* Diabetes and obesity in the offspring of Pima Indian women with diabetes during pregnancy. *Diabetes Care* 1993;**16**(1):310–14.

43. Dabelea D, Hanson R L, Lindsay R S, *et al.* Intrauterine exposure to diabetes conveys risks for type 2 diabetes and obesity: a study of discordant sibships. *Diabetes* 2000;**49**(12):2208–11.

44. Burguet A. Long-term outcome in children of mothers with gestational diabetes. *Diabetes Metab* 2010;**36**(6 Pt 2):682–94.

45. Lawlor D A, Lichtenstein P & Langstrom N. Association of maternal diabetes mellitus in pregnancy with offspring adiposity into early adulthood: sibling study in a prospective cohort of 280 866 men from 248 293 families. *Circulation* 2011;**123**:258–65.

46. Philipps L H, Santhakumaran S, Gale C, *et al.* The diabetic pregnancy and offspring BMI in childhood: a systematic review and meta-analysis. *Diabetologia* 2011;**54**(8):1957–66.

47. Whitaker R C. Predicting preschooler obesity at birth: the role of maternal obesity in early pregnancy. *Pediatrics* 2004;**114**(1):e29–e36.

48. Fraser A, Tilling K, Macdonald-Wallis C, *et al.* Association of maternal weight gain in pregnancy with offspring obesity and metabolic and vascular traits in childhood. *Circulation* 2010;**121**(23):2557–64.

49. Drake A J & Reynolds R M. Impact of maternal obesity on offspring obesity and cardiometabolic disease risk. *Reproduction* 2010;**140**(3):387–98.

50. Whitaker K L, Jarvis M J, Beeken R J, *et al.* Comparing maternal and paternal intergenerational transmission of obesity risk in a large population-based sample. *Am J Clin Nutr* 2010;**91**(6):1560–7.

51. Frayling T M, Timpson N J, Weedon M N, *et al.* A common variant in the FTO gene is associated with body mass index and predisposes to childhood and adult obesity. *Science* 2007;**316**(5826):889–94.

52. Lawlor D A, Davey Smith G, O'Callaghan M, *et al.* Epidemiologic evidence for the fetal overnutrition hypothesis: findings from the mater-university study of pregnancy and its outcomes. *Am J Epidemiol* 2007;**165**(4):418–24.

53. Lawlor D A, Timpson N J, Harbord R M, *et al.* Exploring the developmental overnutrition hypothesis using parental-offspring associations and FTO as an instrumental variable. *PLoS Med* 2008;**5**(3):e33.

54. Patel R, Martin R M, Kramer M S, *et al.* Familial associations of adiposity: findings from a cross-sectional study of 12,181 parental-offspring trios from Belarus. *PLoS One* 2011;**6**(1):e14607.

55. Lake J K, Power C & Cole T J. Child to adult body mass index in the 1958 British birth cohort: associations with parental obesity. *Arch Dis Child* 1997;**77**(5):376–81.

56. Subramanian S V, Ackerson L K & Smith G D. Parental BMI and childhood undernutrition in India: an assessment of intrauterine influence. *Pediatrics* 2010;**126**(3):e663–e671.

57. Smith J, Cianflone K, Biron S, *et al.* Effects of maternal surgical weight loss in mothers on intergenerational transmission of obesity. *J Clin Endocrinol Metab* 2009;**94**(11):4275–83.

58. Oken E, Taveras E M, Kleinman KP, *et al.* Gestational weight gain and child adiposity at age 3 years. *Am J Obstet Gynecol* 2007;**196**(4):322.

59. Moreira P, Padez C, Mourao-Carvalhal I, *et al.* Maternal weight gain during pregnancy and overweight in Portuguese children. *Int J Obes* 2007;**31**(4):608–14.

60. Wrotniak B H, Shults J, Butts S, *et al.* Gestational weight gain and risk of overweight in the offspring at age 7 y in a multicenter, multiethnic cohort study. *Am J Clin Nutr* 2008;**87**(6):1818–24.

61. Oken E, Rifas-Shiman S L, Field A E, *et al.* Maternal gestational weight gain and offspring weight in adolescence. *Obstet Gynecol* 2008;**112**(5):999–1006.

62. Mamun A A, O'Callaghan M, Callaway L, *et al.* Associations of gestational weight gain with offspring body mass index and blood pressure at 21 years of age: evidence from a birth cohort study. *Circulation* 2009;**119**(13):1720–7.

63. Clark P M, Atton C, Law C M, *et al.* Weight gain in pregnancy, triceps skinfold thickness, and blood pressure in offspring. *Obstet Gynecol* 1998;**91**(1):103–7.

64. Godfrey K M, Forrester T, Barker D J, *et al.* Maternal nutritional status in pregnancy and blood pressure in childhood. *Br J Obstet Gynaecol* 1994;**101**(5):398–403.

65. Margetts B M, Rowland M G, Foord F A, *et al.* The relation of maternal weight to the blood pressures of Gambian children. *Int J Epidemiol* 1991;**20**(4):938–43.

66. Laor A, Stevenson D K, Shemer J, *et al.* Size at birth, maternal nutritional status in pregnancy, and blood pressure at age 17: population based analysis. *BMJ* 1997;**315**(7106):449–53.

67. Ludwig D S & Currie J. The association between pregnancy weight gain and birthweight: a within-family comparison. *Lancet* 2010;**376**:984–90.

68. Lawlor D A, Lichtenstein P, Fraser A, *et al.* Does maternal weight gain in pregnancy have long-term effects on offspring adiposity? Sibling study in a prospective cohort of 146,894 men from 135,050 families. *Am J Clin Nutr* 2011; **94**(1):142–8.

69. Soltani H & Fraser R B. A longitudinal study of maternal anthropometric changes in normal weight, overweight and obese women during pregnancy and postpartum. *Br J Nutr* 2000;**84**(1):95–101.

70. Ehrenberg H M, Huston-Presley L & Catalano P M. The influence of obesity and gestational diabetes mellitus on accretion and the distribution of adipose tissue in pregnancy. *Am J Obstet Gynecol* 2003;**189**(4):944–8.

71. Jarvie E, Hauguel-de-Mouzon S, Nelson S M, *et al.* Lipotoxicity in obese pregnancy and its potential role in adverse pregnancy outcome and obesity in the offspring. *Clin Sci (Lond)* 2010;**119**(3):123–9.

72. Crozier S R, Inskip H M, Godfrey K M, *et al.* Weight gain in pregnancy and childhood body composition: findings from the Southampton Women's Survey. *Am J Clin Nutr* 2010;**91**(6):1745–51.

73. Olson C, Strawderman M & Dennison B. Maternal weight gain during pregnancy and child weight at age 3 years. *Mat Child Health J* 2009;**13**(6):839–46.

74. Reynolds R M, Osmond C, Phillips D I W, *et al.* Maternal BMI, parity, and pregnancy weight gain: influences on offspring adiposity in young adulthood. *J Clin Endocrinol Metab* 2010;**95**(12):5365–9.

75. Stuebe A M, Forman M R & Michels K B. Maternal-recalled gestational weight gain, pre-pregnancy body mass index, and obesity in the daughter. *Int J Obes* 2009;**33**(7):743–52.

76. von Kries R, Ensenauer R, Beyerlein A, *et al.* Gestational weight gain and overweight in children: results from the cross-sectional German KiGGS study. *Int J Pediatr Obes* 2010;**6**(1):45–52.

77. Schack-Nielsen L, Michaelsen K F, Gamborg M, *et al.* Gestational weight gain in relation to offspring body mass index and obesity from infancy through adulthood. *Int J Obes* 2009;**34**(1):67–74.

78. Koupil I & Toivanen P. Social and early-life determinants of overweight and obesity in 18-year-old Swedish men. *Int J Obes* 2007;**32**(1):73–81.

10 Influences of maternal obesity on the health of the offspring: a review of animal models

Lucilla Poston, Paul D. Taylor, and Peter Nathanielsz

Introduction

The prevalence of obesity among women worldwide (Figure 1.1; Chapter 1) is a cause for serious concern, not only for the mother's health but also that of her children, whether a result of the immediate risk of complications in pregnancy or from more subtle influences on the developing child (Chapters 9, 11, 12, and 13). In this chapter we provide a summary of the role that animal models have played in contributing to our understanding of potential influences of maternal obesity on offspring health in later life.

As described in Chapter 9, many observational studies in mother/child cohorts have reported an independent association between maternal BMI and offspring BMI in childhood and adulthood [1,2], but the expected predominance of maternal obesity vs. paternal obesity in parent–child obesity relationships is not always apparent [3,4]. Alternative explanations for mother–child associations of obesity are that the child inherits obesogenic genes or that they share similar postnatal environments. There is also some suggestion that maternal obesity is associated with the risk of elevated blood pressure and cardiovascular disease in childhood and beyond, but this is limited to a few reports [5–8]. Intervention studies in obese women before or during pregnancy, with follow-up of the children, are likely to provide the strongest test of the hypothesis that obesity per se causes adverse offspring outcomes. Observational studies of siblings whose mothers achieved weight loss through bariatric surgery certainly provide some support; the sibling born to the mother before surgery is more at risk of obesity than the brother or sister born after maternal weight loss [9]. However, randomized controlled trials of interventions have yet to report and in the meantime the theory that obesity in the pregnant woman directly increases the risk of obesity and related disorders through influences on the unborn child remains to be proven.

Studies in experimental animals have the potential to address relationships between obesity in mother and child while circumventing residual confounding in human cohort studies. Also, since animals age more rapidly than man, the life course from embryo to aged adult is amenable to study in the context of the developmental programming of obesity. Thus the potential influence of maternal obesity on the risk of adulthood disorders is readily testable in animal models. Other practical challenges besetting studies of pregnant women, such as accurate determination of adiposity, controlling for diet, physical activity, and other familial environmental factors, accounting for genetic variability, are all controllable in animal experiments, and protocols can include a more intensive schedule of repeated measurements through the life course. There are potential disadvantages too. Rodents, the most commonly used species, are altricial species, giving birth to several immature pups, which constitute a much larger nutritional demand on the mother than monotocous species. Rodents also deliver at a much earlier stage of development than the human newborn infant. The role of the placenta in nutrient transfer potentially plays an important role, and placental structure and function may vary between species. Placentation shows remarkable heterogeneity from one animal species to another. Some large mammals, e.g., ruminants, show marked structural differences from the hemochorial placenta of the human, mouse, or guinea pig in which maternal blood is in direct contact with the chorion. Larger mammals, such as sheep and non-human primates, deliver more mature offspring with greater relevance to the human, but these species also present practical

Maternal Obesity, ed. Matthew W. Gillman and Lucilla Poston. Published by Cambridge University Press. © Cambridge University Press 2012.

problems for the investigator. For example, practical advantages gained from using larger mammals are offset somewhat by slower maturation to puberty and adulthood, and far greater research costs. It is also important that the relevance to the human condition in animal models is addressed in regard to the dietary composition used to generate obesity and in the avoidance of extremes with little relevance to habitual diets in pregnant women. Based on the premise that biological processes among mammalian species generally observe conservancy of mechanism, here we address the commonalities, and a few dissimilarities, among reports from the different species employed in studying influences of maternal obesity, thereby providing insight into processes likely shared between all mammalian species, including the human.

Species and protocols employed to address long-term influences of maternal obesity on the offspring

The majority of laboratories interested in addressing transgenerational influences of maternal obesity use rodents, generally rats and mice, which grow to maturity in a few months [10–12]. Maternal obesity has been induced by prolonged feeding prior to pregnancy of a purified high-fat diet in which carbohydrates are replaced by fat, or by providing a diet rich in fats with specified addition of sugars, or a "cafeteria diet" of a mix of palatable fat- and sugar-rich foods of unspecified composition [13,14]. Rodents fed on a hypercaloric diet rich in fat tend to reduce their food intake toward the daily caloric requirement, and prolonged fat feeding over several months is required to achieve any increase in fat mass. The addition of simple sugars to a high-fat diet appears to overcome this tight homeostatic control of food intake to affect a more rapid shift toward a positive energy balance [15]. Drawing a parallel with maternal obesity in pregnant women, maternal hyperinsulinemia and glucose intolerance have been reported in rodents as a result of the animals being fed hypercaloric diets, e.g., a fat-rich diet [16,17], a high-fat, high-sugar diet [15,18], or a "cafeteria-style" diet of calorie-rich foods [19,20]. Insulin resistance has also been unequivocally demonstrated by the method of euglycemic hyperinsulinemic clamp in pregnant rats fed a high-calorie diet [19]. Others have reported more modest effects on maternal glucose homeostasis, most likely due to variations in dietary protocol [14].

The influences of maternal dietary caloric excess on the offspring have also been explored, although less frequently, in sheep and in non-human primates. These studies are particularly valuable to enable comparisons between precocial, monotocous species that may more closely resemble human development and the altricial polytocous species more commonly studied. One approach is to evaluate the short-term effects of overfeeding pregnant ewes in the last month of pregnancy until delivery, which has analogy to rapid gestational weight gain in pregnant women [21]. Other studies have aimed to model preconceptual obesity in pregnancy by overfeeding ewes (150% of normal requirements) two months before pregnancy, and until weaning [22], which leads to increased body weight gain during pregnancy and maternal body mass and maternal insulin resistance. Others have achieved obesity by overfeeding ewes for five months until pregnancy is established and then transferring the "obesity" exposed embryos to a non-obese ewe to determine the influences of obesity in the periconceptual period [23]. This design avoids any independent influence of additional weight gain during pregnancy. Studies in non-human primates have investigated the offspring of Japanese macaques that had been fed a fat-rich diet for two to four years (32% of calories from fat whereas controls received 13% from fat) [24]. Some female macaques show resistance to the development of obesity, whereas others become obese on this dietary regime. Understanding the mechanism of this interesting resistance to diet-induced obesity would itself be very valuable. In this macaque model, as well as in obese pregnant baboons, which develop pre-pregnancy adiposity and high circulating triglycerides on a diet providing 45% energy from fat (controls 12%), fetuses showed an approximately 15% birthweight reduction at term compared to offspring of control-fed mothers, which contrasts to the development of macrosomia, predominant among obese pregnant women [25].

The role of the placenta in obese pregnancies

The placenta is the gateway for access of nutrients, metabolites such as hormones, and xenobiotics passing from mother to fetus. As such it is an appropriate starting point in the evaluation of the effects of the maternal uterine environment on the fetus. There have been few studies addressing the impact of maternal obesity on maternal plasma concentrations and flow of both micro- and macronutrients across the placenta to the fetus. Obesity in pregnant women is frequently associated with macrosomia, but we have also reported, using customized birthweight centiles, a high incidence of fetal growth restriction among nulliparous obese pregnant women, which was not entirely explicable by preterm delivery [26]. A recent meta-analysis of women of all parities reported a higher than normal risk of very low birthweight (<1.5 kg) in overweight and obese women [27]. In this analysis this was apparently explicable by a higher incidence of preterm delivery including induced preterm delivery, which may reflect the increased incidence of pre-eclampsia in obese pregnancy.

Diet-induced obesity in the ewe is accompanied by enhanced mRNA expression and protein content of placental fatty acid transfer proteins in mid-gestation, with associated neonatal adiposity [22,28]. However, maternal obesity also heightens the placental inflammatory response in obese ewes at mid-gestation, possibly as a result of increased toll-like receptor 4 (TLR4) expression and free fatty acids [29]. Frias *et al.* [30] have recently reported the influence of maternal fat feeding on placental function in Japanese macaques, which, as mentioned above, resulted in fetal growth restriction. The maternal uterine blood flow volume was reduced, and similarly to the sheep, maternal consumption of the calorie-rich diet increased placental inflammatory cytokines and the expression of TLR4. There was also a reduction in blood flow on the fetal side of the placenta and an increase in frequency of both placental infarctions and stillbirth [30].

Spontaneously obese pregnant baboons show evidence of fetal growth restriction and decreased placental amino acid transport indicating a potential mechanism for the decrease in fetal growth [31]. When healthy female baboons of similar body weight are randomly allocated to a diet of 45% energy from fat compared with the normal control diet of 12% energy from fat for at least nine months prior to and during pregnancy, they exhibit an increase in maternal body fat and triglycerides at term. Fetal methionine and vitamin B_{12}, essential components of the one carbon methylation cycle were reduced, indicating reduced transplacental passage. Fetal and maternal homocysteine are increased indicating dysregulation of the one carbon cycle – a condition that would result in altered methylation status. Interestingly maternal and fetal folate are both increased indicating a folate trap that has been described in other situations [33]. In a

mouse model, however, a maternal high-fat diet (32% energy from fat) results in upregulated placental transport of glucose and neutral amino acids. The outcome is fetal overgrowth compared with fetuses of mothers fed a diet of 11% energy from fat fed for eight weeks before mating and throughout gestation and studied at embryonic day 18.5 [32].

In summary, there is clear evidence for altered placental transfer of key metabolites from mother to fetus in both altricial rodents and precocial animals in the setting of maternal obesity. Differences and similarities exist and demonstrate the need for comparisons between different animal models of obesity.

Phenotypic characteristics of the offspring of obese mothers

Adiposity

Overfeeding during pregnancy and lactation is associated with variable effects on placental and pup weight. Rodent pups born to dams overfed before pregnancy and during pregnancy and the lactation period, do not invariably have a higher birthweight than controls but are generally heavier at weaning if the calorie-enriched diet is fed to the dams over the lactation period as well as during gestation [11]. One group, which attempted to differentiate the effects of pre-pregnancy diet-induced obesity from gestational weight gain reported that pre-pregnancy obesity was associated with lower birthweight, whereas weight gain in pregnancy was associated with increased birthweight [14,34]. The majority of studies have shown that despite being reared on a normal chow diet, the adult offspring of obese dams become heavier than those born to lean dams and that this increase in weight is related to greater adiposity, as directly measured by dual energy X-ray absorptiometry (DXA, previously DEXA) or by weighing of the fat depots ex vivo [17,35–40]. Very few of the animal studies have attempted to define the relative roles of pre-pregnancy obesity and excessive gestational weight gain on the development of adiposity in the offspring, which would have direct relevance to human pregnancy (see Chapter 9). Separating the two, however, introduces a practical challenge in some species, particularly in rodents where a sudden change in diet early in pregnancy to induce rapid gestational weight gain (GWG) may lead to stress and activation of the HPA axis, which may have independent "programming effects." Nevertheless, in the maternal cafeteria model in rats, Langley-Evans *et al.* have reported that the development of adiposity in offspring was most dependent on the pre-pregnancy diet and weight gain rather than GWG [14,34]. The transgenerational (F_0–F_1) transmission of obesity in rodents would thus seem reproducible and occurs in different strains of mice and rats, despite the diverse dietary protocols. This heterogeneity of food composition might suggest that obesity per se rather than elements of the diet is responsible. Distinguishing between the relative influence of maternal obesity and the composition of the obesogenic diet also represents a practical challenge in study design, although in one report "pair feeding" dams on an obesogenic diet to control dam calorie intake led to normalization of fat mass in the offspring, suggesting that maternal obesity is the critical determinant [41]. However, others have suggested that the saturated fat content of the maternal diet may make a contribution [42], with reports that the profile of the unsaturated fatty acids in the maternal diet can influence adiposity in the offspring [43,44].

In rodent offspring, the postnatal period is likely to be one of particular vulnerability to the effects of maternal overnutrition and consequent influences on milk composition. This conclusion was first implied from studies over five decades ago in which a greater fat mass develops as a consequence of the offspring being reared in a smaller than normal litter, when each pup receives a greater share of milk than it would if suckled in a standard size litter [45]. Similarly, overnutrition in the suckling period can also be induced when rat pups are artificially fed a high-carbohydrate diet in early postnatal life (the "pup in a cup" model) and they too develop obesity in adulthood [46]. As a note of caution, these observations may not be readily translatable to early postnatal life in the human infant since rodent pups are delivered at an earlier, less well-developed stage of development. In the infants of obese women, these observations from models of overnutrition in the suckling rat may have greater relevance to the nutritionally enriched environment experienced by the fetus in the third trimester of pregnancy.

Maternal overnutrition similarly induces adiposity in the offspring of larger species including non-human primates. Japanese macaques born to fat-fed mothers, which are underweight at birth, display rapid postnatal growth and develop increased adiposity so that, by six months of age, they are heavier than offspring of normally fed mothers [24]. However, in this species, the offspring phenotype appeared to be unrelated to maternal obesity, but rather to the fat composition of the diet as a proportion of dams that consumed the fat-rich diet were resistant to diet-induced weight gain and the influences on the offspring were independent of weight gain in the mother.

In the sheep model, obese and control ewes increased body weight by 43% and 6%, respectively, from diet initiation (60 days prior to breeding) until mid-pregnancy [47]. Lambs of obese ewes developed greater fat mass [47] but by 19.5 months of age, while body weight and percentage of body fat were similar between groups, insulin sensitivity was reduced in lambs of obese mothers [22]. However, when subjected to a 12-week *ad libitum* feeding challenge at this age, these animals demonstrated an increased appetite, became fatter than controls, and demonstrated elevated plasma leptin and fasted plasma glucose and insulin [22]. Four-month-old lambs, which had developed from embryos only "exposed" to maternal obesity in early pregnancy and then transferred to a lean dam, also develop increased adiposity in later life when compared to controls in which embryo transfer was from a lean dam to another lean dam [23]. These findings imply an influence of maternal obesity at the time of conception, independent of any effect of maternal body fat mass in pregnancy.

None of the models described demonstrate a "perfect match" for obesity in human pregnancy but important characteristics are shared, notably a uniform predisposition to maternal insulin resistance. There is also marked conformity among all species for development of greater adiposity in the offspring. Distinction between predominant influences of the maternal hypercaloric diet, which in most species leads to obesity, or of the increased maternal fat mass per se, remains unresolved and experimentally has proven difficult to unravel. Another area that requires further investigation in animal models is the relationship between maternal overnutrition and fat mass and the milk quality. We (PT and LP) and others have previously reported in rodents that maternal diet-induced obesity in pregnancy and suckling can lead to profound changes in the lipid profile and hormonal content of the milk [15,48,49], which may be critical to the normal development of central pathways of energy balance as discussed below.

Energy intake

In general, the young offspring of obese or fat-fed rodents consume the same amount of food daily as controls, although marked hyperphagia has also been reported [50,51]. In contrast, in adulthood, energy intake is usually higher than that observed in the progeny of lean dams. In other words, a high-level nutritional state in early life either in the in utero or early postpartum periods leads to persistent hyperphagia [15,18,41,50,52]. A similar observation has been made in sheep; when allowed *ad libitum* access to food, 19-month-old offspring of obese ewes consume 10% more food compared to offspring of lean controls [22]. Increased energy intake arising from in utero exposure to nutritional excess therefore provides one explanation for the development of greater adiposity. In rodents, the early postnatal period appears critical as hyperphagia can also be induced by enriching the nutritional plane by rearing pups in small litters [53]. Another potential mechanism leading to obesity is through changes in the central pathways associated with dietary preference and reward, which may lead to passive overconsumption of energy-rich foods. Several investigators have reported a preference for fatty or sugary foods in offspring of rat dams fed a "junk food diet" [35,54] or a fat-rich diet [55], and Sullivan *et al.* recently reported preliminary evidence for a similar food preference in the offspring of the fat-fed Japanese macaque [12]. These studies imply a common period of developmental plasticity in the central pathways of energy balance, which is associated with hypersensitivity to the environmental influences of maternal nutritional excess. Eventually, it would seem that persistent changes in function lead to a state of energy imbalance in the adult offspring.

Translating to the human condition, a unique investigation of a large mother/partner/child cohort (approximately 4000 triads) has recently reported that preference for protein, carbohydrates, and fats seems to be programmed by maternal food intake in pregnancy. Here it was observed that prenatal, but not postnatal, maternal fat intake was associated with fat (and protein) preference in the child [56] although maternal diet during pregnancy was not associated with offspring adiposity or lean mass. The stronger prenatal maternal associations with child dietary intake compared with both paternal and maternal postnatal intake provides some of the first evidence for in utero programming of offspring appetite by maternal intake during pregnancy.

In summary, the animal models show conformity across species in the observation that maternal obesity in utero, and/or during the lactation period, can persistently influence pathways of satiety and food preference in the developing offspring, leading to the predisposition to obesity observed. Aside from the one investigation mentioned above [56], this relationship between maternal diet/obesity and childhood appetite, satiety, and food preference has hitherto seldom been addressed in mother/child cohorts although these studies provide a good rationale for further studies addressing the observations arising from the animal models. Investigation of effects on programming of offspring exercise preferences and metabolic rate would also be of considerable value in determining overall mechanisms that predispose to obesity.

Central pathways of energy balance and dietary preference/reward

The influences of maternal obesity on appetite in the offspring led to a focus on possible mechanistic pathways, notably the hypothalamic networks, which control satiety. The hypothalamus plays a central role in homeostatic pathways of energy balance and is the obvious focus of investigation when probing the origins of offspring hyperphagia. Figure 10.1 shows how the hypothalamus acts as a central coordinating center, integrating afferent signals that provide information on peripheral energy status and sending efferent messages to appropriately modify food intake and energy expenditure. As reviewed in Chapter 11, the intricacies of the neural networks within and between the hypothalamic nuclei are remarkable, and contribute not only to energy balance but also to the many other functions of this complex organ [57–59]. Leptin and insulin not only suppress appetite but also affect long-term energy homeostasis via regionally distinct neuronal pathways to increase energy expenditure via sympathetic stimulation to the metabolically active tissues, notably brown adipose tissue [60]. As discussed in detail in the next chapter (Chapter 11), there is marked agreement from the different models of maternal dietary calorie excess for altered hypothalamic gene expression in the offspring and as recently reviewed [11] these have generally been associated with altered signaling in anorexigenic and orexigenic pathways in a direction that would increase appetite. Figure 10.2 illustrates the hypothalamic regions that have been implicated and their neural connections with afferent and efferent signaling pathways. In one of our laboratories (PT and LP) we have reported that 30-day-old pups of obese dams show evidence for altered neural projections between

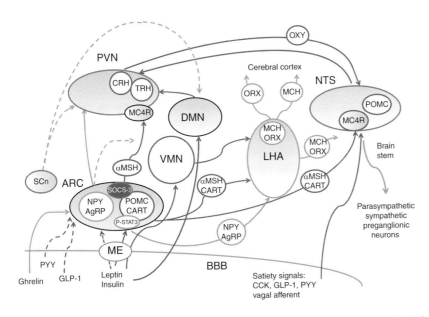

Figure 10.1. Energy balance and hypothalamic regulation. The arcuate nucleus (ARC) is located in the hypothalamus, close to the median eminence (ME) where the blood–brain barrier (BBB) is incomplete allowing blood-borne signals to reach ARC neurons. Leptin, insulin, and ghrelin are the most important hormonal satiety signals and are also actively transported across the BBB where they activate anorexigenic neurons co-expressing alpha melanocyte-stimulating hormone (αMSH) and cocaine- and amphetamine-regulated transcript (CART); and inhibit orexigenic neurons co-expressing agouti-related protein and neuropeptide Y (AgRP and NPY). Both populations of neurons project widely throughout the brain. CART is also expressed in the paraventricular hypothalamic nucleus (PVN) and lateral hypothalamic area (LHA). αMSH is cleaved from the precusor polypeptide pro-opiomelanocortin (POMC) along with other peptides such as B-endorphin and ACTH. The ARC integrates this information together with inputs from brain stem areas and signals other hypothalamic nuclei such as the ventromedial hypothalamic nucleus (VMN), dorsomedial hypothalamic nucleus (DMH), and PVN, to reduce food intake (pathways shown in red). Signals from the ARC to the PVN and the LHA also increase feeding (shown in green). Divergent projections from the orexin-containing neurons (ORX) and melanin-concentrating hormone (MCH) neurons in the LHA, ascend to the cerebral cortex and descend to the brain stem and spinal cord. Oxytocin-containing neurons (OXY) of the PVN innervate vagal preganglionic parasympathetic neurons involved in gastrointestinal control. Hormones from the gastrointestinal tract including cholecystokinin (CCK) and glucagon-like peptide (GLP-1) modulate these processes through shorter term changes in satiety and hunger. Inputs from the suprachiasmatic nucleus to the PVN and DMN also regulate diurnal feeding patterns. The three possible outputs from the hypothalamus that regulate food intake and energy expenditure are: activation of motor neurons via the brain stem; activation of neuroendocrine neurons in the PVN that secrete corticotrophin-releasing hormone (CRH) and thyrotropin-releasing hormone (TRH) to activate the pituitary axes (e.g., hypothalamic–pituitary–adrenal and hypothalamic–pituitary–thyroid axis activation result in secretion of glucocorticoids and thyroid hormone); autonomic nervous system both sympathetic and parasympathetic, e.g., influencing heart rate and thermogenesis in metabolically active tissues. (See figure in color plate section.)

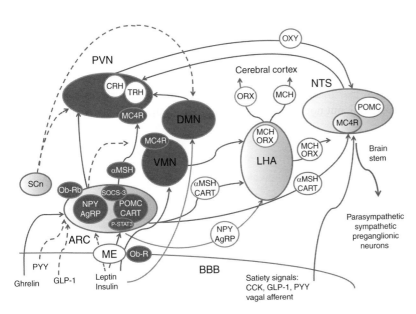

Figure 10.2. Developmental programming of hypothalamic regulation. Areas in red indicate sites susceptible to developmental programming by maternal obesity or neonatal overnutrition. Perhaps not surprisingly those areas most vulnerable to developmental programming lie close to the median eminence (ME) where the blood–brain barrier (BBB) is incomplete allowing blood-borne signals such as leptin to penetrate. Abbreviations as given for Figure 10.1. (See figure in color plate section.)

the arcuate nucleus (ARC) and paraventricular nucleus (PVN) as assessed by immunohistochemical staining of Agouti-related peptide (AgRP)-expressing neurons in the PVN [50], a phenomenon previously reported in adult rats with a genetic predisposition to diet-induced obesity [61]. As discussed in the following chapter, offspring of obese dams show both a behavioral and cell-signaling leptin resistance in the ARC after stimulation with exogenous leptin. Thus the young offspring of obese dams are leptin resistant, and remain leptin resistant and hyperphagic as adults when they also develop obesity [50]. Others have shown gene expression for the MC4 receptor to be upregulated in the ventromedial nucleus (VMN) and that for the leptin receptor (ObR) to be downregulated in the ARC in juvenile obesity-prone rats born to obese mothers, both of which would predispose to increased energy intake [62]. In common with offspring of obese dams, and in accord with a critical window of developmental plasticity in the postnatal period in rodents, several studies have highlighted an important role for postnatal overfeeding in rodents in the "programming" of hypothalamic circuits of energy balance [63,64].

At term, fetuses of obese baboons show evidence of decreased pituitary leptin receptors suggesting that decreased leptin sensitivity may also play a role in the altered development of the non-human primate fetus in the setting of maternal obesity [25]. The fetal

hypothalamus has also been the focus of attention in the Japanese macaque model. When the mothers are fed a high-fat diet, fetuses studied in the final third of pregnancy showed upregulation of pro-opiomelanocortin (POMC) expression and downregulation of AgRP, with an associated increase in pro-inflammatory cytokines and markers of inflammation in the microglia. These abnormalities in the POMC pathway reverse if the mothers' dietary fat intake reverted to normal [65]. Should these abnormalities persist beyond fetal life, as demonstrated in rodents, these aberrant pathways of hypothalamic function may contribute to the increased adiposity of the offspring.

Two recent investigations have probed central mechanisms that could underlie the changes in food preference in the offspring of rat dams fed a fat-rich diet [55] or a "junk food" diet [54] by investigating expression of genes contributing to the central mesolimbic reward pathways (Figure 10.3). In adult offspring of fat-fed dams, which showed a greater preference for sucrose and fat, Vucetic et al. observed an increase in mRNA expression for the dopamine re-uptake transporter (DAT) in the ventral tegmental area, the nucleus accumbens, and the prefrontal cortex [55]. Furthermore, expression of both the μ-opiod receptor and preproenkephalin were increased in the nucleus accumbens, prefrontal cortex, and hypothalamus. Importantly, these authors also showed that

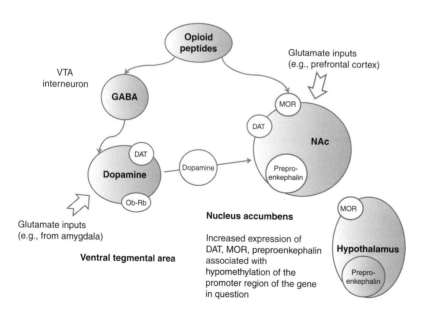

Figure 10.3. Mesolimbic reward pathway. The motivational aspects of feeding involve the dopamine (DA) projections from the ventral tegmental area (VTA) to the D2 receptor-expressing neurons in the nucleus accumbens (NAc). In adult offspring of fat-fed dams, which showed an increased preference for sucrose and fat, Vucetic et al. observed an increase in mRNA expression for the dopamine re-uptake transporter (DAT) in the ventral tegmental area, the nucleus accumbens, and the prefrontal cortex. Expression of both the μ-opiod receptor (MOR) and preproenkaphalin were increased in the nucleus accumbens, prefrontal cortex, and hypothalamus. Increased expression of DAT, MOR, and preproenkephalin was associated with hypomethylation of the promoter region of genes. VTA DA neurons also express receptors for leptin and knock-down of VTA leptin receptors leads to hyperphagia and increased appetite for palatable foods. Thus, central leptin resistance in offspring of obese mice could also lead to increased food intake through dopaminergic pathways.

increased DAT, μ-opiod receptor, and preproen-kephalin expression was associated with hypomethy-lation of the promoter region of each of these genes, thus offering a potential mechanism for persistently altered gene expression and altered food preference (see Chapter 13). Ong and Muhlhausler, in a similar study, demonstrated that DAT mRNA expression was higher than controls in the offspring of "junk food"-fed dams, which exhibited higher fat intake from weaning compared to offspring of lean dams. In contrast to the previous study, μ-opioid receptor mRNA expression was lower. The common observation of increased DAT expression would imply that there may be a reduction in the availability of the neurotransmitter dopamine at the synapse, which in turn may affect the appetitive drive. These observations provide strong evidence that perinatal exposure to calorie-rich diets results in altered development of the central reward system [54].

In summary, experimental work in rodents and non-human primates has strongly implicated hypothalamic pathways of energy balance in the development of obesity in the offspring of obese/fat-fed animals. In addition, studies in rodents suggest that the pathways that lead an animal to prefer high-calorie foods appear to be permanently activated.

The humoral link between maternal nutritional excess and modification of central pathways of energy balance

The hypothesis currently addressed by many experimenters in animal models of maternal overnutrition, is that a humoral influence resulting from maternal obesity leads to permanent changes in hypothalamic function during a critical period of developmental plasticity. Two hormones have been implicated, leptin and insulin, and in the non-human primate, an increased inflammatory response, involving cytokine-induced activation of the hypothalamic–pituitary–adrenal (HPA) axis [65].

Leptin has been identified as playing a major role in the normal development of the rodent hypothalamus in early postnatal life by Bouret and colleagues, and this fascinating discovery is elegantly reviewed by Bouret in Chapter 11. As might be anticipated, if leptin is key to the development of the hypothalamic neural circuitry, manipulation of neonatal leptin status might be expected to permanently alter hypothalamic function. Indeed, maternal dietary restriction in rodents

lowers neonatal leptin and this leads to persistent change in energy balance and an obese phenotype [66,67], and in neonates from semi-starved mothers leptin-replacement therapy during the critical period of hypothalamic development (postnatal day 3–13) rescues this obese phenotype [68]. However, the effect of leptin treatment is highly dependent on the nutritional state of the mother, and in normal animals neonatal leptin treatment can cause permanent leptin resistance [69] and promote the obese phenotype [66]. Hence any suggestion that leptin supplementation in formula feeds may be obesity-protective in infants, should be viewed with extreme caution.

Kirk et al. have reported a changed profile of the physiological neonatal leptin "surge" in the offspring of obese mice in which there was an exaggeration in the early increase in the pup's leptin concentration [50]. The leptin was hypothesized to originate in the adipose tissue of the pup, as there was an association with increased expression of the leptin (Ob) gene in adipose tissue over the same time course. Further studies from one of our laboratories (PT, LP) have shown that administration of leptin to the neonatal pups to mimic the surge leads to the development of leptin resistance and increased appetite in weanling animals and thence to adiposity in later life, supporting the hypothesis that leptin plays a permissive role in the generation of obesity [70]. A recent publication on the offspring of obese sheep reports a reduced and early postnatal leptin surge [71]. It remains to be demonstrated whether precocial species demonstrate a fetal leptin surge in addition to this postnatal surge that is similar to that seen in the rodent.

Maternal and neonatal hyperinsulinemia has been similarly implicated as a possible modulator of the developing offspring hypothalamus in animal models [72]. In studying the influences of maternal diabetes on the developing offspring using models of maternal diabetes, Plagemann and colleagues proposed that fetal hyerpinsulinemia may contribute to dysfunction of pathways critical to normal development of the neuronal hypothalamic networks central to energy balance, thus permanently increasing food intake and thereby contributing to adulthood obesity and insulin resistance [53]. This group had shown acquired malformations of the VMN in juvenile and adult offspring of diabetic dams (chemically-induced), as well as increased immunopositivity of the orexigenic peptides NPY and AgRP in the ARC, and decreased expression of the anorexigenic melanocyte-stimulating hormone (αMSH). Daily injection of insulin from days 8–11 postpartum led to increased weight and diabetes susceptibility in later life. Whether insulin plays an equally important role in the offspring of obese dams has yet to be formally assessed, but as we and others have shown the rat dams to be insulin resistant [19] a degree of neonatal hyperinsulinemia would be anticipated.

Energy expenditure

There are fewer reports on energy expenditure in offspring of obese dams. Reduced locomotor activity has been observed in the offspring of obese mice employing remote radiotelemetry [15] whereas others have reported increased locomotor activity to behavioral stimulants in offspring from dams fed a saturated fat diet [73]. Persistently altered mitochondrial function acquired early in life could influence energy balance [74] and abnormalities in mitochondrial function have been identified in skeletal muscle from offspring of obese dams, which may have widespread implications for energy homeostasis [75]. Further studies are clearly needed to properly address this "other half" of the energy balance equation.

Behavior

Behavioral traits other than those related to feeding and physical activity may be adversely affected by prenatal exposure to a fat-rich diet. In the offspring of fat-fed Japanese macaques, Sullivan *et al.* have observed perturbations in the serotonergic system of the brain associated with increased anxiety-like traits [12]. There is also a report that suggests maternal obesity impairs special learning performance in young mouse offspring [76]. Recently, we (PT, LP) have investigated "open field" responses to address locomotor and exploratory behavior in offspring of obese mice and have demonstrated evidence of hyperactivity traits compared to controls [77]. These two studies demonstrate potential commonalities.

Adipocyte development and function

As reviewed in Chapter 12, adipocyte function may be permanently affected by nutritional status in early life. In our laboratory (PT, LP) we have shown that adult offspring of obese mice demonstrate an increase in adipocyte size and increased mRNA expression of genes involved in adipocyte differentiation (beta-adrenoceptor 2 and 3, 11 β HSD1, and PPARγ 2) [15]. In a study in which pre-pregnancy maternal obesity was induced

by feeding female rats with a fat-rich diet from weaning to breeding 90 days later, and through pregnancy and lactation, male offspring showed increased fat mass, serum triglycerides, and leptin at 150 days of postnatal life associated with increased fat cell size [78]. Others report altered fat tissue expression of pro-adipogenic and lipogenic genes in offspring of obese rats (PPARγ, Pref-1, Wisp 2, SREBP1, AcCoA, FAS, FAT) [79]. These observations may imply that early life exposure to maternal obesity leads to continued expansion beyond neonatal life of the adipocyte precursor pool, which would contribute to the development of obesity in a situation of positive energy balance.

Metabolic dysfunction in offspring of obese animals

In common with several of the models of maternal diabetes, the offspring of obese rodents frequently develop insulin resistance, with some animals eventually becoming diabetic [15,17,18,40]. In the liver, altered expression of key components of the insulin-signaling pathway was observed in the offspring of obese mice. Expression of IRS-1 protein was decreased while phosphorylation of IRS-1 at Ser 307, an inhibitory signal of insulin action, was increased. Reduced liver IRS expression and hyper-phosphorylation of IRS serine residues are key factors in the development of insulin resistance and type 2 diabetes, and insulin resistance is an early defect in the pathogenesis of non-alcoholic fatty liver disease [48]. In 19.5-month-old offspring of obese sheep, when subjected to a 12-week ad lib feeding challenge at this age, the increased adiposity compared to controls was associated with elevated plasma leptin and fasted plasma glucose and insulin [22]. In 22-month-old offspring, skeletal muscle downstream insulin signaling was lower than in control lambs as shown by reduction in the phosphorylation of protein kinase B (AKT1), mammalian target of rapamycin (MTOR), and 4-E binding protein 1 (EIF4EBP1). More intramuscular adipocytes were observed in OB compared to Con offspring muscle, and the expression of peroxisome proliferator-activated receptor (PPAR) gamma (PPARγ), an adipocyte marker, was also higher, which was consistent with the higher intramuscular triglyceride content [80].

In rodents and in macaques, the developing liver seems highly susceptible to the influences of maternal high-fat feeding/obesity leading to a phenotype with marked similarity to non-alcoholic fatty liver disease in humans. In the fetal macaque in the third trimester, there is evidence that exposure to a maternal fat-rich diet leads to hepatic fat deposition, upregulation of gluconeogenic enzymes, and a three-fold increase in the hepatic triglyceride concentration with evidence of hepatic oxidative stress. These abnormalities were reversed when the mothers consumed a normal low-fat diet, but were not dependent on the development of obesity in the mothers, some of which remained lean. There was also preliminary evidence at postnatal day 180 for persistent elevation of liver triglycerides [24]. A recent study by Suter et al., detailed in Chapter 13, has implicated epigenetic modification in the etiology of altered gene expression and generation of the liver phenotype [81]. Adult offspring of obese mice also demonstrate markers of hepatic steatosis; Oben et al. have reported lipid deposition, an increase in triglycerides and markers of inflammation, as well as evidence for fibrosis [48]. These abnormalities were exaggerated in the offspring from normal dams cross-fostered to obese dams fed a fat- and sugar-rich diet, suggesting that nutrition in the postnatal period in rodents may be critical to development of this phenotype. In human pregnancy, as in the macaque, because of these different stages of development at birth, this may translate to a period of vulnerability in the third trimester. In another study, in which the dams were fed a high-fat diet alone, a similar adult offspring phenotype was observed and was exaggerated by a high-fat dietary challenge in adulthood [82]. Here, hepatic mitochondrial dysfunction was reported in tandem with markers of inflammation, increased lipogenesis, and oxidative stress. In summary, the developing liver in all species studied seems highly susceptible to the influences of maternal obesity and/or an obesogenic diet.

Cardiovascular function

Cardiovascular function of the progeny may also be compromised by maternal obesity. Several studies in mother–child cohorts have reported an association between maternal BMI or gestational weight gain and childhood blood pressure [6,8,83,84]. Investigation of the ovine maternal obesity model suggests early compromise of the developing cardiovascular system; fetal hearts develop an impaired heart-rate-left-ventricular-developed pressure product in response to high workload stress. Phosphorylation of AMP-activated protein kinase (AMPK), a cardioprotective-signaling pathway, was reduced while the stress-signaling pathway, p38

MAPK, was upregulated. Also, phosphorylation of c-Jun N-terminal kinase (JNK) and insulin receptor substrate-1 (IRS-1) at Ser 307 were increased, associated with lower downstream PI3K-Akt activity indicating impaired cardiac insulin signaling [85]. If these changes persist into adult life they would predispose offspring to insulin resistance and cardiac dysfunction. Cardiac development can also be compromised by increased fibrogenesis and the total collagen concentration was greater in the myocardium when compared to offspring of obese dams [86].

In rodents, adult offspring of diet-induced obese mice develop hypertension as demonstrated using the method of radio telemetry, which enables continuous measurement of blood pressure in conscious unrestrained animals [15]. In isolated resistance arteries studied in vitro using a myograph, endothelial dysfunction was observed in three-month-old animals. At this age the mice have increased adiposity compared to controls and this study could not distinguish between a primary defect in blood pressure or one secondary to increased adiposity. However, in the rat, a species in which it is technically possible to measure blood pressure in weanling animals, blood pressure was higher in offspring of obese dams than controls before the development of greater fat mass. Mean arterial blood pressure was also raised at 90 days of age, and by 180 days, and the hypertension was associated with a loss in diurnal variation. Young offspring of the obese dams also showed an enhanced pressor response to restraint stress, and supranormal renal noradrenaline content and renin mRNA expression. Since these findings were indicative of increased sympathetic outflow, spectral analysis of the blood pressure tracings was undertaken, which revealed increased low-frequency oscillations in 30- and 90-day-old offspring compared to controls, indicative of increased sympathetic tone. There was also evidence of altered baroreceptor sensitivity as assessed by recording pressor and dilatory responses to noradrenaline and sodium nitroprusside, respectively [69]. These observations suggest the hypertension in the offspring of the obese dams is of sympathetic origin. Since central sympathetic efferents have origins in the hypothalamus and the brain stem and leptin increases blood pressure by increasing central efferent sympathetic tone, this elevation in blood pressure may arise from perturbation of central leptin sensitivity in early life. The young offspring of obese rats demonstrated an enhanced pressor response to leptin when compared to controls. However, they were less responsive to leptin-induced appetite suppression [69]. This apparent paradox of "selective leptin resistance" is similar to that observed in obese adult rodents and explicable on the basis that the cardiovascular and appetite regulatory actions of leptin may occur in different hypothalamic neurons [87]. To date, there has been no investigation of cardiovascular function in adult offspring of obese sheep or non-human primates.

The studies of cardiovascular function in animal models of maternal obesity have been largely confined to rodents, except for one study in the fetuses of obese ewes. Similar studies in non-human primates would be valuable in determining whether these observations were pertinent across species. Nonetheless, these reports have provided sufficient interest to prompt investigation of blood pressure and blood pressure variability in the children of obese mothers in several ongoing mother–child cohort studies.

Interventions to improve outcomes in offspring of obese animals: informing strategies for human pregnancy?

The alarming rise in obesity among pregnant women worldwide has prompted the need to develop effective interventions to improve pregnancy outcome, and potentially to reduce the longer term adverse outcomes in the offspring; as reviewed in Chapter 14 and a recent review [88], there is as yet no effective intervention.

While the influences of leptin and insulin on the developing brain are likely to be of importance in the later stages of development, some evidence suggests that the unwanted offspring outcomes resulting from exposure to maternal obesity and accompanying high-energy obesogenic diets prior to and during pregnancy, may result from periconceptional influences. It is thus important to evaluate the ability of altered dietary intake and energy expenditure commencing before conception to improve outcomes. In a model of pre-pregnancy maternal obesity resulting from feeding female rats with a high-fat diet from weaning and through pregnancy and lactation, transferring the mothers to normal chow for one month before mating partially reversed the increased body fat and fat cell size seen in male adult offspring [78]. Others have shown that pair feeding fat-fed dams throughout pregnancy to the same caloric dietary intake as controls successfully prevents development of the offspring adult phenotype [41]. A second approach has involved feeding antioxidants to dams fed a diet rich in saturated

fat. In common with a previous study Igosheva *et al.* [89] reported evidence of oxidative stress in preimplantation embryos, and also in fetuses, and newborns of Western diet-fed rats. The addition of an antioxidant supplement to the maternal diet decreased adiposity and normalized glucose tolerance leading the authors to conclude that inflammation and oxidative stress appear to play key roles in the development of increased adiposity in the offspring of the Western diet-fed pregnant dam and that restoration of the antioxidant balance during pregnancy in the Western diet-fed dam is associated with decreased adiposity in offspring [79].

Given the potential role of leptin and insulin in the development of the offspring phenotype, further studies are required in which protocols specifically address interventions to reduce fat mass and improve glucose homeostasis.

Summary

This chapter highlights the substantial and compelling evidence from animal models to support the hypothesis that maternal obesity in pregnancy may have deleterious influences on the offspring. Animal models that enable detailed scrutiny of the different stages of development and investigation of cellular pathways have identified potentially important mechanistic pathways, notably the plasticity of the central mechanisms of energy balance and reward, which provide an entirely novel approach to the developmental origins of obesity. They have also highlighted the vulnerability of the developing liver and cardiovascular system. Nevertheless, while it is necessary to undertake a variety of different dietary challenges to reflect the complexity of the human situation there remains a need for some standardization of protocols between laboratories to demonstrate reproducibility of phenotype in the offspring. The future will also inevitably lead to better understanding of the interaction between the genes and the environment, for which these models are eminently suitable.

References

1. Salsberry P J & Reagan P B. Dynamics of early childhood overweight. *Pediatrics* 2005;**116(6)**:1329–38.

2. Whitaker R C. Predicting preschooler obesity at birth: the role of maternal obesity in early pregnancy. *Pediatrics* 2004;**114(1)**:e29–36.

3. Lawlor D A, Timpson N J, Harbord R M, *et al.* Exploring the developmental overnutrition hypothesis

using parental-offspring associations and FTO as an instrumental variable. *PLoS Med* 2008;**5**(3):e33.

4. Patel R, Martin R M, Kramer M S, *et al.* Familial associations of adiposity: findings from a cross-sectional study of 12,181 parental-offspring trios from Belarus. *PLoS One.* 2011;**6**(1):e14607.

5. Forsen T, Eriksson J G, Tuomilehto J, *et al.* Mother's weight in pregnancy and coronary heart disease in a cohort of Finnish men: follow up study. *BMJ* 1997;**315**(7112):837–40.

6. Boney C M, Verma A, Tucker R & Vohr B R. Metabolic syndrome in childhood: association with birth weight, maternal obesity, and gestational diabetes mellitus. *Pediatrics* 2005;**115**(3):e290–6.

7. Lawlor D A, Najman J M, Sterne J, *et al.* Associations of parental, birth, and early life characteristics with systolic blood pressure at 5 years of age: findings from the Mater-University study of pregnancy and its outcomes. *Circulation* 2004;**110**(16):2417–23.

8. Mamun A A, O'Callaghan M, Callaway L, *et al.* Associations of gestational weight gain with offspring body mass index and blood pressure at 21 years of age: evidence from a birth cohort study. *Circulation* 2009;**119**(13):1720–7.

9. Smith J, Cianflone K, Biron S, *et al.* Effects of maternal surgical weight loss in mothers on intergenerational transmission of obesity. *J Clin Endocrinol Metab* 2009;**94**(11):4275–83.

10. Armitage J A, Khan I Y, Taylor P D, Nathanielsz P W & Poston L. Developmental programming of the metabolic syndrome by maternal nutritional imbalance: how strong is the evidence from experimental models in mammals? *J Physiol* 2004;**561**(Pt 2):355–77.

11. Remmers F & Delemarre-van de Waal H A. Developmental programming of energy balance and its hypothalamic regulation. *Endocr Rev* 2011;**32**(2):272–311.

12. Sullivan E L, Smith M S & Grove K L. Perinatal exposure to high-fat diet programs energy balance, metabolism and behavior in adulthood. *Neuroendocrinology* 2011;**93**(1):1–8.

13. Bayol S A, Simbi B H & Stickland N C. A maternal cafeteria diet during gestation and lactation promotes adiposity and impairs skeletal muscle development and metabolism in rat offspring at weaning. *J Physiol* 2005;**567**(3):951–61.

14. Akyol A, Langley-Evans S C & McMullen S. Obesity induced by cafeteria feeding and pregnancy outcome in the rat. *Br J Nutr* 2009;**102**(11):1601–10.

15. Samuelsson A M, Matthews P A, Argenton M, *et al.* Diet-induced obesity in female mice leads to offspring hyperphagia, adiposity, hypertension, and insulin resistance: a novel murine model of developmental programming. *Hypertension* 2008;**51**(2):383–92.

16. Taylor P D, Khan I Y, Lakasing L, *et al.* Uterine artery function in pregnant rats fed a diet supplemented with animal lard. *Exp Physiol* 2003;**88**(3):389–98.

17. Srinivasan M, Katewa S D, Palaniyappan A, Pandya J D & Patel M S. Maternal high-fat diet consumption results in fetal malprogramming predisposing to the onset of metabolic syndrome-like phenotype in adulthood. *Am J Physiol Endocrinol Metab* 2006;**291**(4):e792–9.

18. Nivoit P, Morens C, Van Assche F A, *et al.* Established diet-induced obesity in female rats leads to offspring hyperphagia, adiposity and insulin resistance. *Diabetologia* 2009;**52**(6):1133–42.

19. Holemans K, Caluwaerts S, Poston L & Van Assche F A. Diet-induced obesity in the rat: a model for gestational diabetes mellitus. *Am J Obstet Gynecol.* 2004;**190**(3):858–65.

20. Chen H, Simar D, Lambert K, Mercier J & Morris M J. Maternal and postnatal overnutrition differentially impact appetite regulators and fuel metabolism. *Endocrinology* 2008;**149**(11):5348–56.

21. Muhlhausler B S, Duffield J A & McMillen I C. Increased maternal nutrition increases leptin expression in perirenal and subcutaneous adipose tissue in the postnatal lamb. *Endocrinology* 2007;**148**(12):6157–63.

22. Long N M, George L A, Uthlaut A B, *et al.* Maternal obesity and increased nutrient intake before and during gestation in the ewe results in altered growth, adiposity, and glucose tolerance in adult offspring. *J Anim Sci* 2010;**88**(11):3546–53.

23. Rattanatray L, MacLaughlin S M, Kleemann D O, *et al.* Impact of maternal periconceptional overnutrition on fat mass and expression of adipogenic and lipogenic genes in visceral and subcutaneous fat depots in the postnatal lamb. *Endocrinology* 2010;**151**(11):5195–205.

24. McCurdy C E, Bishop J M, Williams S M, *et al.* Maternal high-fat diet triggers lipotoxicity in the fetal livers of nonhuman primates. *J Clin Invest* 2009;**119**(2):323–35.

25. Li C, Xie L, Choi J, *et al.* Fetal baboon pituitary leptin and leptin receptor (Ob-R) are both down regulated by maternal nutrient excess (MN). *Reproductive Sciences* 2011;**18**:165A.

26. Rajasingam D, Seed P T, Briley A L, Shennan A H, Poston L. A prospective study of pregnancy outcome and biomarkers of oxidative stress in nulliparous obese women. *Am J Obstet Gynecol* 2009;**200**(4):395e1–9.

27. McDonald S D, Han Z, Mulla S & Beyene J. Overweight and obesity in mothers and risk of preterm birth and low birth weight infants: systematic review and meta-analyses. *BMJ* 2010;**341**:c3428.

28. Ma Y, Zhu M J, Uthlaut A B, *et al.* Upregulation of growth signaling and nutrient transporters in cotyledons of early to mid-gestational nutrient restricted ewes. *Placenta* 2010;**31**(5):387–91.

29. Zhu M J, Du M, Nathanielsz P W & Ford S P. Maternal obesity up-regulates inflammatory signaling pathways and enhances cytokine expression in the mid-gestation sheep placenta. *Placenta* 2011;**32**(3):255–63.

30. Frias A E, Morgan T K, Evans A E, *et al.* Maternal high-fat diet disturbs uteroplacental hemodynamics and increases the frequency of stillbirth in a nonhuman primate model of excess nutrition. *Endocrinology* 2011;**152**(6):2456–64.

31. Farley D, Tejero M E, Comuzzie A G, *et al.* Feto-placental adaptations to maternal obesity in the baboon. *Placenta* 2009;**30**(9):752–60.

32. Jones H N, Woollett L A, Barbour N, *et al.* High-fat diet before and during pregnancy causes marked up-regulation of placental nutrient transport and fetal overgrowth in C57/BL6 mice. *FASEB J* 2009;**23**(1):271–8.

33. Nathanielsz P W, Wu G, Ford S P, *et al.* Dysregulation of one carbon cycle (1CC) metabolites by maternal nutrient excess (MNE) in baboon pregnancy. *Reprod Sci* 2011;**18**(3 Suppl):334A

34. Akyol A, McMullen S & Langley-Evans S C. Glucose intolerance associated with early-life exposure to maternal cafeteria feeding is dependent upon post-weaning diet. *Br J Nutr* 2011:1–15.

35. Bayol S A, Farrington S J & Stickland N C. A maternal 'junk food' diet in pregnancy and lactation promotes an exacerbated taste for 'junk food' and a greater propensity for obesity in rat offspring. *Br J Nutr* 2007;**98**(4):843–51.

36. Chang G Q, Gaysinskaya V, Karatayev O & Leibowitz S F. Maternal high-fat diet and fetal programming: increased proliferation of hypothalamic peptide-producing neurons that increase risk for overeating and obesity. *J Neurosci* 2008;**28**(46):12107–19.

37. Dunn G A & Bale T L. Maternal high-fat diet promotes body length increases and insulin insensitivity in second-generation mice. *Endocrinology* 2009;**150**(11):4999–5009.

38. Ferezou-Viala J, Roy A F, Serougne C, *et al.* Long-term consequences of maternal high-fat feeding on hypothalamic leptin sensitivity and diet-induced obesity in the offspring. *Am J Physiol Regul Integr Comp Physiol* 2007;**293**(3):R1056–62.

39. Levin B E & Govek E. Gestational obesity accentuates obesity in obesity-prone progeny. *Am J Physiol* 1998;**275**(4/2):R1374–9.

40. Shankar K, Harrell A, Liu X, *et al.* Maternal obesity at conception programs obesity in the offspring. *Am J Physiol Regul Integr Comp Physiol* 2008;**294**(2):R528–38.

41. White C L, Purpera M N & Morrison C D. Maternal obesity is necessary for programming effect of high-fat diet on offspring. *Am J Physiol Regul Integr Comp Physiol* 2009;**296**(5):R1464–72.

42. Carmody J S, Wan P, Accili D, Zeltser L M & Leibel R L. Respective contributions of maternal insulin resistance and diet to metabolic and hypothalamic phenotypes of progeny. *Obesity (Silver Spring)* 2011;**19**(3):492–9.

43. Dong Y M, Li Y, Ning H, *et al.* High dietary intake of medium-chain fatty acids during pregnancy in rats prevents later-life obesity in their offspring. *J Nutr Biochem* 2010;**22**(8):791–7.

44. Korotkova M, Ohlsson C, Gabrielsson B, Hanson L A, Strandvik B. Perinatal essential fatty acid deficiency influences body weight and bone parameters in adult male rats. *Biochim Biophys Acta* 2005;**1686**(3):248–54.

45. Cryer A & Jones H M. The development of white adipose tissue. Effect of litter size on the lipoprotein lipase activity of four adipose-tissue depots, serum immunoreactive insulin and tissue cellularity during the first year of life in male and female rats. *Biochem J* 1980;**186**(3):805–15.

46. Patel M S, Srinivasan M & Laychock S G. Metabolic programming: role of nutrition in the immediate postnatal life. *J Inherit Metab Dis* 2009;**32**(2):218–28.

47. Ford S P, Zhang L, Zhu M, *et al.* Maternal obesity accelerates fetal pancreatic beta-cell but not alpha-cell development in sheep: prenatal consequences. *Am J Physiol Regul Integr Comp Physiol* 2009;**297**(3):R835–43.

48. Oben J A, Mouralidarane A, Samuelsson A M, *et al.* Maternal obesity during pregnancy and lactation programs the development of offspring non-alcoholic fatty liver disease in mice. *J Hepatol* 2010;**52**(6):913–20.

49. Del Prado M, Delgado G & Villalpando S. Maternal lipid intake during pregnancy and lactation alters milk composition and production and litter growth in rats. *J Nutr* 1997;**127**(3):458–62.

50. Kirk S L, Samuelsson A M, Argenton M, *et al.* Maternal obesity induced by diet in rats permanently influences central processes regulating food intake in offspring. *PLoS One* 2009;**4**(6):e5870.

51. Chen H & Morris M J. Differential responses of orexigenic neuropeptides to fasting in offspring of obese mothers. *Obesity (Silver Spring)* 2009;**17**(7):1356–62.

52. Chen H, Simar D & Morris M J. Hypothalamic neuroendocrine circuitry is programmed by maternal obesity: interaction with postnatal nutritional environment. *PLoS One* 2009;**4**(7):e6259.

53. Plagemann A & Harder T. Hormonal programming in perinatal life: leptin and beyond. *Br J Nutr* 2008; 1–2.

54. Ong Z Y & Muhlhausler B S. Maternal "junk-food" feeding of rat dams alters food choices and development of the mesolimbic reward pathway in the offspring. *FASEB J* 2011;**25**(7):2167–79.

55. Vucetic Z, Kimmel J, Totoki K, Hollenbeck E & Reyes T M. Maternal high-fat diet alters methylation and gene expression of dopamine and opioid-related genes. *Endocrinology*. 2010;**151**(10):4756–64.

56. Brion M J, Ness A R, Rogers I, *et al.* Maternal macronutrient and energy intakes in pregnancy and offspring intake at 10 y: exploring parental comparisons and prenatal effects. *Am J Clin Nutr* 2010;**91**(3):748–56.

57. Elmquist J K, Elias C F & Saper C B. From lesions to leptin: hypothalamic control of food intake and body weight. *Neuron* 1999;**22**(2):221–32.

58. Spiegelman B M & Flier J S. Obesity and the regulation of energy balance. *Cell* 2001;**104**(4):531–43.

59. Cone R D. Anatomy and regulation of the central melanocortin system. *Nat Neurosci* 2005;**8**(5):571–8.

60. Haynes W G, Morgan D A, Walsh S A, Mark A L & Sivitz W I. Receptor-mediated regional sympathetic nerve activation by leptin. *J Clin Invest* 1997;**100**(2):270–8.

61. Bouret S G, Gorski J N, Patterson C M, *et al.* Hypothalamic neural projections are permanently disrupted in diet-induced obese rats. *Cell Metab* 2008;**7**(2):179–85.

62. Gorski J N, Dunn-Meynell A A & Levin B E. Maternal obesity increases hypothalamic leptin receptor expression and sensitivity in juvenile obesity-prone rats. *Am J Physiol Regul Integr Comp Physiol* 2007;**292**(5):R1782–91.

63. Glavas M M, Kirigiti M A, Xiao X Q, *et al.* Early overnutrition results in early-onset arcuate leptin resistance and increased sensitivity to high-fat diet. *Endocrinology* 2010;**151**(4):1598–610.

64. Patel M S & Srinivasan M. Metabolic programming due to alterations in nutrition in the immediate postnatal period. *J Nutr* 2010;**140**(3):658–61.

65. Grayson B E, Levasseur P R, Williams S M, *et al.* Changes in melanocortin expression and inflammatory pathways in fetal offspring of nonhuman primates fed a high-fat diet. *Endocrinology* 2010;**151**(4):1622–32.

66. Vickers M H, Gluckman P D, Coveny A H, *et al.* The effect of neonatal leptin treatment on postnatal weight gain in male rats is dependent on maternal nutritional status during pregnancy. *Endocrinology* 2008;**149**(4):1906–13.

67. Yura S, Itoh H, Sagawa N, *et al.* Role of premature leptin surge in obesity resulting from intrauterine undernutrition. *Cell Metab* 2005;**1**(6):371–8.

68. Vickers M H, Gluckman P D, Coveny A H, *et al.* Neonatal leptin treatment reverses developmental programming. *Endocrinology* 2005;**146**(10):4211–16.

69. Samuelsson A M, Morris A, Igosheva N, *et al.* Evidence for sympathetic origins of hypertension in juvenile offspring of obese rats. *Hypertension* 2010;**55**(1):76–82.

70. Samuelsson A-M, Clark J, Shattock M J, *et al.* Postnatal leptin administration in naïve rat pups leads to leptin resistance, hypertension and gender specific myocardial dysfunction. *J Dev Orig Health Dis* 2:S12.

71. Long N M, Ford S P & Nathanielsz P W. Maternal obesity eliminates the neonatal lamb plasma leptin peak. *J Physiol* 2011;**589**(6):1455–62.

72. Poston L. Developmental programming and diabetes – the human experience and insight from animal models. *Best Pract Res Clin Endocrinol Metab* 2010;**24**(4):541–52.

73. Brenneman D E & Rutledge C O. Effect of dietary lipid on locomotor activity and response to psychomotor stimulants. *Psychopharmacology (Berl)* 1982;**76**(3):260–4.

74. Symonds M E, Sebert S P, Hyatt M A & Budge H. Nutritional programming of the metabolic syndrome. *Nat Rev Endocrinol* 2009;**5**(11):604–10.

75. Shelley P, Martin-Gronert M S, Rowlerson A, *et al.* Altered skeletal muscle insulin signaling and mitochondrial complex II-III linked activity in adult offspring of obese mice. *Am J Physiol Regul Integr Comp Physiol* 2009;**297**(3):R675–81.

76. Tozuka Y, Kumon M, Wada E, *et al.* Maternal obesity impairs hippocampal BDNF production and spatial learning performance in young mouse offspring. *Neurochem Int* 2010;**57**(3):235–47.

77. Fernandes M, Grayton H, Poston L, *et al.* Prenatal exposure to maternal obesity leads to hyperactivity in offspring. *Molecular Psychiatry* 2011, doi:10.1038/mp.2011.164.

78. Zambrano E, Martinez-Samayoa P M, Rodriguez-Gonzalez G L & Nathanielsz P W. Dietary intervention prior to pregnancy reverses metabolic programming in male offspring of obese rats. *J Physiol* 2010;**588**(10):1791–9.

79. Sen S & Simmons R A. Maternal antioxidant supplementation prevents adiposity in the offspring of Western diet-fed rats. *Diabetes* 2010;**59**(12):3058–65.

80. Yan X, Huang Y, Zhao J X, *et al.* Maternal obesity-impaired insulin signaling in sheep and induced lipid accumulation and fibrosis in skeletal muscle of offspring. *Biol Reprod*. 2011;**85**(1):172–8.

81. Suter M, Bocock P, Showalter L, *et al.* Epigenomics: maternal high-fat diet exposure in utero disrupts peripheral circadian gene expression in nonhuman primates. *FASEB J* 2011;**25**(2):714–26.

82. Bruce K D, Cagampang F R, Argenton M, *et al.* Maternal high-fat feeding primes steatohepatitis in adult mice offspring, involving mitochondrial dysfunction and altered lipogenesis gene expression. *Hepatology* 2009;**50**(6):1796–808.

83. Oken E, Rifas-Shiman S L, Field A E, Frazier A L & Gillman M W. Maternal gestational weight gain and offspring weight in adolescence. *Obstet Gynecol* 2008;**112**(5):999–1006.

84. Wen X, Triche E W, Hogan J W, Shenassa E D & Buka S L. Prenatal factors for childhood blood pressure mediated by intrauterine and/or childhood growth? *Pediatrics*;**127**(3):e713–21.

85. Wang J, Ma H, Tong C, *et al.* Overnutrition and maternal obesity in sheep pregnancy alter the JNK-IRS-1 signaling cascades and cardiac function in the fetal heart. *FASEB J* 2010;**24**(6):2066–76.

86. Huang Y, Yan X, Zhao J X, *et al.* Maternal obesity induces fibrosis in fetal myocardium of sheep. *Am J Physiol Endocrinol Metab* 2010;**299**(6):e968–75.

87. Rahmouni K, Morgan D A, Morgan G M, Mark A L & Haynes W G. Role of selective leptin resistance in diet-induced obesity hypertension. *Diabetes* 2005;**54**(7):2012–18.

88. Dodd J M, Grivell R M, Crowther C A & Robinson J S. Antenatal interventions for overweight or obese pregnant women: a systematic review of randomised trials. *BJOG* **117**(11):1316–26.

89. Igosheva N, Abramov A Y, Poston L, *et al.* Maternal diet-induced obesity alters mitochondrial activity and redox status in mouse oocytes and zygotes. *PLoS One* 2010;**5**(4):e10074.

Developmental origins of obesity: energy balance pathways – appetite

The role of developmental plasticity of the hypothalamus

Sebastien G. Bouret

Introduction

The perinatal environment exerts profound effects on the structure and function of the mammalian central nervous system (CNS). Although certain experiences are essential for orderly brain development to proceed, the occurrence of some harmful experiences can also have deleterious consequences on the developing brain. Over the past decade, we have learned how maternal diet modifies the fetal and postnatal genome substantially and contributes to deleterious health outcomes for the developing offspring [1–3]. There is also compelling evidence that obesity and high-fat feeding during pregnancy and lactation can have lasting consequences on brain development and behavior. For example, children born to obese mothers have a higher risk of having symptoms of attention-deficit/hyperactivity disorder (ADHD) than children of normal weight mothers [4]. Similarly, in rodents the consumption of a high-fat diet during pregnancy and lactation impairs hippocampal development with lasting consequences on spatial learning performance in the offspring [5,6]. Accumulating evidence also indicates that maternal and early postnatal obesity also perturbs the development of CNS pathways that are involved in energy balance regulation. This chapter will review the wide scope of structural and molecular changes that have been observed in specific brain regions involved in appetite regulation, in particular the hypothalamus, when individuals are exposed to an obesogenic environment during perinatal life.

Anatomy and development of hypothalamic circuits that are involved in energy balance

Hypothalamic circuits controlling energy balance

Our current understanding of the physiological mechanisms that underlie hunger and satiety is scarcely 20 years old (see [7,8] for review). In 1994, the discovery of leptin, a hormone secreted by fat cells that acts on the brain to blunt feeding behavior and permits energy expenditure, led to a paradigm shift in our understanding with the realization that our subconscious motivation to eat can be powerfully and dynamically regulated by hormonal signals. This discovery was followed by the discovery of ghrelin in 2000, a hormone secreted from the stomach to promote hunger. The brain sites of action of these hormones have been extensively mapped. In particular, leptin and ghrelin act within complex neuronal networks in the hypothalamus that are responsible for the regulation of energy balance (see [9,10] for review; Figure 11.1). In these neuronal networks, neurons of the arcuate nucleus of the hypothalamus are of primary importance. One subpopulation of arcuate neurons co-expresses neuropeptide Y (NPY) and Agouti-related peptide (AgRP), which act as major orexigenic signals. Another subset of arcuate neurons produces pro-opiomelanocortin (POMC) and cocaine- and amphetamine-regulated transcript peptide (CART) and represents an important anorectic

Maternal Obesity, ed. Matthew W. Gillman and Lucilla Poston. Published by Cambridge University Press. © Cambridge University Press 2012.

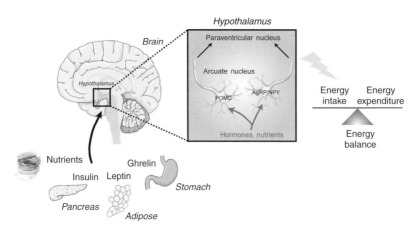

Figure 11.1. Organization of hypothalamic pathways regulating appetite. Highly simplified schematic diagrams to illustrate possible routes and neuronal populations relaying metabolic signals, such as leptin, ghrelin, insulin, and nutrients, from the periphery to the brain. Two distinct populations of neurons in the arcuate nucleus of the hypothalamus – one co-expressing neuropeptide Y (NPY) and Agouti-related protein (AgRP), and the other expressing pro-opiomelanocortin (POMC) – represent major routes for the regulation of body weight by peripheral signals. These neurons send direct projections to discrete populations of neurons, including in the paraventricular nucleus of the hypothalamus, to control energy balance. This figure was created in part using illustrations from "Servier Medical Art" with permission. (See figure in color plate section.)

regulator. Both AgRP/NPY and POMC neurons are direct targets of leptin and ghrelin. These anatomically distinct populations of arcuate neurons send overlapping projections to other sites that are implicated in the control of feeding, such as the paraventricular and dorsomedial nuclei of the hypothalamus and the lateral hypothalamic area. Additionally, nutrients, such as glucose and fatty acids, directly regulate the activity and function of various populations of hypothalamic neurons [11].

Partly because of its direct access to metabolic hormones and nutrients, the hypothalamus appears as a potential privileged site for the perinatal programming effects of maternal obesity and postnatal overnutrition. However, before assessing the influence of maternal obesity on hypothalamic development and function, we must have a good understanding of the time lines of normal hypothalamic development in species that are used for the study of metabolic programming, such as rodents and non-human primates.

Time lines of normal hypothalamic development

The complex patterns of neuronal wiring in the adult hypothalamus depend on a series of developmental events that establish a framework on which functional circuits can be built. The cellular processes that are involved in the formation of a functioning hypothalamus fall into two major categories: the determination of cell numbers and the determination of neuronal connectivity.

The first important period for hypothalamic development is the period when hypothalamic neurons are born. Cells that compose hypothalamic nuclei, including neurons, derive primarily from precursors that originate in the proliferative zone surrounding the lower portion of the third ventricle. This proliferative zone is also known as the neuroepithelium of the third ventricle. Birth-dating studies that have employed the administration of the thymidine analog BrdU or [3H] thymidine at various stages of embryonic development indicate that hypothalamic neuronal proliferation occurs primarily during mid-gestation (i.e., between E10 and E14) in rodents [12,13]. Hypothalamic appetite-regulating neurons acquire their cell identity rapidly after these neurons are born. For example, birth-dating experiments reveal that the peak birth date of POMC neurons in the arcuate nucleus is E11–E12, and neurons in the arcuate nucleus also first express POMC mRNA at E11–E12 [14]. The expression of both orexigenic (NPY, AgRP) and anorexigenic (POMC, CART) neuropeptide mRNAs continues to increase in the arcuate nucleus during the postnatal period and reach maximal expression levels by the third week of postnatal life [15]. Part of the complex process of hypothalamic development also includes the proper migration of neurons from their sites of origin (i.e., the proliferative zone of the third ventricle) to their final positions in the mature hypothalamus. This developmental process occurs primarily during late gestation in rodents.

The second important developmental period for hypothalamic development in rodents is during the first weeks of postnatal life when neurons send their axonal projections to their target sites. Although arcuate neurons are generated during mid-gestation, axonal projections from these neurons to their down-stream target sites do not start to develop in rodents until the end of the first postnatal week. Axonal tracing approaches and immunohistochemical labeling show that, in both mice and rats, projections from the arcuate nucleus, and particularly, projection pathways derived from NPY/AgRP neurons, are immature at birth and develop mainly during the second week of life [16,17]. In contrast to the development of projections from the arcuate nucleus, efferents from the dorsomedial nucleus to the paraventricular nucleus and lateral hypothalamic area are fully established by the first week of postnatal life [16]. Similarly, projections from the ventromedial nucleus also develop prior to projections from the arcuate nucleus; by P10, fibers from the ventromedial nucleus supply strong inputs to the lateral hypothalamic area, but at this age, the lateral hypothalamus is almost devoid of fibers from the arcuate nucleus [16].

It is also important to raise awareness about species differences and that the normal ontogeny of hypothalamic development in rodents differs markedly from human and non-human primates. First, the regional development of the rodent hypothalamus proceeds on a time line of days vs. weeks to months in human and non-human primates. Second, although rodents exhibit considerable postnatal hypothalamic development, human and non-human primates undergo considerably more prenatal maturation of hypothalamic structures. Therefore, whereas the hypothalamus appears largely immature until near the weaning period in rodents, hypothalamic maturation occurs primarily during intrauterine life in primates, including humans [18]. For example, hypothalamic cell proliferation is initiated during the first quarter of gestation in humans, and the development of hypothalamic axonal projections (precisely, the projections from arcuate AgRP/NPY neurons) occurs as early as gestational day 100 (i.e., late second trimester of gestation) in non-human primates [19,20]. Therefore different species may exhibit different periods of vulnerability to an obesogenic environment based on the temporal and regional maturation patterns of the hypothalamus.

Influence of maternal obesity on hypothalamic regulation and development

Various hypothalamic regulatory processes can be influenced by maternal obesity, including changes in the hypothalamic expression of appetite regulators, perturbations in the hypothalamic response to metabolic hormones, and alterations of the architecture of the hypothalamic neural circuits. Disruption of one or more of these biological processes can lead to long-term hypothalamic dysfunctions and, ultimately, to improper metabolic regulation.

Influence of maternal obesity on appetite-regulated gene expression

One approach to study the influence of maternal obesity on hypothalamic development and function is through experimental animal models. Maternal high-fat diet feeding during pregnancy is probably the most widely used approach for studying the consequences of maternal obesity in rodents. Offspring born to obese females fed a high-fat diet (45% to 60% of calories from fat) during gestation only or during both gestation and lactation become progressively overweight, hyperphagic, and glucose intolerant, and they display an increase in adiposity [21,22]. Using this experimental approach, myriad studies have indicated that maternal obesity is associated with an elevated ratio of orexigenic to anorexigenic neuropeptide expression in the hypothalamus. For example, maternal high-fat feeding during pregnancy causes an overall increase in the expression of orexigenic neuropeptides, such as NPY and AgRP, and a decrease in the expression of anorexigenic neuropeptides, such as POMC and CART [22]. The elevated ratio of orexigenic to anorexigenic neuropeptides may explain the increased drive to eat in perinatally malprogrammed animals. However, the application and generalization of the results of mRNA studies warrant a good degree of caution until the relationships between mRNA and protein levels is well characterized.

Because hypothalamic pathways continue to develop postnatally in rodents, reduction of litter size in either rats or mice has proven extremely fruitful for the study of perinatal overfeeding on hypothalamic development and function. Since the 1950s, manipulations of litter size have been used to control nutrient intake and growth rates in rodent neonates [23]. Animals that are raised in small litters display accelerated growth during the pre-weaning period, and these animals remain heavier and fatter throughout life [24,25]. Also, postnatally overfed animals show accelerated and exacerbated weight gain when fed a high-fat diet [25]. Notably, postnatal overfeeding affects the neuronal response to appetite-regulating neuropeptides. For example, paraventricular neurons of chronically overfed pups display reduced electrophysiological responses to arcuate neuropeptides, such as NPY, AgRP, αMSH, and CART [26].

The changes in neuropeptide gene expression that are observed in animals exposed to overfeeding during pre- or postnatal life reflect an acquired mechanism that originates from a malprogramming of hypothalamic neuropeptidergic systems during early life rather than being a consequence of metabolic dysfunctions, such as overweight and hyperphagia, during adult life. Supporting this idea, changes in neuropeptide gene expression are often observed in early embryonic life and/or during the first postnatal weeks, i.e., prior to the development of overweight and hyperphagia [22,27,28].

Maternal obesity and sensitivity of hypothalamic neurons to hormonal signals

Resistance to the regulatory action of leptin is a hallmark of obesity in adult individuals. For example, most forms of obesity are associated with elevated levels of circulating leptin and a diminished response of the hypothalamus to the appetite-suppressing effects of leptin [29,30]. Intriguingly, animals that are born to obese dams display similar disruptions in leptin signaling and secretion prior to the development of the obese phenotype. Offspring that are born to mothers fed a high-fat diet show abnormally high levels of leptin as early on as P7 and a blunted response to the anorectic effects of leptin [21]. This diminished response to leptin is associated with a reduced ability of leptin to induce pSTAT3, which is a marker of leptin receptor activation, in arcuate neurons [21]. These observations argue that the reduced anorectic response to leptin in animals born to obese dams is, at least in part, a centrally mediated phenomenon.

Leptin and insulin resistance have also been described in arcuate neurons of adult rats subjected to chronic postnatal overnutrition [24,31]. Electrophysiological studies from brain slices indicate that the arcuate neurons of rats that are raised in small litters are less inhibited by leptin and insulin, and some of these neurons are partially activated by these hormones [24,31]. A likely mechanism underlying this hormonal resistance is an alteration in receptor expression and/or signaling. For example, a downregulation of hypothalamic leptin receptor mRNA has been described in several animal models of nutritional programming, including small litters and maternal obesity [22,32].

Structural influences of maternal obesity on hypothalamic appetite-related networks

A number of studies have shown structural alterations in the hypothalamus of animals exposed to an obesogenic environment during perinatal life. These alterations range from the determination of cell numbers to the establishment of neuronal connectivity (Figure 11.2). Fetuses exposed to a maternal high-fat diet and obesity

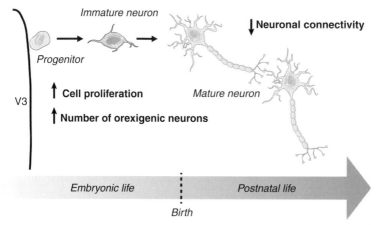

Figure 11.2. Exposure to an obesogenic environment during perinatal life induces marked effects on neuronal wiring in the hypothalamus. The formation of hypothalamic neural circuits occurs in two major phases: one phase (that includes cell proliferation, neuronal migration, and cell fate) during which the numbers of neurons composing the hypothalamus will be established; and another phase during which neuronal connectivity (that includes axon growth and synapse formation) will be established. Exposure to an obesogenic environment (such as maternal obesity and/or postnatal overnutrition) appears to influence each of these developmental events and results in a higher number of orexigenic neurons and disrupted hypothalamic neural projections. This figure was created in part using illustrations from "Servier Medical Art" with permission. (See figure in color plate section.)

during pregnancy in rats display enhanced cell pro-liferation in the neuroepithelium (i.e., the embryonic brain structure that ultimately generates hypothalamic neurons), which results in higher numbers of hypothalamic neurons that contain galanin, enkephalin, dynorphin, melanin-concentrating hormone, and orexin, each of which are orexigenic neuropeptides [33]. In general, rodent studies indicate that the adverse effects of a maternal obesogenic environment on hypothalamic cell numbers are similar when they occur either during gestation or during gestation and/or lactation. For example, offspring of high-fat diet mothers cross-fostered with control mothers during lactation exhibit similar changes in orexigenic cell numbers and metabolic outcomes compared with pups raised by high-fat diet mothers during pregnancy and lactation [33]. Similarly, raising pups in small litters results in a higher number of hypothalamic neurons that produce orexigenic neuropeptides [34].

Exposure of neonates to an obesogenic environment during development also impacts hypothalamic axonal connectivity; animals born to dams fed a high-fat diet have a disrupted development of neural projections that contain AgRP [21]. Notably, a similar disruption in the development of AgRP-containing fibers is observed in the hypothalamus of non-human primate fetuses from obese mothers [35].

Leptin as a likely hormonal mediator of hypothalamic malprogramming that is induced by perinatal obesity

As noted above, maternal obesity induces a plethora of structural and molecular changes in the hypothalamus.

ARH->PVH projections in ob/ob neonates

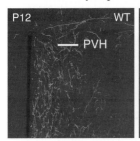
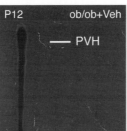
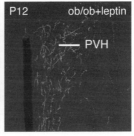

ARH->PVH projections in ob/ob adults

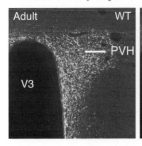
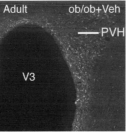
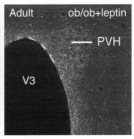

Leptin-induced axon growth

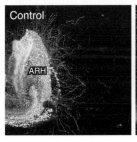
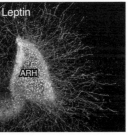

Figure 11.3. Neuroprogramming actions of the adipocyte-derived hormone leptin. In addition to its regulatory role in adults, leptin is an important signal for the development of hypothalamic circuits that control energy homeostasis. Neural projections from the arcuate nucleus (ARH) to the paraventricular nucleus of the hypothalamus (PVH) are disrupted in leptin-deficient (ob/ob) mice. Moreover, leptin appears to act primarily during neonatal critical periods to exert its neurodevelopmental effects. Although daily injections of ob/ob neonates with leptin rescue a normal pattern of innervation by arcuate neurons of the paraventricular nucleus, injections of the hormone in mature animals remain largely ineffective in restoring a normal pattern of arcuate projections. In addition, the application of leptin to isolated explants of the arcuate nucleus induces neurite extension, which suggests that leptin acts directly on arcuate neurons to promote axon growth. Reproduced with permission from [36]. (See figure in color plate section.)

However, the precise biological mechanisms that underlie the malprogramming effects of a perinatal obesogenic environment on hypothalamic organization and function remain largely unknown. Nevertheless, maternal obesity induces a wide range of hormonal changes in both the dams and neonates, and evidence that has accumulated during the past few years indicates that changes in perinatal leptin levels in pups born to obese dams [21] represent a likely cause for the malprogramming effects of maternal obesity on hypothalamic development (Figure 11.3). The first report that variations in leptin levels are associated with marked changes in hypothalamic neural development came from a study in leptin-deficient (ob/ob) mice. Neuroanatomical approaches have revealed that the density of acuate axons innervating the paraventricular nucleus is severely reduced in ob/ob neonates compared to wild type animals [36]. In addition, leptin treatment of ob/ob neonates restores a normal pattern of arcuate connectivity; however, the same leptin treatment in adults does not reverse the abnormalities in arcuate projections in ob/ob mice [36], which suggests that leptin acts primarily during a restricted neonatal period to exert its developmental effects on arcuate neural projections. These observations indicate that leptin represents a powerful neurotrophic signal that promotes the formation of projections from the arcuate nucleus. In vitro studies showing that leptin treatment increases the density and length of axons from the arcuate nucleus further support this hypothesis [36]. Importantly, the developmental actions of leptin contribute to the ultimate phenotype of the organism [37,38], which suggests the potential importance of leptin-regulated arcuate circuit formation to future energy balance. Together, these observations suggest that leptin is well positioned to participate in developmental responses to nutritional and metabolic changes, such as the changes observed during maternal obesity. Further work will be required to establish a functional role for leptin in central programming of obesity in humans, and the results from these studies may provide opportunities for primary prevention and treatments.

Genetic predispositions to obesity

Despite an obvious relationship between obesity and a Western lifestyle, it is also clear that different individuals exposed to the same obesogenic environments display different responses to obesity predispositions.

In addition to environmental factors, genetic predispositions are important determinants for obesity risk and can synergistically interact with a Western dietary pattern in determining obesity risk. In that regard, the model of diet-induced obesity developed by Levin [39] is particularly well suited for the study of the underlying biological processes that contribute to the development of obesity in humans because Levin's diet-induced obese rats share several features with human obesity, including polygenic inheritance. This animal model is also useful for the study of the relative contribution of genetic vs. environmental factors in metabolic programming. In this model, the offspring of mothers that are genetically predisposed to diet-induced obesity are obese, hyperphagic, and glucose intolerant when fed a high-energy diet compared to offspring born to diet-resistant dams [40,41].

Influence of genetic predispositions to obesity on hypothalamic development

Although it is clear that nutrition-induced maternal obesity influences the degree to which the hypothalamic nuclei, including the arcuate nucleus, develop, it is also evident that the architecture of various hypothalamic pathways can be influenced by genetic background (Figure 11.4). For example, the diet-induced obese rats that inherited obesity as a polygenic trait display reduced central leptin sensitivity as early as P10, i.e., before they develop obesity [42]. This early reduction in leptin sensitivity in diet-induced obese rats exerts profound consequences on the architecture of the hypothalamic neurocircuitry. Compared with diet-resistant rats, diet-induced obese rats have a diminished density of arcuate projections in the paraventricular nucleus, which is caused by the inability of leptin to promote neurite outgrowth directly from arcuate neurons [42]. In this particular rat model, genetic background seems to prevail over environmental factors to influence the formation of arcuate projections. For example, although maternal nutrition clearly influences the development of hypothalamic neural projections in non-genetically obese animals [21], it does not affect the architecture of arcuate axonal projections in genetically diet-induced obese rats [42]. The disruption of arcuate neural projections is not the only structural abnormality that is observed in diet-induced obese rats. These animals also display abnormal dendrite morphology in the ventromedial nucleus [43]. Whether these defects are caused

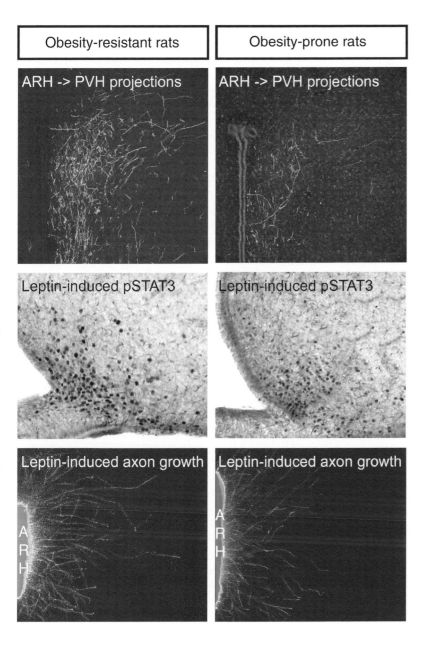

Figure 11.4. Effects of genetic predispositions to obesity on the neurotrophic response to leptin. Compared with diet-resistant (DR) rats, rats that have obesity inherited as a polygenic trait (diet-induced obese, DIO rats) display an abnormal development of arcuate neural projections to the paraventricular nucleus of the hypothalamus (PVH) that appears to be the result of diminished responsiveness of arcuate neurons to the neurotrophic actions of leptin during postnatal development.

by reduced leptin sensitivity, however, remains to be established.

Plasticity of hypothalamic feeding circuits in animals genetically predisposed to obesity

It is important to recognize that the hypothalamus continues to remodel and change not just early in development but throughout the entire period of development and even during adulthood. However, both the degree and the nature of adult hypothalamic neuroplasticity may be influenced by perinatal environmental experiences and genetically programmed events. For example, a significant remodeling of synapses has been reported in the rat hypothalamus [44]. However, adult rats born to diet-induced obese dams display increased inhibitory inputs to POMC neurons compared to animals born to obesity-resistant, diet-resistant rats [44]. In addition, when fed a high-fat diet, diet-induced obese rats exhibit a loss of synapses, but diet-resistant rats show an increase in POMC synaptic coverage [44]. These observations indicate that adult nutrition can affect hypothalamic plasticity by causing a synaptic rearrangement of synaptic inputs on arcuate neurons, but that this neuroplastic response is greatly dependent on genetic predispositions to obesity.

Conclusions

In the midst of a staggering obesity epidemic, there is a need to better understand the influence of this pathological condition on perinatal development. Epidemiological and clinical studies have provided valuable information on the role played by maternal obesity and early postnatal overnutrition in increasing the susceptibility for the development of diseases in adult life, including obesity and diabetes. Animal models have also been useful in identifying organizational and regulatory changes that occur within key systems that are involved in metabolic regulation. They showed that exposure to an obesogenic environment during critical periods of life has lasting effects on the development and organization of hypothalamic circuits that regulate body weight and energy balance. These observations have led us to the recognition that developmental malprogramming of neuroendocrine systems by maternal and/or postnatal obesity may represent a likely cause for obesity risk in later life. However, if we want to ameliorate and perhaps reverse the metabolic programming of the fetus and/or neonate, it will also be important that we have a better understanding of the cellular and molecular mechanisms that underlie this environment-dependent malprogramming. Similarly, to design optimal interventional studies, it will be important to increase our knowledge about the periods of maximal vulnerability of the hypothalamus in response to changes in the perinatal nutritional and hormonal environment. In addition, the present state of knowledge about neuroendocrine programming in humans is still imprecise, and there is an urgent need for an in-depth characterization of critical periods for hypothalamic development in various species including humans.

References

1. Oken E & Gillman, M W. Fetal origins of obesity. *Obes Res* 2003;**11**:496–506.

2. McMillen I C & Robinson J S. Developmental origins of the metabolic syndrome: prediction, plasticity, and programming. *Physiol Rev* 2005;**85**:571–633.

3. Taylor P D & Poston L. Developmental programming of obesity in mammals. *Exp Physiol* 2007;**92**:287–98.

4. Rodriguez A, Miettunen J, Henriksen T B, *et al.* Maternal adiposity prior to pregnancy is associated with ADHD symptoms in offspring: evidence from three prospective pregnancy cohorts. *Int J Obes* 2008;**32**:550–7.

5. Tozuka Y, Kumon M, Wada E, *et al.* Maternal obesity impairs hippocampal BDNF production and spatial learning performance in young mouse offspring. *Neurochem Int* 2010;**57**:235–47.

6. Niculescu M D & Lupu D S. High fat diet-induced maternal obesity alters fetal hippocampal development. *Int J Dev Neuroscience* 2009;**27**:627–33.

7. Elmquist J K, Maratos-Flier E, Saper C B & Flier J S. Unraveling the central nervous system pathways underlying responses to leptin. *Nat Neurosci* 1998;**1**:445–50.

8. Nogueiras R, Tschoep M H & Zigman J M. Central nervous system regulation of energy metabolism. *Ann N Y Acad Sci* 2008;**1126**:14–19.

9. Dickson S L. Neuroendocrinology briefings. *J Neuroendocrinol* 2002;**14**:83–4.

10. Elmquist J K, Coppari R, Balthasar N, Ichinose M & Lowell B B. Identifying hypothalamic pathways controlling food intake, body weight, and glucose homeostasis. *J Comp Neurol* 2005;**493**:63–71.

11. Levin B E. Metabolic sensing neurons and the control of energy homeostasis. *Physiol Behav* 2006;**89**:486–9.

12. Markakis E A. Development of the neuroendocrine hypothalamus. *Front Neuroendocrinol* 2002;**23**:257–91.

13. Bouret S G. Development of hypothalamic neural networks controlling appetite. *Forum Nutr* 2010;**63**:84–93.

14. Padilla S L, Carmody J S & Zeltser L M. POMC-expressing progenitors give rise to antagonistic neuronal populations in hypothalamic feeding circuits. *Nat Med* 2010;**16**:403–5.

15. Cottrell E C, Cripps R L, Duncan J S, *et al.* Developmental changes in hypothalamic leptin receptor: relationship with the postnatal leptin surge and energy balance neuropeptides in the postnatal rat. *Am J Physiol Regul Integr Comp Physiol* 2009;**296**:R631–9.

16. Bouret S G, Draper S J & Simerly R B. Formation of projection pathways from the arcuate nucleus of the hypothalamus to hypothalamic regions implicated in the neural control of feeding behavior in mice. *J Neurosci* 2004;**24**:2797–805.

17. Grove K L, Allen S, Grayson B E & Smith M S. Postnatal development of the hypothalamic neuropeptide Y system. *Neurosci* 2003;**116**:393–406.

18. Koutcherov Y, Mai J K, Ashwell K W & Paxinos G. Organization of human hypothalamus in fetal development. *J Comp Neurol* 2002;**446**:301–24.

19. Keyser A. *Development of the Hypothalamus in Mammals.* (New York: Marcel Dekker Inc,1979).

20. Grayson B E, Allen S E, Billes S K, *et al.* Prenatal development of hypothalamic neuropeptide systems in the nonhuman primate. *Neuroscience* 2006;**143**:975–86.

21. Kirk S L, Samuelsson A-M, Argenton M, *et al.* Maternal obesity induced by diet in rats permanently influences central processes regulating food intake in offspring. *PLoS ONE* 2009;**4**:e5870.

22. Chen H, Simar D & Morris M J. Hypothalamic neuroendocrine circuitry is programmed by maternal obesity: interaction with postnatal nutritional environment. *PLoS ONE* 2009;**4**:e6259.

23. Kennedy G C. The development with age of hypothalamic restraint upon the appetite of the rat. *J Endocrinol* 1957;**16**:9–17.

24. Davidowa H & Plagemann A. Decreased inhibition by leptin of hypothalamic arcuate neurons in neonatally overfed young rats. *Neuroreport* 2000;**11**:2795–8.

25. Glavas M M, Kirigiti M A, Xiao XQ, *et al.* Early overnutrition results in early-onset arcuate leptin resistance and increased sensitivity to high-fat diet. *Endocrinology* 2010;**151**:1598–610.

26. Davidowa H, Li Y & Plagemann A. Altered responses to orexigenic (AgRP, MCH) and anorexigenic (a-MSH, CART) neuropeptides of paraventricular hypothalamic neurons in early postnatally overfed rats. *Eur J Neurosci* 2003;**18**:613–21.

27. Gupta A, Srinivasan M, Thamadilok S & Patel M S. Hypothalamic alterations in fetuses of high fat diet-fed obese female rats. *J Endocrinol* 2009;**200**:293–300.

28. Morris M J & Chen H. Established maternal obesity in the rat reprograms hypothalamic appetite regulators and leptin signaling at birth. *Int J Obes* 2008;**33**:115–22.

29. Enriori P J, Evans A E, Sinnayah P & Cowley M A. Leptin resistance and obesity. *Obesity* 2006;**14**:254S–8S.

30. Myers M G, Cowley M A & Műnzberg H. Mechanisms of leptin action and leptin resistance. *Ann Rev Physiol* 2008;**70**:537–56.

31. Davidowa H & Plagemann A. Insulin resistance of hypothalamic arcuate neurons in neonatally overfed rats. *Neuroreport* 2007;**18**:521–4.

32. Chen H & Morris M J. Differential responses of orexigenic neuropeptides to fasting in offspring of obese mothers. *Obesity* 2009;**17**:1356–62.

33. Chang G-Q, Gaysinskaya V, Karatayev O & Leibowitz S F. Maternal high-fat diet and fetal programming: increased proliferation of hypothalamic peptide-producing neurons that increase risk for overeating and obesity. *J Neurosci* 2008;**28**:12107–19.

34. Plagemann A, Harder T, Rake A, *et al.* Observations on the orexigenic hypothalamic neuropeptide Y-system in neonatally overfed weanling rats. *J Neuroendocrinol* 1999;**11**:541–6.

35. Grayson B E, Levasseur P R, Williams S M, *et al.* Changes in melanocortin expression and inflammatory pathways in fetal offspring of nonhuman primates fed a high-fat diet. *Endocrinology* 2010;**151**:1622–32.

36. Bouret S G, Draper S J & Simerly R B. Trophic action of leptin on hypothalamic neurons that regulate feeding. *Science* 2004;**304**:108–10.

37. Vickers M H, Gluckman P D, Coveny A H, *et al.* Neonatal leptin treatment reverses developmental programming. *Endocrinology* 2005;**146**:4211–16.

38. Attig L, Solomon G, Ferezou J, *et al.* Early postnatal leptin blockage leads to a long-term leptin resistance and susceptibility to diet-induced obesity in rats. *Int J Obes* 2008;**32**:1153–60.

39. Levin B E, Dunn-Meynell A A, Balkan B & Keesey R E. Selective breeding for diet-induced obesity and resistance in Sprague–Dawley rats. *Am J Physiol Regul Integr Comp Physiol* 1997;**273**:R725–30.

40. Ricci M R & Levin B E. Ontogeny of diet-induced obesity in selectively bred Sprague–Dawley rats. *Am J Physiol Regul Integr Comp Physiol* 2003;**285**:R610–18.

41. Levin B E, Dunn-Meynell A A, Ricci M R & Cummings D E. Abnormalities of leptin and ghrelin regulation in obesity-prone juvenile rats. *Am J Physiol Endocrinol Metab* 2003;**285**:e949–57.

42. Bouret S G, Gorski J N, Patterson C M, *et al.* Hypothalamic neural projections are permanently disrupted in diet-induced obese rats. *Cell Metab* 2008;**7**:179–85.

43. LaBelle D R, Cox J M, Dunn-Meynell A A, Levin B E & Flanagan-Cato L M. Genetic and dietary effects on dendrites in the rat hypothalamic ventromedial nucleus. *Physiol Behav* 2009;**98**:511–16.

44. Horvath T L, Sarman B, García-Cáceres C, *et al.* Synaptic input organization of the melanocortin system predicts diet-induced hypothalamic reactive gliosis and obesity. *Proc Natl Acad Sci USA* 2010;**107**:14875–80.

12

Adipose tissue development and its potential contribution to later obesity

Shalini Ojha, Helen Budge, and Michael E. Symonds

Introduction

The early life environment may persistently influence the development of adipose tissue, thereby predisposing the offspring to obesity. There is substantial development within the adipose tissue depots from early fetal life through weaning to puberty [1]. These periods are associated with critical windows of vulnerability to the environment and lifestyle. Importantly, these windows differ greatly between species and are dependent on the maturity of the adipose tissue at birth [2].

The majority of animal species have only very limited adipose tissue stores at birth, which may relate to the high energy costs associated with deposition of fat as opposed to protein [3]. In addition, fetal adipose tissue tends to be primarily brown fat, which is characterized as being uniquely able to rapidly generate heat due to the presence of uncoupling protein (UCP)1 [4–6], with thermal production being as high as 300 W/kg compared to 1 W/kg in all other tissues [7,8]. One notable exception is the human infant, which not only has appreciable brown fat stores but also large amounts of white subcutaneous fat [9]. Consequently, the newborn is capable of both generating large amounts of heat around its internal organs following cold exposure to the extrauterine environment, and of minimizing heat loss due to the insulatory properties of white fat.

Our current understanding of adipose tissue development has been transformed over the past few years due to the discovery that brown adipocytes can share a common lineage with skeletal muscle rather than with white adipocytes [4,10]. In addition, brown adipose tissue is retained throughout the life cycle in humans, in small amounts located primarily within the supraclavicular region [4–6]. In adult humans, however, only 40 to 50 g of brown adipose tissue would be required

to contribute 20% of the total daily energy expenditure [11,12].

In view of these substantial advances and challenges to our understanding of adipose tissue biology, there is currently only a limited amount of information available that can provide insights into the potential mechanisms involved in the developmental pathway to obesity [8]. Our understanding in this area is further challenged by the very different responses of adipose tissue seen in small compared with large mammals both during fetal and postnatal development [13]. These reflect, in part, their need to swiftly adapt to changes in the prevailing thermal environment, responses that differ greatly between depots, at least in large mammals [14]. In this chapter, we review the limited information available, which suggests that the early life nutritional environment can influence adipocyte biology and influence the risk of obesity in later life.

Maternal diet and glucose supply to the fetus

Glucose is a major metabolic substrate determining fat accumulation in the fetus, and direct or indirect promotion of glucose supply to the fetus increases fat deposition [15]. Maternal carbohydrate metabolism is highly sensitive to food intake but maternal endocrine responses have the potential to maintain normal glucose concentrations even during dietary manipulation [16]. Under conditions of suboptimal nutrition, these responses will reduce maternal metabolic requirements and promote fat mobilization, ensuring that the mother remains normoglycemic [16,17]. Under conditions of maternal nutritional excess maternal fat depots increase and normoglycemia is maintained unless, in the face of continued caloric excess and development of obesity, as described in Chapters 5 and 15, more extreme insulin resistance leads to failure of glucose homeostasis and potentially to gestational diabetes. However, although there is an important linear association between maternal glucose tolerance and neonatal adiposity at birth [18], the fetal response to increased maternal food intake may not be solely mediated by changes in glucose supply as excess of other nutrients also plays an important role.

The maternal nutritional environment can have a major impact on long-term metabolic health of the offspring [19]. The effects of targeted undernutrition in human populations have been demonstrated from the Dutch Winter Famine of 1944–45, when exposure to famine in early gestation did not affect birthweight but increased the risk of obesity and cardiovascular disease in adulthood, while late gestation exposure reduced birthweight and increased the predisposition to type 2 diabetes mellitus in middle age [20]. Conversely, the association between maternal obesity and the potential for fetal overnutrition and obesity in later life is supported by the increase in birthweight with maternal body mass index (BMI) [21]. A strong relationship between birthweight and later development of obesity, and relationships between maternal BMI and offspring obesity, are reviewed in Chapter 9. As recently highlighted by the Centre for Maternal and Child Enquiries [21] and detailed in Chapters 6 and 9, the consequences of raised maternal BMI are not restricted to larger offspring but include increased risk of miscarriage, preterm birth, and other neonatal complications – outcomes which tend to be enhanced with maternal diabetes. These adverse outcomes are likely to be mediated by the higher maternal glucose, free fatty acid, and triglyceride concentrations to which the mother and fetoplacental unit is exposed. All the resulting effects on adipose tissue mass and its subtypes in the offspring have yet to be well described. In sheep, at least, offspring benefit from increases in brown, rather than white, adipose tissue in response to nutrient excess [22]. To gain a better understanding of how changes in maternal diet or other early life factors can increase risk of later obesity it is necessary to consider the normal ontogeny of adipose tissue development.

The ontogeny of adipose tissue in early life

Adipose tissue is a unique organ as it is the only one that is capable of seemingly unlimited growth, a process that can occur as a result of either increasing cell number or size [23]. The importance of early life events in establishing subsequent adipocyte distribution, size, and function is indicated by the findings that white adipocyte progenitor cells become committed to the adipose lineage during the late fetal/early postnatal period. At least in mice there is also a marked expansion of this pool in early postnatal life [24]. Adipose tissue cell number, but not size, can therefore be set in early life [25]. Indeed, adipose tissue cellularity is set in childhood and adolescence after which adipocyte number remains stable through adulthood, even following weight loss. The precise mechanisms by which a developmental increase in cell number occurs early in life remain to be clarified. Children who become obese in early life display a marked increase in adipose tissue cell size, and their fat depots differ from those of non-obese children. When adults lose weight, cell volume is reduced but cell number appears to be unchanged, suggesting that the foundations of obesity are laid down in early life [25].

In both humans and sheep, a species frequently used to interrogate early life origins of obesity, adipose tissue first appears in mid-gestation and accumulates over the final third of gestation [26]. Other adaptations that act to promote both the appearance and subsequent recruitment of UCP1 occur concomitantly. These include increased sympathetic innervation, β-adrenergic receptor density, and catecholamine concentrations [15]. Birth then results in a surge of UCP1 synthesis in precocial species such as sheep [27]. This is followed by a gradual loss of UCP1 to undetectable levels by one month of age in central fat depots [28], a process that takes approximately nine months in human subjects [29]. The extent to which brown adipose tissue development may differ within those depots, such as in the supraclavicular region, which are retained into adult life has yet to be examined. Interestingly, in view of the common origin of brown adipocytes and skeletal muscle [30], a close link between functional brown adipose tissue and muscle volume has recently been suggested in children and adolescents [31].

Importantly, fetal adipose tissue in sheep has both brown and white fat characteristics. It is made up of both multilocular and unilocular adipocytes [32] and demonstrates an ontogenic rise in leptin secretion, a characteristic of white adipose tissue [27,33]. As UCP1 abundance declines in perirenal adipose tissue in early postnatal life, other potentially related markers are also lost [29]. These include the key transcription factors peroxisome proliferator-activated receptor (PPAR)α and PPAR coactivator 1α [34], and glucose regulated protein 78, an endoplasmic reticulum chaperone crucial for protein synthesis [35]. These changes mark the loss of brown adipose tissue and, simultaneously, there is substantial rise in the amount of white adipose tissue accompanied by increased abundance of UCP2, which peaks around 30 days after birth [36] and could have a role in the transition from brown to white adipose tissue.

Role of glucocorticoids in the development of adipose tissue

The growth of adipose tissue is influenced by glucocorticoids, which control adipocyte differentiation, metabolism, and gene expression [23]. Glucocorticoids are key intermediaries of stress responses and mediate part of the programming of offspring hypothalamo–pituitary–adrenal (HPA) axes. Obese pregnant mothers have increased concentrations of inflammatory cytokines [37] and exposure of the developing fetus to such pro-inflammatory influences is a potential mechanism by which maternal high-fat intake affects brain development and energy homeostasis [38].

The action of glucocorticoids on adipose tissue is mediated by the glucocorticoid receptor (GR) and types 1 and 2 of the enzyme 11-β-hydroxysteriod dehydrogenase (11βHSD). 11βHSD1 is an 11-oxoreductase, which catalyses the conversion of inactive cortisone to bioactive cortisol and amplifies the action of glucocorticoid at the level of glucocorticoid receptor [39]. 11βHSD2 acts in reverse and catalyzes the inactivation of cortisol to cortisone [40]. The ontogeny of glucocorticoid action is therefore very different in adipose tissue compared with most other tissues during perinatal life [23]. In most organs, birth is accompanied by a pronounced peak in glucocorticoid receptor abundance, which occurs in response to the peak in fetal plasma cortisol that precedes parturition [41]. Then, as the newborn effectively adapts to the thermal and metabolic stress of the extrauterine environment both plasma cortisol concentrations and glucocorticoid receptor abundance fall in parallel as summarized in Figure 12.1. Adipose tissue is an exception, as an increase in glucocorticoid receptor gene expression continues up to puberty [23] and is paralleled by an increase in plasma cortisol as shown in Figure 12.1 [42]. In young sheep, both glucocorticoid receptor and 11βHSD1 expression increase with postnatal age

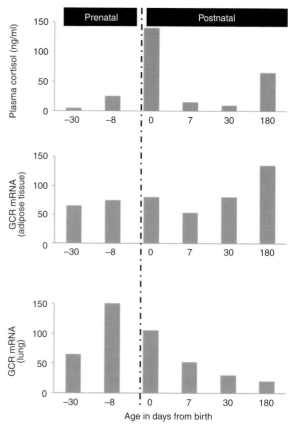

Figure 12.1. Mean ovine fetal and postnatal concentrations of plasma cortisol and glucocorticoid receptor gene expression according to age. Plasma cortisol levels increase in late fetal life to peak at delivery and then fall in the postnatal period as the newborn adapts to the extrauterine environment. Glucocorticoid receptor gene expression rises in adipose tissue while it falls in other tissues such as lungs (GR mRNA, glucocorticoid receptor mRNA expressed as a percentage of 18S rRNA expression). Adapted from Fowden *et al.* 1989 [90], Bispham *et al.* 2003 [16], and Gnanalingham *et al.* 2005 [23].

and fat mass, whereas 11βHSD2 shows an inverse relationship with perirenal fat mass [23]. Thus adipocyte sensitivity to glucocorticoids is maintained and elevated levels of glucocorticoid receptors and 11βHSD1 impact on adipose tissue development and possibly on the development of visceral adiposity. These findings are of particular interest as 11βHSD1 gene expression is similarly raised with adult obesity [43,44].

The extent to which increased glucocorticoid action in early life within adipose tissue has the potential to promote later obesity has not been fully established. In rodents, corticosterone (the analogue to cortisol in humans) levels are raised in mothers fed a high-fat diet [45]. Maternal high-fat diet and obesity may also impact changes in the HPA axis by elevated levels of cytokines and corticosterone [46]. The influences of glucocorticoids could be related to the divergent effects on brown and white adipose tissue function. For example, dexamethasone administration to the mother in late gestation promotes brown fat thermogenesis in the newborn [47] at the same time as reducing maternal food intake [48]. More information from animal models is available in relation to the influence of maternal nutrient restriction in early and mid-gestation in sheep, which also increases glucocorticoid receptor and 11βHSD1 expression and reduces expression of 11βHSD2 in ovine perirenal adipose tissue at term, changes that persist up to six months of age [23]. These adaptations have no effect on fat mass either when the offspring are raised in a normal or low-activity environment, although in the low-activity condition pronounced insulin resistance is apparent [1]. In contrast, late gestational nutrient restriction of the mother reduces both birthweight and fat mass in conjunction with decreased glucocorticoid receptor and 11βHSD1 gene expression, whereas 11βHSD2 is raised both at birth and 30 days of age [23]. These changes would predispose to adipocyte expansion and to obesity. The extent to which glucocorticoid action could be reset in other fat depots remains to be explored but a linear relationship between changes in endocrine sensitivity and obesity onset is not readily apparent.

The role of leptin in the development of adipose tissue

Leptin is an important peripheral and neuroendocrine signal, which has impact on adipose tissue development and formation of metabolic pathways. It acts on the ventromedial nucleus of the hypothalamus to reduce appetite and increase energy expenditure when white adipose tissue stores increase. In addition, it has several peripheral actions and a facilitative role in insulin–glucose metabolism through its further impact on adipose tissue development [49]. In rodents, a high-fat diet in pregnancy increases leptin levels at birth accompanied by increase in body and fat-pad weights followed by increased abundance of leptin receptors in the hypothalamus [50]. Offspring of diet-induced obese rats show an enhanced and lengthened leptin surge with an increase in leptin expression in abdominal white adipose tissue [51]. Such alteration in CNS leptin signaling does not cause obesity in early life but such a lasting impairment may be the precursor of leptin resistance

related to obesity in adults [52]. In humans, the fetus in a pregnancy complicated with maternal diabetes is hyperglycemic and hyperinsulinemic and has high cord-blood leptin concentrations [53] in parallel with increased adiposity [54]. There is growing evidence that leptin is associated with various pathophysiologies in obesity and that maternal nutrient excess alters leptin at critical periods of development inducing permanent effects on adipose tissue regulation. See Chapter 11 for more information on critical periods of leptin action.

Other markers of adipose tissue development

Another critical transcription factor that can determine adipocyte lineage is PPAR. Its different isoforms regulate adipose tissue mass through changes in adipokine secretion, together with the stimulation of lipoprotein lipase and glycerol-3-phosphate dehydrogenase [55]. Therefore PPAR has a role in fatty acid oxidation and an increased abundance could promote lipid deposition within fetal adipose tissue depots. PPARγ has a critical role in regulation of adipocyte differentiation. When expression is low, cells fail to differentiate into adipocytes and when expression is increased, PPARγ can induce adipogenesis in growing fibroblast cell lines [56]. CCAAT/enhancer-binding proteins (C/EBP) are also involved in the differentiation of adipocytes. C/EBP β and δ are induced very early in adipocyte differentiation and activate PPARγ to initiate differentiation of pre-adipocytes while C/EBPα is activated after PPARγ to aid in the terminal adipocyte differentiation [57].

The role of insulin and insulin-like growth factor (IGF)-1 in the differentiation of adipocytes is also of great interest. These appear to act through signal transcription factors of which insulin receptor signal (IRS)-1 and 2 are the most ubiquitous. IRS-1 and IRS-2 deficient cells have no ability to differentiate into adipocytes and their expression dramatically decreases the expression of C/EBPα and PPARγ [58]. Therefore insulin and IGF-1 appear to have an essential role in the terminal differentiation of adipocytes.

Information from animal models of obesity

There is accumulating evidence for both short- and longer term effects of excess maternal weight gain obtained from rodent studies. Some of these studies include consumption of a isocaloric diet where fat content is increased five- to ten-fold while protein and, to a much greater extent, carbohydrate content are substantially reduced [59]. The effect of consumption of such diets is likely to be different from that seen following overnutrition in humans, in which increased fat intake may not be so dramatic. The adverse maternal outcomes following consumption of this type of diet prior to mating include defects in ovarian function and, subsequently, blastocyst survival rates are reduced due to abnormal embryonic cellular differentiation [60]. Maternal obesity at conception and overnutrition during pregnancy can program rapid weight gain in offspring exposed to a high-fat diet on weaning [61]. Offspring changes include increases in markers of adipogenesis [62]. These may contribute to the adverse adipose tissue development seen prior to development of increased body weight in the offspring.

A number of models of dietary-induced obesity during pregnancy have been developed, primarily in rodents. In the majority of these, there is no effect of maternal obesity on birthweight. This finding may reflect placental adaptations that could limit the increase in fetal nutrient supply in response to the types of unbalanced diets used in these studies [63] or altered body composition with higher fat mass and lower lean mass as suggested in Figure 12.2. In addition, as obesity in some studies in larger species is induced with fewer variations in the composition and quality of the diet eaten, the metabolic and endocrine adaptations seen within some models would be expected to be very different to those occurring in humans. For example, the five-fold increase in plasma insulin up to 25 μU/ml and raised cortisol [64] seen in pregnant sheep that rapidly become obese prior to conception indicate pronounced maternal metabolic stress, changes that are more pronounced than those expected in humans.

A gestational diet rich in animal fat and sugar, a pattern potentially closer to that consumed by some obese humans, induces increased gene expression of PPARγ, greater percentage of large adipocytes, and insulin resistance in offspring of female mice [65] suggesting maternal diet-induced long-term adverse consequences in the offspring. To further mimic human situations, when a high-fat diet is provided to both male and female mice over several generations there is a gradual increase in adipose tissue mass and plasma levels of markers of metabolic syndrome such as insulin, leptin, TNFα, and resistin [66]. This hypertrophy and hyperplasia of adipose tissue occurs without any significant change in total food or energy intake and is accompanied by a steady increase in inflammatory markers. The association of a pro-inflammatory state to high risk of developing obesity is well recognized. For example, higher levels of systemic inflammatory markers and increased neurohormonal activity are present even in non-obese children of obese parents [67]. Macrophage numbers are increased in adipose tissue in obesity [68] as are other markers of chronic inflammation [69] and such an inflammatory state may even be intrinsic to adipose tissue particularly when insulin

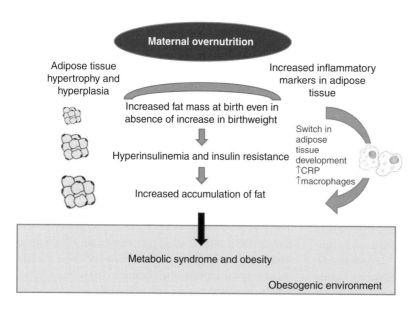

Figure 12.2. Maternal obesity and nutrient excess in pregnancy induce changes in adipocyte differentiation including hypertrophy and hyperplasia, and upregulation of inflammatory markers. These changes may lead to insulin resistance and hyperinsulinism, and ultimately to metabolic syndrome and obesity, especially in an obesogenic environment.

resistance precedes the development of obesity and metabolic syndrome [70], as illustrated in Figure 12.2.

Effects of types of fat in the maternal diet

Other changes may be influenced by the composition of fat in the diet rather than just how much of it is consumed by the mother. Rats fed a diet rich in N6 polyunsaturated fatty acids (PUFA) produce offspring with an increased proportion of total body and abdominal fat with increase in hepatic triglyceride concentrations and hepatic insulin resistance [71]. In contrast, other studies emphasize the effects of essential fatty acid deficiency in the maternal diet on altered leptin expression and adiposity in the offspring [72]. Diets rich in PUFA may reduce inflammatory markers although N6 PUFAs and increased N6:N3 may be inflammatory [73]. Fatty acids with N6 structure such as arachidonic acid promote maturation of adipocytes while N3 fatty acids such as docosahexaenoic acid induce lipolysis, inhibit adipocyte differentiation, and promote apoptosis [74]. The fatty acid supply to the fetus is mainly determined by the maternal lipid profile. In non-human primates, a high N6:N3 ratio in maternal diet, reflective of current trends in some Western diets in humans, is mimicked in the fetal circulation with evidence of enhanced apoptosis in fetal liver [75]. In rodents, diets rich in N6 PUFA increase body weight while a diet rich in N3

PUFA decreases it [76,77]. Similarly, observational studies in humans show an inverse relationship of maternal N3 PUFA intake and birthweight for gestational age [78] and offspring adiposity at three years of age, while a higher N6:N3 ratio in the maternal diet is associated with higher child adiposity at three years of age [79], a possible precursor of a lifetime of obesity and metabolic syndrome, as shown is Figure 12.3. There is increasing interest in this area with a view to reducing the risks of childhood obesity. A randomized trial of supplementation of N3 PUFA and reduction of N6:N3 PUFA in maternal diet is currently in progress [80]. Thus the proportion and quality of fat and other macronutrients in maternal diet rather than merely the total calorie intake have important implications for the offspring, an observation that is vital in view of the current trend of easy availability and possibly increased abundance of trans fats in the human diet.

Information from animal models of maternal nutrient deprivation

Maternal nutrient restriction appears to increase PPARα, as well as UCP2, expression [81] and this could be indicative of greater white, as opposed to brown, fat deposition as both are characteristics of white adipose tissue. Similarly in a rodent model, uteroplacental insufficiency-induced growth restriction induces an increase in adipose tissue PPARγ expression and is

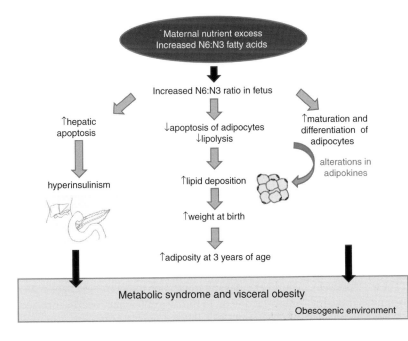

Figure 12.3. Fatty acid composition of maternal diet may influence offspring outcome. Increased N6:N3 ratio induces changes in the liver, in adipocyte differentiation, and maturation, which can increase lipid deposition in early life leading to obesity and metabolic syndrome later in adulthood.

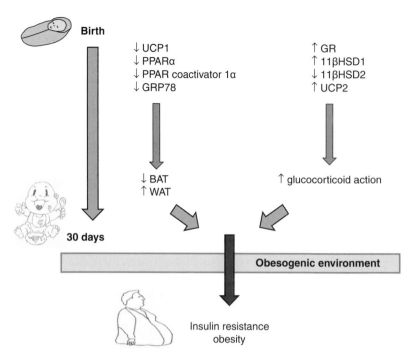

Figure 12.4. Ontogeny of ovine adipose tissue in early life – with loss of brown adipose tissue (BAT) markers, rise in white adipose tissue (WAT) markers, and an increase in glucocorticoid action. These changes interact with an obesogenic environment to produce insulin resistance and may contribute to obesity in later life. (UCP, uncoupling protein; PPARα, peroxisome proliferator-activated receptor-α; GR, glucocorticoid receptor; 11βHSD, 11-β-hydroxysteriod dehydrogenase; GRP78, glucose-regulated protein 78.)

associated with increased visceral adiposity in males [82]. At the same time, macrophage infiltration within adipose tissue could be enhanced, thereby inhibiting the actions of insulin. Changes in other markers of inflammation after birth could further facilitate such a process as the potential actions of both toll-like receptor 4 (TLR4), a component of the innate immune system that induces the paracrine loop between macrophages and adipocytes, and CD68, which is a macrophage marker, are increased over the first month of life [35]. Consequently, targeted changes of the in utero nutritional environment could contribute to early perturbations in glucose/insulin signaling as observed in the metabolic syndrome, even in the absence of any absolute changes in adipose tissue mass [35].

Gene expression for IL-18, a pro-inflammatory cytokine, is also suppressed in adolescent offspring born to nutrient-restricted sheep [35] and this could potentially reduce appetite suppression, thereby promoting positive energy balance. Offspring of nutrient-restricted sheep in late gestation have lower fat mass at birth, catch up and restore fat content by one month of age, and then go on to show increased fat mass by one year of age. This is accompanied by an increase in gene expression for both TLR4 and CD68. These responses indicate a switch in adipose tissue development in early postnatal life, which could determine later fat mass

(Figure 12.4). Ultimately, increasing fat mass accompanied by macrophage infiltration with inflammation renders adipose tissue insulin resistant and the metabolic syndrome may result, at least, if exposure to an obesogenic environment occurs [83].

Influence of gender on body composition and obesity onset

Across most mammalian species adult females possess more brown and white fat than aged-matched males [84,85]. Furthermore, as rodent females are more active than males [59], important programmed consequences in the regulation of body weight occur with female rodents usually being smaller but fatter than their male counterparts and attaining their mature body weight early in life [86]. They may therefore exhibit an important number of differences in energy balance regulation. For example, it has recently been shown that tyrosine phosphatase epsilon (RPTPe), a phosphatase which downregulates insulin receptors, acting through a resetting of hypothalamic leptin signaling, may preferentially regulate body mass in non-pregnant adult female, but not adult male, rodents [87]. This difference only becomes apparent when they are challenged with a high-fat diet or, in the case of females, ovariectomized. The extent to which castration and increasing age may cause a similar difference in males remains to be established. Further evidence for the effects of gender is now emerging. For example, when pregnant female rats and their offspring are fed a diet rich in fat, sugar, and salt, female offspring show increased adiposity with earlier onset of hyperglycemia, hyperinsulinemia, and hyperlipidemia [88], while an imbalance of N6:N3 PUFA ratio in the maternal diet increases blood pressure and serum triglyceride concentrations only in male offspring [89].

Conclusion

There has been a significant increase in maternal and childhood obesity over the past decade. Both animal experiments and human epidemiological data suggest that there is a substantial role for early life experiences in the programming of adipose tissue function and distribution. Increasing knowledge in this area may inform preventive measures to break the cycle of obesity and its accompanying adverse health and social consequences.

References

1. Sebert S P, Hyatt M A, Chan L L, *et al.*, Maternal nutrient restriction between early and midgestation and its impact upon appetite regulation after juvenile obesity. *Endocrinology*, 2009;**150**(2):634–41.

2. Symonds M E & Budge H. Nutritional models of the developmental programming of adult health and disease. *Proc Nutr Soc* 2009;**68**(2):173–8.

3. Budge H & Symonds M E. Fetal and neonatal nutrition – lipid and carbohydrate requirements and adaptations to altered supply at birth. In Kurjak A & Chervenak FA (eds.) *Textbook of Perinatal Medicine.* (CRC Press: Boca Raton, 2006), pp. 1007–16.

4. Cannon B & Nedergaard J. Developmental biology: neither fat nor flesh. *Nature* 2008;**454**(7207):947–8.

5. Cypess A M & Kahn C R. The role and importance of brown adipose tissue in energy homeostasis. *Curr Opin Pediatr* 2010;**22**(4):478–84.

6. Cypess A M & Kahn C R. Brown fat as a therapy for obesity and diabetes. *Curr Opin Endocrinol Diabetes Obes* 2010;**17**(2):143–9.

7. Power G. Biology of temperature: the mammalian fetus. *J Dev Physiol* 1989;**12**:295–304.

8. Symonds M E, Budge H, Perkins A C *et al.*, Adipose tissue development – impact of the early life environment. *Prog Biophys Mol Biol* 2011;**106**(1):300–6.

9. Symonds M E & Lomax M A. Maternal and environmental influences on thermoregulation in the neonate. *Proc Nutr Soc* 1992;**51**:165–72.

10. Seale P, Kajimura S & Spiegelman B M. Transcriptional control of brown adipocyte development and physiological function – of mice and men. *Genes Dev* 2009;**23**(7):788–97.

11. Rothwell N J & Stock M J. A role for brown adipose tissue in diet-induced thermogenesis. *Nature* 1979;**281**(5726):31–5.

12. Rothwell N J & Stock M J. Luxuskonsumption, diet-induced thermogenesis and brown fat: the case in favour. *Clin Sci (Lond)* 1983;**64**(1):19–23.

13. Symonds M E, Stephenson T, Gardner D S, *et al.* Long-term effects of nutritional programming of the embryo and fetus: mechanisms and critical windows. *Reprod Fertil Dev* 2007;**19**(1):53–63.

14. Cannon B, Connoley E, Obregon M-J, *et al.* Perinatal activation of brown adipose tissue. In Kunzel W & Jesen A (eds.) *The Endocrine Control of the Fetus.* (Berlin: Springer Verlag, 1988), pp. 306–20.

15. Symonds, M E, Mostyn A, Pearce S, *et al.* Endocrine and nutritional regulation of fetal adipose tissue development. *J Endocrinol* 2003;**179**(3):293–9.

16. Bispham J, Gopalakrishnan G S, Dandrea J, *et al.* Maternal endocrine adaptation throughout pregnancy to nutritional manipulation: consequences for maternal plasma leptin and cortisol and the programming of fetal adipose tissue development. *Endocrinology* 2003;**144**(8):3575–85.

17. Symonds M E, Sebert S P & Budge H. The impact of diet during early life and its contribution to later disease: critical checkpoints in development and their long-term consequences for metabolic health. *Proc Nutr Soc* 2009;**68**(4):416–21.

18. HAPO Study Cooperative Research Group. Hyperglycemia and Adverse Pregnancy Outcome (HAPO) Study: associations with neonatal anthropometrics. *Diabetes* 2009;**58**(2):453–9.

19. McMillen I C & Robinson J S. Developmental origins of the metabolic syndrome: prediction, plasticity, and programming. *Physiol Rev* 2005;**85**(2):571–633.

20. Roseboom T J, van der Meulen J H, Ravelli A C, *et al.* Effects of prenatal exposure to the Dutch famine on adult disease in later life: an overview. *Twin Res* 2001;**4**(5):293–8.

21. Centre for Maternal and Child Enquiries (CMACE). Maternal obesity in the UK: Findings from a national project. (London: CMACE, 2010).

22. Budge H, Bispham J, Dandrea J, *et al.* Effect of maternal nutrition on brown adipose tissue and prolactin receptor status in the fetal lamb. *Pediatr Res* 2000;**47**:781–6.

23. Gnanalingham M G, Mostyn A, Symonds M E, *et al.* Ontogeny and nutritional programming of adiposity in sheep: potential role of glucocorticoid action and

uncoupling protein-2. *Am J Physiol Regul Integr Comp Physiol* 2005;**289**(5):R1407–15.

24. Tang W, Zeve D, Suh J M, *et al*. White fat progenitor cells reside in the adipose vasculature. *Science* 2008;**322**(5901):583–6.

25. Spalding K L, Arner E, Westermark P O, *et al*. Dynamics of fat cell turnover in humans. *Nature* 2008;**453**(7196):783–7.

26. Symonds M E, Mostyn A & Stephenson T. Cytokines and cytokine-receptors in fetal growth and development. *Biochem Soc Trans* 2001;**29**:33–7.

27. Budge H, Dandrea J, Mostyn A, *et al*. Differential effects of fetal number and maternal nutrition in late gestation on prolactin receptor abundance and adipose tissue development in the neonatal lamb. *Pediatr Res* 2003;**53**(2):302–8.

28. Clarke L, Buss D S, Juniper D T, *et al*. Adipose tissue development during early postnatal life in ewe-reared lambs. *Exp Physiol* 1997;**82**(6):1015–27.

29. Lean M E. Brown adipose tissue in humans. *Proc Nutr Soc* 1989;**48**(2):243–56.

30. Seale P, Bjork B, Yang W, *et al*. PRDM16 controls a brown fat/skeletal muscle switch. *Nature* 2008;**454**(7207):961–7.

31. Gilsanz V, Chung S A, Jackson H, *et al*. Functional brown adipose tissue is related to muscle volume in children and adolescents. *J Pediatr* 2011;**158**(5):722–6.

32. Yuen B S, Owens P C, Muhlhausler B S, *et al*. Leptin alters the structural and functional characteristics of adipose tissue before birth. *FASEB J* 2003;**17**(9):1102–4.

33. Symonds M E, Pearce S, Bispham J, *et al*. Timing of nutrient restriction and programming of fetal adipose tissue development. *Proc Nutr Soc* 2004;**63**(3):397–403.

34. Lomax M A, Sadiq F, Karamanlidis G, *et al*. Ontogenic loss of brown adipose tissue sensitivity to beta-adrenergic stimulation in the ovine. *Endocrinology* 2007;**148**(1):461–8.

35. Sharkey D, Symonds M E & Budge H. Adipose tissue inflammation: developmental ontogeny and consequences of gestational nutrient restriction in offspring. *Endocrinology* 2009;**150**(8):3913–20.

36. Mostyn A, Wilson V, Dandrea J, *et al*. Ontogeny and nutritional manipulation of mitochondrial protein abundance in adipose tissue and the lungs of postnatal sheep. *Br J Nutr* 2003;**90**(2):323–8.

37. Stewart F M, Freeman D J, Ramsay J E. *et al*. Longitudinal assessment of maternal endothelial function and markers of inflammation and placental function throughout pregnancy in lean and obese mothers. *J Clin Endocrinol Metab* 2007;**92**(3):969–75.

38. Sullivan E L, Smith M S & Grove K L. Perinatal exposure to high-fat diet programs energy balance, metabolism and behavior in adulthood. *Neuroendocrinology* 2011;**93**(1):1–8.

39. Bamberger C M, Schulte H M & Chrousos G P. Molecular determinants of glucocorticoid receptor function and tissue sensitivity to glucocorticoids. *Endocr Rev* 1996;**17**(3):245–61.

40. Stewart P M & Krozowski Z S. 11 beta-Hydroxysteroid dehydrogenase. *Vitam Horm* 1999;**57**:249–324.

41. Gnanalingham M G, Mostyn A, Dandrea J, *et al*. Ontogeny and nutritional programming of uncoupling protein-2 (UCP2) and glucocorticoid receptor (GCR) mRNA in the ovine lung. *J Physiol* 2005;**565**(1):159–69.

42. Sebert S P, Dellschaft N S, Chan L L, *et al*. Maternal nutrient restriction during late gestation and early postnatal growth in sheep differentially reset the control of energy metabolism in the gastric mucosa. *Endocrinology* 2011;**152**(7):2816–26.

43. Engeli S, Bohnke J, Feldpausch M, *et al*. Regulation of 11beta-HSD genes in human adipose tissue: influence of central obesity and weight loss. *Obes Res* 2004;**12**(1):9–17.

44. Paulmyer-Lacroix O, Boullu S, Oliver C, *et al*. Expression of the mRNA coding for 11beta-hydroxysteroid dehydrogenase type 1 in adipose tissue from obese patients: an in situ hybridization study. *J Clin Endocrinol Metab* 2002;**87**(6):2701–5.

45. Taylor P D, Khan I Y, Lakasing L, *et al*. Uterine artery function in pregnant rats fed a diet supplemented with animal lard. *Exp Physiol* 2003;**88**(3):389–98.

46. Grayson B E, Kievit P, Smith M S, *et al*. Critical determinants of hypothalamic appetitive neuropeptide development and expression: species considerations. *Front Neuroendocrinol* 2010;**31**(1):16–31.

47. Clarke L, Heasman L & Symonds M E. Influence of maternal dexamethasone administration on thermoregulation in lambs delivered by caesarean section. *J Endocrinol* 1998;**156**:307–14.

48. Gnanalingham M, Hyatt M, Bispham J, *et al*. Maternal dexamethasone administration and the maturation of perirenal adipose tissue of the neonatal sheep. *Organogenesis* 2008;**4**(3):188–94.

49. Bouret S G. Early life origins of obesity: role of hypothalamic programming. *J Pediatr Gastroenterol Nutr* 2009;**48**(Suppl 1):S31–8.

50. Gorski J N, Dunn-Meynell A A & Levin B E. Maternal obesity increases hypothalamic leptin receptor expression and sensitivity in juvenile obesity-prone rats. *Am J Physiol Regul Integr Comp Physiol* 2007;**292**(5):R1782–91.

51. Kirk S L, Samuelsson A M, Argenton M, *et al*. Maternal obesity induced by diet in rats permanently influences central processes regulating food intake in offspring. *PLoS One* 2009;**4**(6):e5870.

52. Ferezou-Viala J, Roy A F, Serougne C, *et al.* Long-term consequences of maternal high-fat feeding on hypothalamic leptin sensitivity and diet-induced obesity in the offspring. *Am J Physiol Regul Integr Comp Physiol* 2007;**293**(3):R1056–62.

53. Ainge H, Thompson C, Ozanne S E, *et al.* A systematic review on animal models of maternal high fat feeding and offspring glycaemic control. *Int J Obes (Lond)* 2011;**35**(3):325–35.

54. McMillen I C, Adam C L & Muhlhausler B S. Early origins of obesity: programming the appetite regulatory system. *J Physiol* 2005;**565**(Pt 1):9–17.

55. Reddy J K & Hashimoto T. Peroxisomal beta-oxidation and peroxisome proliferator-activated receptor alpha: an adaptive metabolic system. *Annu Rev Nutr* 2001;**21**:193–230.

56. Altiok S, Xu M & Spiegelman B M. PPARgamma induces cell cycle withdrawal: inhibition of E2F/DP DNA-binding activity via down-regulation of PP2A. *Genes Dev* 1997;**11**(15):1987–98.

57. Fasshauer M, Klein J, Kriauciunas K M, *et al.* Essential role of insulin receptor substrate 1 in differentiation of brown adipocytes. *Mol Cell Biol* 2001;**21**(1):319–29.

58. Miki H, Yamauchi T, Suzuki R, *et al.* Essential role of insulin receptor substrate 1 (IRS-1) and IRS-2 in adipocyte differentiation. *Mol Cell Biol* 2001;**21**(7):2521–32.

59. Symonds M E, Sebert S & Budge H. The obesity epidemic: from the environment to epigenetics – not simply a response to dietary manipulation in a thermoneutral environment. *Frontiers in Epigenomics* 2011;**2**, doi:10.3389/fgene.2011.00024.

60. Minge C E, Bennett B D, Norman R J, *et al.* Peroxisome proliferator-activated receptor-gamma agonist rosiglitazone reverses the adverse effects of diet-induced obesity on oocyte quality. *Endocrinology* 2008;**149**(5):2646–56.

61. Shankar K, Harrell A, Liu X, *et al.* Maternal obesity at conception programs obesity in the offspring. *Am J Physiol Regul Integr Comp Physiol* 2008;**294**(2):R528–38.

62. Shankar K, Kang P, Harrell A, *et al.*, Maternal overweight programs insulin and adiponectin signaling in the offspring. *Endocrinology* 2010;**151**(6):2577–89.

63. Symonds M E, Heasman L, Clarke L, *et al.* Maternal nutrition and disproportionate placental to fetal growth. *Biochem Soc Trans* 1998;**26**:91–6.

64. Wang J, Ma H, Tong C, *et al.* Overnutrition and maternal obesity in sheep pregnancy alter the JNK-IRS-1 signaling cascades and cardiac function in the fetal heart. *FASEB J* 2010;**24**(6):2066–76.

65. Samuelsson A M, Matthews P A, Argenton M, *et al.* Diet-induced obesity in female mice leads to offspring hyperphagia, adiposity, hypertension, and insulin resistance: a novel murine model of developmental programming. *Hypertension* 2008;**51**(2):383–92.

66. Massiera F, Barbry P, Guesnet P, *et al.* A Western-like fat diet is sufficient to induce a gradual enhancement in fat mass over generations. *J Lipid Res* 2010;**51**(8):2352–61.

67. Lieb W, Pencina M J, Lanier K J, *et al.* Association of parental obesity with concentrations of select systemic biomarkers in nonobese offspring: the Framingham Heart Study. *Diabetes* 2009;**58**(1):134–7.

68. Weisberg S P, McCann D, Desai M, *et al.* Obesity is associated with macrophage accumulation in adipose tissue. *J Clin Invest* 2003;**112**(12):1796–808.

69. Wellen K E & Hotamisligil G S. Obesity-induced inflammatory changes in adipose tissue. *J Clin Invest* 2003;**112**(12):1785–8.

70. Yessoufou A, Moutairou K & Khan N A. A model of insulin resistance in mice, born to diabetic pregnancy, is associated with alterations of transcription-related genes in pancreas and epididymal adipose tissue. *J Obes* 2011;**2011**:654–967.

71. Buckley A J, Keseru B, Briody J, *et al.* Altered body composition and metabolism in the male offspring of high fat-fed rats. *Metabolism*, 2005;**54**(4):500–7.

72. Korotkova M, Gabrielsson B, Hanson L A, *et al.* Maternal essential fatty acid deficiency depresses serum leptin levels in suckling rat pups. *J Lipid Res* 2001;**42**(3):359–65.

73. Egger G & Dixon J. Inflammatory effects of nutritional stimuli: further support for the need for a big picture approach to tackling obesity and chronic disease. *Obes Rev* 2010;**11**(2):137–49.

74. Kim H K, Della-Fera M, Lin J, *et al.* Docosahexaenoic acid inhibits adipocyte differentiation and induces apoptosis in 3T3-L1 preadipocytes. *J Nutr* 2006;**136**(12):2965–9.

75. Grant W F, Gillingham M B, Batra A K, *et al.* Maternal high fat diet is associated with decreased plasma n-3 fatty acids and fetal hepatic apoptosis in nonhuman primates. *PLoS One* 2011;**6**(2):e17261.

76. Korotkova M, Gabrielsson B, Lonn M, *et al.* Leptin levels in rat offspring are modified by the ratio of linoleic to alpha-linolenic acid in the maternal diet. *J Lipid Res* 2002;**43**(10):1743–9.

77. Massiera F, Saint-Marc P, Seydoux J, *et al.* Arachidonic acid and prostacyclin signaling promote adipose tissue development: a human health concern? *J Lipid Res* 2003;**44**(2):271–9.

78. Oken E, Kleinman K P, Olsen S F, *et al.* Associations of seafood and elongated n-3 fatty acid intake with

fetal growth and length of gestation: results from a US pregnancy cohort. *Am J Epidemiol* 2004;**160**(8):774–83.

79. Donahue S M, Rifas-Shiman S L, Gold D R, *et al.* Prenatal fatty acid status and child adiposity at age 3 y: results from a US pregnancy cohort. *Am J Clin Nutr* 2011;**93**(4):780–8.

80. Hauner H, Vollhardt C, Schneider K T, *et al.* The impact of nutritional fatty acids during pregnancy and lactation on early human adipose tissue development. Rationale and design of the INFAT study. *Ann Nutr Metab* 2009;**54**(2):97–103.

81. Bispham J, Gardner D S, Gnanalingham M G, *et al.* Maternal nutritional programming of fetal adipose tissue development: differential effects on messenger ribonucleic acid abundance for uncoupling proteins and peroxisome proliferator-activated and prolactin receptors. *Endocrinology* 2005;**146**(9):3943–9.

82. Joss-Moore L A, Wang Y, Campbell M S, *et al.* Uteroplacental insufficiency increases visceral adiposity and visceral adipose PPARgamma2 expression in male rat offspring prior to the onset of obesity. *Early Hum Dev* 2010;**86**(3):179–85.

83. Budge H, Sebert S, Sharkey D, *et al.* Session on 'Obesity'. Adipose tissue development, nutrition in early life and its impact on later obesity. *Proc Nutr Soc* 2009;**68**(3):321–6.

84. Pearce S, Casteilla L, Gualillo O, *et al.* Differential effects of age and gender on the postnatal

responsiveness of brown adipose tissue to prolactin administration in rats. *Exp Physiol* 2003;**88**(4):527–31.

85. Au-Yong I T, Thorn N, Ganatra R, *et al.* Brown adipose tissue and seasonal variation in humans. *Diabetes* 2009;**58**(11):2583–7.

86. Symonds M E. Integration of physiological and molecular mechanisms of the developmental origins of adult disease: new concepts and insights. *Proc Nutr Soc* 2007;**66**(3):442–50.

87. Rousso-Noori L, Knobler H, Levy-Apter E, *et al.* Protein tyrosine phosphatase epsilon affects body weight by downregulating leptin signaling in a phosphorylation-dependent manner. *Cell Metab* 2011;**13**(5):562–72.

88. Bayol S A, Simbi B H, Bertrand J A, *et al.* Offspring from mothers fed a 'junk food' diet in pregnancy and lactation exhibit exacerbated adiposity that is more pronounced in females. *J Physiol* 2008;**586**(13):3219–30.

89. Korotkova M, Gabrielsson B G, Holmang A, *et al.* Gender-related long-term effects in adult rats by perinatal dietary ratio of n-6/n-3 fatty acids. *Am J Physiol Regul Integr Comp Physiol* 2005;**288**(3):R575–9.

90. Fowden A L, Harding R, Ralph M M, *et al.* Nutritional control of respiratory and other muscular activities in relation to plasma prostaglandin E in the fetal sheep. *J Dev Physiol* 1989;**11**(4):253–62.

Chapter

13

Maternal diet and nutritional status and risk of obesity in the child: the role of epigenetic mechanisms

Melissa A. Suter and Kjersti M. Aagaard-Tillery

Introduction

Other chapters in this volume address the possibilities that maternal gestational weight gain, maternal obesity, and gestational diabetes influence the risk of obesity in the developing offspring through adverse influences of the intrauterine environment during periods of developmental plasticity. In this chapter we review the literature, which suggests that epigenetic modulation of gene expression is likely to serve as one of the more promiscuous molecular mechanisms with which these maternal and early developmental footprints are cast. Together with other potential mechanisms (e.g., establishment and perturbation of the microbiome) layered epigenomic regulation, genomic instability, and molecular and developmental biology are altering our understanding as to how the developmental origins of obesity and associated metabolic disease take their roots.

Epigenetic modifications and the developmental origins of health and disease

While genomic DNA is the template of our heredity, it is the coordination and regulation of its expression that results in the wide complexity and diversity seen among organisms. In the "postgenomic era," investigators have begun to appreciate higher order architectural features of the genome, which include not only single nucleotide variance in gene regulatory regions (e.g., single nucleotide polymorphisms, or SNPs), but also genomic structural variation (i.e., copy number imbalance through large insertions or deletions). Collectively, structural rearrangements acting in concert with allelic

polymorphisms contribute to the *genomic* landscape from which disease phenotypes arise.

It is becoming increasingly evident that *epigenomics* plays an equally important and possibly more prevalent role in the development of common and complex diseases [1,2]. The term, first coined by Conrad Waddington, refers to "the interactions between genes and their products which bring phenotype into being" [1]. In sum, it is the study of how changes in gene activity during development cause specific phenotypes to emerge over the lifetime of the individual [1,2]. Epigenetic mechanisms are believed to be stably inherited during cell division, and yet modifiable by interaction with the environment [1]. The epigenetic code is "written" on top of the DNA sequence, and may act as a mechanism to provide a memory of previous gene expression. Epigenetic mechanisms identified and well characterized at the molecular level include DNA methylation of CpG dinucleotides, post-translational histone modifications, and RNA-associated gene silencing. While alterations in CpG methylation and histone modifications have been characterized with respect to an obesogenic phenotype, there remains a dearth of information on the role RNA-associated gene silencing plays in the development of obesity. Epigenetics has also been implicated in learning and memory [3], cancer transformation [4], and, most relevant to this chapter, the developmental origins of health and disease.

The drastic increase in the worldwide incidence of obesity in the past three decades cannot be explained by changes in the genome [5]. Although the study of specific alleles has yielded many genetic candidates implicated in the etiology of obesity, changes in human genotype do not occur at such a rapid rate to account for the increased prevalence of obesity worldwide.

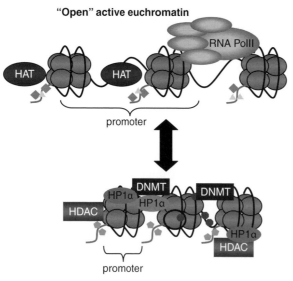

"Open" active euchromatin

HAT

HAT

RNA PolII

promoter

◆ H3K4me3
▲ H3K14ac
⬟ H3K9me3
● DNA methylation

DNMT

HP1α
HP1α

DNMT

HDAC

HP1α

HDAC

promoter

"Closed" silenced heterochromatin

Figure 13.1. Characteristics of chromatin structure. Chromatin is organized into euchromatin, which is associated with active gene expression, and tightly compacted heterochromatin, which is associated with gene silencing. Histone modifications such as lysine acetylation (H3K14ac) and H3K4me3 are traditionally associated with euchromatin. Heterochromatin is traditionally enriched for H3K9me3 and DNA methylation as well as other non-histone-associated chromatin proteins such as HP1α. (See figure in color plate section.)

Environmental influences must be paramount, and recent attention has focused on prenatal influences. The idea that in utero experiences can influence post-natal phenotypes is not novel. However, the idea that experiences in utero are involved in the etiology of obesity and metabolic syndrome in adulthood provides a potential mechanism to help explain the alarming increase and anticipation in the rate and onset of obesity, and is quickly becoming an integral field for mechanistic studies.

Epigenetic modifications

Chromatin structure

During the mitotic phase of the cell cycle, chromosomes are in their most condensed form. The cell uses many mechanisms to maintain compaction and organization of the information contained in DNA. In all eukaryotic organisms, the most fundamental level of DNA organization occurs at the level of the nucleosome. Two copies of four histone proteins, H2A, H2B, H3, and H4, constitute the histone octamer. Around this octamer, DNA wraps approximately 1.7 times to form the nucleosome [6]. DNA replication, transcription, and damage repair all must contend with these potential spatial inhibitions in the chromatin structure.

While nucleosomes represent the "building blocks" for the formation of higher order chromatin structure, histones maintain an epigenetic code that has a role in the regulation of gene expression, DNA replication, recombination, and repair [7–9]. Each of these processes has been demonstrated in eukaryotic models to employ post-translational modifications of chromatin structure in their regulation. As schematically depicted in Figure 13.1, histones have a protruding charged 15–38 amino acid N-terminus ("histone tail"), which helps dictate nucleosome assembly into higher order chromatin structure. The ability to store information appears to reside in the amino-terminal histone tails of the four core histones, which are exposed on the nucleosome surface and are subject to enzyme-catalyzed post-translational modifications of select amino acids, including lysine acetylation, lysine and arginine methylation, serine or threonine phosphorylation, lysine ubiquitination, lysine sumoylation, or glutamine ADP ribosylation (reviewed further below). Although the histone tail modifications have been the most highly characterized, the globular (i.e., non-"tail") portion of the histones also contain amino acid residues, which are subject to modification.

The study of epigenetic modifications in the development of obesity is a new and burgeoning field. Using animal models of maternal obesity, changes in fetal phenotype are being characterized [10,11]. Changes in fetal hepatic histone modifications associated with maternal high-fat diet have recently been discovered [12,13]. However, before we can begin to understand the implications of these epigenetic changes, more work remains to be done.

Histone modifications

Chromatin is organized within the eukaryotic genome into nucleosomes. The histones that form the nucleosome core are subject to various post-translational modifications such as phosphorylation, acetylation, methylation, and ubiquitylation. These modifications are essential for proper heterochromatin formation, gene silencing, gene expression, and DNA damage repair. Although most modifications characterized occur within the N-terminal domains of H3 and H4, which extrude from the nucleosome surface, some reside within the histone globular domains within the nucleosome core. Methylation of distinct lysine and arginine residues along with hypoacetylation of lysine residues are markers of transcriptionally silent genes [8–9]. Together, these data suggest that histone modifications are extremely dynamic and highly regulated, and are therefore likely to play an essential role in environmentally-induced disease susceptibility. Their role in the developmental origins of adult disease is currently an important issue in biomedical research.

Although highly studied [7,14], the role of these histone modifications is still poorly understood. Modifications may recruit downstream effectors such as DNA damage repair proteins, transcription factors, and heterochromatin-associated factors. Like DNA methylation, these modifications are inherited through subsequent cell cycles and are modifiable with interaction with the environment. Similarly, although specific modifications are associated with specific chromatin states, there are many exceptions to the rule. Histone modifications are dynamic. Cells have enzymes that can acetylate histones as well as enzymes that remove the acetyl group. Therefore post-translational modifications added to the histone proteins are, in effect, reversible.

Histone lysines can be mono-, di-, or trimethylated. Methylation of histone H3 lysine 4 (H3K4) has been highly characterized from yeast to man. Through the high-throughput analysis afforded by chromatin immunoprecipitation (ChIP) followed by massively parallel sequencing (ChIP-seq), the localization of each form of methylated H3K4 has been mapped in *Saccharomyces cerevisiae* and mammalian cells [21]. Localization of trimethylation of H3K4 (H3K4me3) appears to be evolutionarily conserved. H3K4me3 maps to the 5′ end of active genes and shows correlation with PolII localization and gene activation. However, mono- and dimethylation do not share the same pattern in yeast and mammals. Methylation of histones, per se, does not necessarily correlate with gene activation. Trimethylation of lysine 9 of histone H3 (H3K9me3) as well as H3K27 trimethylation both appear to localize to silenced genes [22].

Localization of acetylated histones has also been characterized throughout the genome. Most studies have focused on acetylation of both lysines 9 and 14 of histone H3 (H3K9/14ac) or acetylation of the four lysines within the H4 histone "tail" (K5, 8, 12, 16) [22]. Similar to H3K4me3, acetylated histones are found near the transcription start site of active genes [23]. Acetylated histones are also found within the coding regions of active genes. Where histone methylation can be associated with either silenced or active genes (depending on the lysine residue methylated) histone acetylation is generally associated only with active genes [23].

DNA methylation

The contribution of DNA methylation to gene expression is still not fully understood. In mammals, DNA is methylated on the C5 position of cytosine residues. This is most prevalent for "CpG dinucleotides," or a cytosine residue immediately 5′ to a guanine. Although 70% to 80% of CpGs within the adult mammalian genome are methylated, the methylation status of cytosines within the largely unmethylated "CpG islands" is of great interest in relation to gene expression [14]. CpG islands are GC-rich stretches of the genome, which traditionally lie within the promoter and upstream enhancer region of genes. Alterations of methylation within these CpG islands are associated with changes in gene expression. Such alterations may be of upmost importance to cell survival, as genome-wide changes in DNA methylation are reported in various cancers [15]. However, whether these methylation changes are implicated in the cause of cancer or an effect thereof, remains to be elucidated. DNA methylation patterns are heritable through the mitotic cell cycle; following DNA replication the newly synthesized strand will re-establish the methylation patterns of the parental strand. However, these patterns can be altered by environmental exposures throughout the life of the cell. It is therefore a good candidate for study of epigenetic reprogramming in the developmental origins of health and disease.

DNA methylation during germ cell formation, fertilization, and development has been well characterized in the mouse model system. Although both the

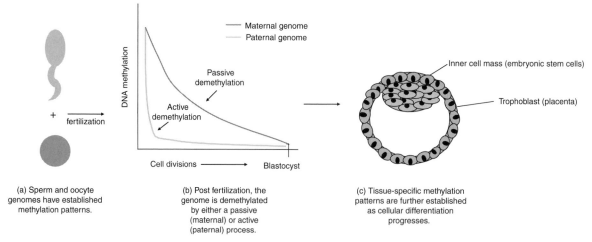

Figure 13.2. Establishment of DNA methylation in a fertilized egg. Sperm and egg genomes are methylated before fertilization. After fertilization the genome is demethylated, excluding imprinted genes. The paternal genome is demethylated in an active process, of which the molecular mechanisms remain unknown. The maternal genome is demethylated in a passive manner, through cell-cycle replication without methylation of the newly synthesized strand. Once the embryo reaches the blastocyst stage the methylation patterns of the trophoblast begin to change from that of the inner cell mass. The trophoblast gives rise to the placental tissue and the cells within the inner cell mass will establish distinct methylation patterns as they begin to differentiate. (See figure in color plate section.)

paternal and maternal genomes within a fertilized zygote are demethylated, the time frame and mechanism of the demethylation are completely different. The paternal genome is demethylated in an active, replication-independent process within hours of fertilization (Figure 13.2) [16]. The maternal genome undergoes a passive, replication-dependent demethylation with the progression of the mitotic cell cycle [17]. The exact mechanism of paternal genome demethylation, and subsequently how the maternal genome avoids this demethylation, is still under investigation. Following this rapid demethylation, methylation patterns are re-established, which appears to be essential for proper development.

Genome-wide methylation patterns contribute to cellular pluripotency [18]. As differentiation of cells begins after implantation, *de novo* methylation occurs in a gene-specific fashion. Promoter methylation aids in silencing pluripotency-associated genes such as *Oct4*, while demethylation occurs to allow genes that have not been expressed in development to be expressed in adulthood (see review in [18]).

As well as an established role in gene regulation during development, DNA methylation is essential in maintaining proper expression of imprinted genes. About 80 genes in humans and mice are regulated by genomic imprinting [19]. Imprinted genes are expressed in a parent-of-origin specific pattern and

are established in the germ line. Because primordial germ cells undergo active demethylation, the parent-of-origin specific methylation patterns must be re-established later in development. For male germ cells, imprinted regions are established in fetal stages, while patterns in female gametes are established after birth [19]. Imprinted genes are traditionally clustered in large chromosomal regions and parent-of-origin expression is dependent on specific methylation patterns in imprinting control regions [19].

Imprinting disorders and obesity

Imprinting

Mendelian genetics led scientists to hypothesize that each copy of a specific gene is equally expressed from the paternal and maternal genomes. The discovery of IGF-2, a gene that is expressed in a parent-of-origin-specific fashion, alerted scientists to the fact that some genes are marked for differential expression between the paternal and maternal genomes [24]. Proper establishment of imprinted genes is essential for proper embryonic development [25]. Importantly, the establishment of the parent-of-origin specificity for imprinting is through methylation of CpG sites within imprinting control regions on the relevant chromosomes [26]. Prader–Willi syndrome is an imprinting

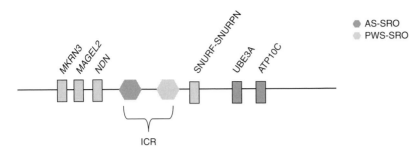

Figure 13.3. The imprinted region on chromosome 15 implicated in Prader–Willi syndrome. On chromosome 15 there is an imprinted region that contains genes that are expressed from either the maternally (pink) or paternally (blue) inherited chromosome. Parent-of-origin expression is controlled by an imprinting control region. Alterations of expression of UBE3A distinctly correlates with Angelman syndrome.

Alterations in expression of the four paternally expressed genes has been implicated in the development of Prader–Willi syndrome. (See figure in color plate section.)

disorder, which yields striking evidence for epigenetic mechanisms in the etiology of obesity.

Prader–Willi syndrome and obesity

Prader–Willi syndrome is a developmental disorder characterized by low birthweight followed by hyperphagia and obesity in childhood [27]. Prader–Willi syndrome arises from a disruption of a parent-of-origin expression of alleles located within a 2 Megabase (MB) region of chromosome 15 (15q11q13) [27]. Mapping and characterization of this region has helped to elucidate the epigenetic mechanisms involved in the etiology of Prader–Willi syndrome.

Within this 2 MB region lies a cluster of imprinted genes. Two of these genes, *UBE3A* and *ATP10C*, are expressed exclusively from the maternally-derived chromosome [27]. Disruption of expression of *UBE3A* from the maternal chromosome is responsible for development of the developmental disorder Angelman syndrome, in which obesity is not part of the phenotype. However, the specific genes or chromosome region responsible for Prader–Willi syndrome is not as well defined. Prader–Willi syndrome results from loss of expression of the paternally derived genes within this chromosomal region (Figure 13.3), and control of expression of these genes is in part regulated by an imprinting control region. Expression of the paternally-derived genes *MKRN3*, *NDN*, and *SNURF-SNRPN* is regulated through DNA methylation; the promoter region of these genes is unmethylated on the paternally-derived chromosome and methylated and therefore silenced on the maternally-derived chromosome [27]. Although many *genetic* anomalies can account for loss of parent-of-origin expression, including deletion of this region from the paternally-derived chromosome, or maternal

uniparental disomy of chromosome 15, Prader–Willi syndrome has also been found to be caused by aberrant DNA methylation within the imprinting control region on chromosome 15 [27–29]. Therefore alteration of an epigenetic modification (DNA methylation) is involved in the development of Prader–Willi syndrome, a disorder characterized by both hyperphagia and obesity.

The Prader–Willi syndrome associated region on chromosome 15 is not the only imprinted region implicated in the etiology of obesity. Aberrant DNA methylation within the differentially methylated region of the *GNAS* gene on chromosome 20 (20q13.11) is associated with development of pseudohypoparathyroidism type 1b (PHP1b) [30]. Familial PHP1b is a maternally transmitted syndrome characterized by obesity and resistance to parathyroid hormone and thyroid stimulating hormone [30]. However, sporadic cases of PHP1b have been reported due to a loss of methylation within the differentially methylated region of the maternally derived chromosome, with no apparent genetic changes [31, 32]. Again, alterations of DNA methylation patterns (imprinting) without a known genetic abnormality are associated with an obesogenic phenotype. However, it is not known if aberrant imprinting is implicated in the current obesity epidemic [33].

Summary

Prader–Willi syndrome is a developmental disorder caused by aberrant DNA methylation within the imprinting control region on chromosome 15. Patients with Prader–Willi syndrome exhibit hyperphagia and obesity, linking epigenetic alterations (i.e., loss of a specific DNA methylation pattern) with the development of obesity.

The in utero environment, epigenetic changes, and obesity

Metastable epialleles: further evidence for an epigenetic link to obesity

A unique mouse model system, the Agouti yellow mouse, is helping to further the understanding of in utero exposures and the adult onset of obesity at a molecular level. These mice contain a "metastable epiallele" and a distinct phenotypic readout. A metastable epiallele is an allele which is differentially expressed in genetically identical individuals, due to changes in the surrounding DNA methylation [34]. Evidence derived from the study of these metastable epialleles shows that DNA methylation in the offspring can be altered due to maternal dietary constraints. Furthermore, these specific epigenetic changes are associated with increased incidence of obesity in adulthood. These unique epialleles offer a molecular approach to determining the epigenetic changes that correlate with obvious phenotypic readouts.

Seventy to eighty percent of CpGs within the genome are methylated. Specifically, repetitive elements found throughout the genome are traditionally packaged into heterochromatin, complete with hypermethylation of the CpGs to silence these genomic regions. Metastable epialleles, however, are repeat regions that are not fully methylated. Methylation of the viable yellow Agouti (A^{vy}) allele, a well-characterized metastable epiallele, has been used to study epigenetic alterations in offspring due to altered in utero environments.

The A^{vy} allele arose from the insertion of a murine transposon immediately upstream of the transcription start site of the Agouti gene. The Agouti gene codes for a paracrine signaling molecule, which causes follicular melanocytes to produce a yellow rather than black pigment. This element contains a promoter whose differential methylation status regulates constitutive transcription (see review [35]). Specifically, methylation status of nine critical CpG sites within this promoter determine the expression level of the Agouti gene and expression is inversely correlated with methylation: increased methylation silences transcription while lack of methylation promotes transcription. Expression from the Agouti locus can then be measured by the simple phenotypic output of coat color of the mouse. When the promoter is hypermethylated the gene is silenced, and the mouse has a brown coat color (pseudoagouti). When unmethylated, the mouse has a yellow coat color. Partial methylation results in an intermediate coat color; mottled yellow-brown, due to the expression in some cells while others are silenced. Expression of the Agouti gene is also correlated with an increase in body weight in mice.

Experiments with mice containing the A^{vy} allele have shown direct evidence of alterations in maternal diet leading to increased body weight of the offspring, concomitant with methylation changes in the fetal Agouti promoter [36–39]. Supplementation of the maternal diet with methyl donors essential for the one carbon metabolism pathway, such as folic acid and vitamin B_{12}, increases promoter methylation in the offspring A^{vy} locus, silencing transcription. Offspring exposed to methyl donor supplementation in utero show a darker coat color and decreased body weight compared to offspring of mothers who did not receive the supplementation [36,37]. Methyl donor supplementation has even been shown to prevent a transgenerational inheritance of obesity in the Agouti model [38].

Methylation of this locus was also altered if the maternal diet was supplemented with genestein, the major phytoestrogen in soy, leading to a shift towards psuedoagouti and protection of the offspring from developing obesity [39]. It was recently reported that these metastable epialleles also show variable histone modifications between yellow and pseudoagouti [40]. In mice where the gene is silenced (pseudoagouti) the promoter region shows an increase in H4K20me3. The promoter region of mice with an active Agouti gene show an increase in levels of H3K9/14ac, as well as acetylated H4 (K5, 8, 12, and 19). No differences of H3K4me3 levels were seen [40].

Metastable epialleles and in utero environmental exposures

The Agouti mouse model has been useful to determine the epigenetic mechanisms associated with obesity due to exposure to the endocrine disruptor bisphenol A (BPA), a compound found, until recently, in many plastics including those used for infant feeding. Reports have linked in utero exposure to BPA with increased adiposity and weight in the offspring in rodent models [41–43]. In mice subjected to antenatal BPA exposure (low dose, chronic exposure), the offspring A^{vy} allele was hypomethylated in three different germ layers. The level of methylation changes could be reversed to that of controls with supplementation of the maternal diet with methyl donors such as folic acid or genestein [44].

Summary

Site-specific changes in DNA methylation occur in response to varying in utero environments. In utero exposure to maternal dietary supplements, genestein, or endocrine-disrupting chemicals such as BPA can lead to altered DNA methylation and histone modification enrichment within specific metastable epiallales. This altered methylation status is associated with the adult onset of obesity in offspring exposed in utero.

Exposure to famine: the Dutch "Hunger Winter" of 1944–45

Studies of the Dutch famine have greatly increased our understanding of the effects of in utero exposure to maternal diet constraints on birthweight and adult metabolic diseases. Unlike most famines, the Dutch famine occurred during a defined time period. In late 1944 and early 1945, areas of northern and western Holland were subject to a Nazi-imposed embargo on food supplies entering the region. Combined with the embargo, canals were frozen further halting the flow of food supplies to the Dutch inhabitants. During this famine, the average citizen's daily calorie ration was approximately 500 calories per day, causing upwards of 18 000 people to die of starvation during the Hunger Winter [20]. Yet, throughout the famine, the Dutch health care system did not fail. Meticulous records were kept on patients, including women who were pregnant during this time of starvation. Because of this, the period when the fetus was exposed to starvation (periconceptually, early gestation, late gestation) can be reliably established and has been the subject of the sentinel studies further discussed in this volume. Now that these individuals are far into adulthood, researchers have been able to determine phenotypic outcome based on in utero exposure to starvation, using siblings who were not exposed to the famine as a control.

Studies have shown that people exposed to the Dutch famine in utero were more likely to have glucose intolerance, obesity, and an artherogenic/athlerosclerotic lipid profile, compared with unexposed siblings [45,46]. Individuals exposed early in gestation do not show a change in birthweight compared with unexposed individuals, and yet show a three-fold increase in coronary heart disease in adulthood [45].

Similar findings of a predisposition to adult metabolic disease have been found studying individuals exposed in utero and early childhood to famine in Nigeria. Famine struck millions of Biafran peoples during the Nigerian Civil War (1967–1970). Forty years following the famine, individuals exposed to the famine prenatally are showing hypertension, impaired glucose tolerance, increased waist circumference, and overweight phenotypes compared with individuals born after the famine [47].

These adult phenotypes beg the question of how the memory of in utero experience is maintained. Among the many hypotheses offered to explain the longevity of famine exposure memory are epigenetic mechanisms. Are certain marks set in utero which help to program the emergence of a phenotype 40 to 50 years after the environmental exposure? As genomic and epigenomic technologies are expanding at a rapid pace, the ability to further delve into this hypothesis is becoming more feasible.

The first report of epigenetic changes in adults exposed in utero to the Dutch famine was changes in the site-specific methylation patterns of insulin growth factor-2 (*IGF-2*). *IGF-2* is a maternally-imprinted gene with a well-characterized differentially methylated region in the promoter. Periconceptual famine exposure is associated with hypomethylation of five CpG sites within the *IGF-2* differentially methylated region when compared with unexposed siblings [48]. In a follow-up to this study, the methylation status of 15 genes was probed in the same cohort to determine if changes in DNA methylation are seen throughout the genome. Six out of fifteen loci showed a difference in methylation associated with famine exposure [49]. Of these six genes, DNA methylation was increased in the imprinted genes *GNASAS* and *MEG3* and the non-imprinted *IL10*, *ABCA1*, and *LEP* proximal promoters. A decrease in promoter methylation was found for the gene *INSIGF*. These studies show that DNA methylation patterns in adults exposed to famine in utero differ from their unexposed siblings 60 years later [49].

As a third and recent study examining the role of methylation as an arbitrator or predictor of later-in-life disease, Godfrey *et al.* recently employed MassARRAY® technology to screen for the methylation status of 68 CpGs in the 5′ upstream region in gDNA extracted from umbilical cord tissue in apparently healthy neonates from two large-scale prospective cohorts [50]. Each cohort was followed for nine years, and they ultimately identified highly variable meCpG site-specific variation, which tracked with adiposity variance, and then related that to maternal diet and additional subject variables (gender, birthweight, gestational age) in regression analyses. Of note, the investigators observed an association between RXRA promoter methylation with fat mass at nine years of age as well as lower maternal carbohydrate intake in the first trimester of pregnancy. While the results of this study are provocative, there are some methodologic points worthy of consideration (i.e., use of umbilical cord tissue, which is an abundant source of mesenchymal stem cells). In addition, it is of interest that their intra-individual variation in meCpG variation was in fact greater than their inter-individual or cohort variation, and test of interaction models were not systematically applied. Moreover, there was neither substantive validation of the findings, nor an attempt to correlate with gene expression changes. At a physiologic level, it is of further note that these authors observed that low maternal carbohydrate intake significantly correlated with RXRA methylation variance and future adiposity [50]. This is noteworthy in and of itself, for as discussed both in this chapter and others in the volume, the predominance of evidence to date has indicated that triglyceride levels, maternal pre-pregnancy BMI, and glycemic index are strong predictors of infant adiposity and future risk of obesity. Nevertheless, this study will serve as a likely pivotal study in our advancing understanding of genomic methylation as both predictor and arbitrator of future risk.

Maternal protein restriction

Decades of research in animal models has revealed that in utero exposure to a maternal low-protein diet can lead to permanent changes in offspring metabolism, blood pressure, and adiposity [47–51]. In an effort to discern whether it is overall caloric restriction vs. protein restriction per se, alternate models of a perturbed gestational milieu have been explored. For example, rat and mouse models of maternal low-protein diet exposure have been useful in characterizing epigenetic and metabolic changes in the offspring. In utero exposure to maternal low-protein diet leads to decreased body weight of offspring, as well as a predisposition to hypertension, and altered glucose metabolism [51]. Bertram et al. has reported in a rat model that glucocorticoid receptor gene expression is increased at least two-fold in the liver, kidney, lung, and brain of fetuses exposed to maternal low protein in utero [52]. This increase in

expression is maintained into adult life compared with unexposed controls [52]. PPARα expression is also altered in rat liver with maternal low-protein exposure [53]. The glucocorticoid receptor, as well as PPARα, is epigenetically regulated by maternal low-protein diet exposure. PPARα is important for lipid and carbohydrate homeostasis, and GR for blood pressure regulation. Lillycrop et al reported that in the rat liver, the promoter region of the glucocorticoid receptor, $GR1_{10}$, shows a 33% decrease in methylation and expression of GR is increased by 84% in offspring exposed to maternal low protein [53, 54]. Expression of the DNA methyltransferase, Dnmt1, is also lower in maternal low-protein offspring. Further characterization of $GR1_{10}$ reveals altered histone modification patterns in maternal low-protein offspring, with an increase in H3K9 acetylation and a decrease in H3K9 di- and tri-methylation [53]. It is well characterized within a rat model of maternal protein restriction that offspring are susceptible to type 2 diabetes [55]. It has recently been shown that the offspring exposed to maternal low protein have alterations in both DNA and histone methylation within the Hnf4a gene in islet cells. This gene has been implicated in the etiology of type 2 diabetes [56].

Interventions to alleviate the adverse phenotypes of maternal low-protein exposure may be mediated by epigenetic alterations. For example, offspring exposed to a maternal low-protein diet supplemented with folic acid, a common component in prenatal vitamins and an essential part of the one carbon metabolism pathway, do not show a propensity to hypertension in adulthood [57]. On a molecular level, the offspring also did not show a difference in promoter methylation in the GR or PPARα promoters compared with control diet animals [53]. It appears that the supplementation helped to revert both the phenotypic and epigenetic changes of maternal low protein. Timing of folic acid supplementation is important. If folic acid is given to protein-restricted offspring in the juvenile period (postnatal days 35–40), rather than during gestation, changes in metabolism and epigenotype are not normalized [58].

One study reported that maternal low-protein exposure increases the expression of the transcription factor CCAAT/enhancer-binding protein (C/EBPβ) in the skeletal muscle of female offspring in a rat model, but not male [59]. Analysis of the C/EBPβ promoter revealed increased acetylated histones H3 and H4 in the females and not males. A study of genes that are involved in predisposition to hypertension showed gene-specific changes in expression accompanied by altered promoter methylation [60]. The angiotensin receptor, AT1b, shows increased mRNA and protein levels in the adrenal gland in one-week-old rats exposed to MLP. This increased expression is accompanied by a decrease in promoter methylation. However, changes in gene expression due to maternal low-protein exposure are not always concomitant with changes in DNA methylation. The glucokinase gene in rats is reduced in six-month-old maternal low-protein rat liver, yet there is no differential promoter methylation between control or maternal low-protein exposed animals [61].

One intriguing aspect of the maternal low-protein rat model system was the discovery that the adverse phenotypes are transmitted transgenerationally. Exposure to the maternal low-protein diet during gestation, leads to high blood pressure and insulin resistance in the subsequent F1 generation, even when the F1 is on a control diet postweaning. Their offspring (the F2 generation) have also been reported to have high blood pressure and insulin resistance in adulthood. In fact, disruptions in glucose homeostasis have even been reported in the F3 generation [62–64]. Study of the adult male F2 liver showed decreased PPARα and GR promoter methylation [63]. The methylation status of the hepatic promoters was passed through a transgenerational model even though the F2 generation was never exposed in utero to the low-protein diet and consumed only a control diet in adulthood. Transgenerational inheritance patterns are provocative evidence for an epigenetic, rather than genetic, mode of phenotypic transmission.

Summary

In utero exposure to a maternal low-protein diet increases the likelihood that the exposed offspring will develop type 2 diabetes, hypertension, increased adiposity, and high blood pressure. These pathologies are accompanied not only by changes in gene expression profiles in liver, kidney, lung, and brain, but epigenetic changes such as altered gene-specific DNA methylation and changes in histone modifications.

Maternal obesity and high-fat diet exposure

As reviewed in other chapters in this volume, it appears that one way maternal obesity begets offspring obesity is through intrauterine processes. However, distinguishing effects of behavioral factors associated with obesity (e.g., energy intake) from obesity per se is not

an easy undertaking. Along with reports of the effects of maternal undernutrition, protein restriction, and intrauterine growth restriction, studies of maternal overnutrition and high-caloric density are becoming of immense importance for their potential to elucidate the reasons for the current epidemic of obesity. In a non-human primate model of maternal obesity, fetal offspring exhibit the pathology of non-alcoholic fatty liver disease in utero [11]. These results have also been seen in a mouse model of maternal obesity [65]. In a rat model of maternal obesity, although pups from obese dams did not weigh more than those from lean dams, they gained greater body weight and body fat when fed a high-fat diet (HFD) postweaning than those from lean dams [66]. Exposure to a high-fat diet in utero in animal models can make offspring more susceptible to type 2 diabetes, altered leptin sensitivity, hypertension, and obesity [67–70].

Various epigenetic changes have been associated with exposure to a maternal high-fat diet, with histone modifications serving as a cornerstone to these observations. As one such example, in a non-human primate model of maternal obesity, we have demonstrated that fetuses exposed to a maternal high-fat diet in utero have increased levels of hepatic H3K14 acetylation, concomitant with decreased levels of HDAC1 protein, mRNA, and activity; these changes persist postnatally [12]. Employing techniques of chromatin immunoprecipitation (ChIP) followed by differential display PCR, we have identified the peripheral circadian regulator *Npas2* (a transcription factor essential in maintaining oscillatory circadian rhythms) as a fetal gene reprogrammed by H3K14ac in high-fat diet exposed animals, but not by maternal obesity per se. Of interest, although no differences were seen in *Npas2* promoter DNA methylation, promoter H3K14ac occupation was increased in high-fat diet exposed fetal animals; this was not true for offspring carried by an obese mother whose diet had been reverted to the control diet during gestation. This alteration in promoter occupancy was further associative at a molecule-specific level with alterations in gene expression of *Npas2* in high-fat diet exposed animals [13]. A postweaning high-fat diet also significantly disrupted *Npas2* expression even without high-fat diet exposure in utero.

Because alterations and disruptions of circadian rhythms are correlated with obesity and cardiovascular disease, the contribution of maternal diet to reprogramming the fetal circadian rhythm is of interest in furthering our understanding of current childhood

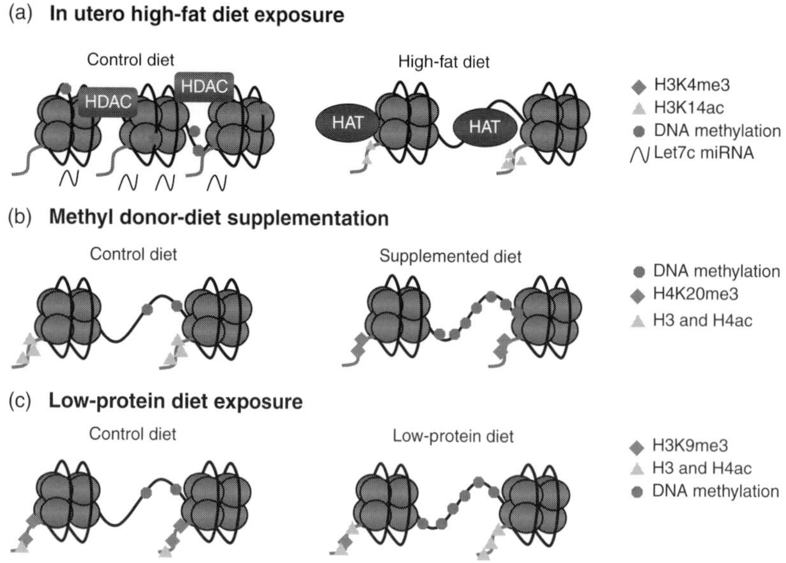

(a) **In utero high-fat diet exposure**

(b) **Methyl donor-diet supplementation**

(c) **Low-protein diet exposure**

Figure 13.4. Alterations in chromatin structure associated with different in utero constraints. (a) In utero exposure to a high-fat diet is associated with an increase in fetal H3K14ac in non-human primates, as well as a decrease in Let7c miRNA in 15-week-old mice. (b) In utero exposure to a methyl-supplemented maternal diet is associated with an increase in DNA methylation as well as H4K20me3, and decreased histone acetylation in the Agouti mouse model system. (c) Low-protein diet exposure is associated with an increase in histone acetylation as well as DNA methylation and a decrease in H3K9me3 in a rodent model system. (See figure in color plate section.)

obesity trends. Glucose and lipid homeostasis are known to display circadian variation, and a high-fat diet in a murine model amplifies the diurnal variation in glucose tolerance in a *Clock*-dependent fashion. Similar to glucose homeostasis, characterization of peripheral *Clock* family members in liver and adipose tissue demonstrate robust and coordinated expression of the circadian oscillation system as well as *Clock*-controlled downstream effectors [71]. Temporally restricted feeding or alterations in diet content (caloric dense/high fat) results in a coordinated phase-shift in circadian expression of the major oscillator genes and their downstream targets in adipose tissues [71,72]. Our evidence served as a fundamental description that the peripheral circadian metabolic clock in the developing non-human primate fetus can be altered in utero by virtue of maternal dietary exposure, as evidenced by our observed changes in circadian gene expression patterns in fetal liver.

Investigators have shown that DNA methylation changes have been reported in a mouse model of offspring exposed to a high-fat diet in utero. Male mice aged 18 to 24 weeks exposed in utero to a maternal high-fat diet showed an increased preference for glucose and fat. Gene expression changes were reported in the brain including alterations in dopamine re-uptake transporter (DAT), μ-opiod receptor (MOR), and preproenkephalin (PENK). Global and gene-specific DNA methylation patterns in the brain were altered in high-fat diet exposed animals [73]. High-fat diet exposure altered gene expression, epigenetic marks, and food preference in animals maintained on a control diet.

Summary

In utero exposure to varying maternal constraints such as high-fat diet, calorie restriction, or protein restriction has been found to be associated with the adult onset of obesity. These exposures are also associated with changes in DNA methylation and histone modifications in the offspring. The molecular mechanisms behind the development of obesity and the association with epigenetic changes are a field that is just beginning to be explored (Figure 13.4).

Epigenetic changes associated with paternal diet

Most studies investigating the developmental origins of disease focus on maternal factors influencing fetal outcome. Specifically, phenotypic outcomes have been characterized for altered conditions in utero such as maternal diet constraints, placental malperfusion, or toxin exposure, which could affect the development of gene programming. Recently, studies on the effect of the paternal diet on offspring susceptibility to adult metabolic diseases have begun to emerge. The effect of these exposures precludes the effect of exposure in utero, and points to a potential for epigenetic reprogramming in paternal gametes, which is transmitted to the offspring.

Epidemiological studies have shown that excessive food availability during the "slow growth stage" (8 to 12 years old) in *grandfathers* is associated with diabetes and cardiovascular disease in *grandsons* [74]. The off-spring of male mice exposed to calorie restriction in utero show reduced birthweight and impaired glucose tolerance [75].

A study of adult male rats showed that the female offspring of fathers who were fed a high-fat diet exhibited impaired glucose tolerance in adulthood and developed a diabetic-like condition [76]. Paternal high-fat diet altered the expression of 642 genes in the pancreatic islet cells of adult female offspring, concomitant with gene-specific changes in CpG promoter methylation.

A study using a mouse model system of paternal protein restriction determined that offspring exhibit altered hepatic gene expression, lipid and cholesterol biosynthesis, and modest changes in CpG methylation dependent on paternal diet [77]. The authors showed that although they did see widespread modest changes in CpG methylation, changes in promoter methylation did not globally correlate with changes in gene expression. However, a substantial increase in methylation upstream of a single specific gene, PPARα, was observed. The authors hypothesize that although global changes in methylation are not seen, this single change in methylation status of a transcription factor may account for changes in gene expression of many genes.

Summary

The contribution of a father's diet to the offspring phenotype is an exciting, albeit new, field of investigation. New studies are showing that paternal diet does indeed influence offspring metabolism. Studies in rodents show that a paternal high-fat diet is associated with a diabetic phenotype in the offspring, accompanied by epigenetic changes in the offspring. However, few publications of the contribution of paternal diet to offspring metabolism are available and much work remains to be done.

Intrauterine growth restriction

The association between intrauterine growth restriction (IUGR), small for gestational age (SGA) infants, and adult metabolic morbidities has been well characterized. Intrauterine growth restriction has been linked to central obesity, insulin resistance, hypertension, and dyslipidemia, among other metabolic symptoms [76]. Many organs and systems are ultimately involved in the emerging phenotype including adipose tissue, liver, β-cells, and the kidney. Poor fetal growth can lead to an increase in visceral adiposity in adulthood [78,79]. The establishment of an animal model of IUGR in rats using bilateral artery ligation has helped to investigate the epigenetic changes that occur in the various organs affected by IUGR and the predisposition to obesity.

Many studies using the rodent IUGR model have studied epigenetic changes in the liver associated with growth restriction. Global epigenetic changes occur in the liver as well as gene-specific changes in IUGR animals. Overall histone H3 lysine acetylation at residues 9, 14, and 18 are increased at day 0 and remain high in day 21 males [78]. In day 21 females the levels of K9 and K18 acetylation decrease. Concomitant with an increase in lysine acetylation, a decrease in the protein and mRNA levels of HDAC1 are also seen in day 0 liver, but there is no difference seen by day 21. Genes important in maintaining metabolism, PPARγ, PGC-1, and CPT1, are altered in IUGR animals [79,80]. These changes in expression are associated with an increase in acetylation of H3K9 in the promoters of PGC-1 and a decrease of acetylation in the CPT1 promoter [80].

Further hepatic epigenetic changes associated with IUGR include differential acetylation of H3K9 and H3K14, and alteration in DNA methylation in the DUSP5 promoter concomitant with alterations in mRNA levels of DUSP5 [81]. Similar results have been reported for the IGF-1 gene. Intrauterine growth restriction decreases serum IGF-1 levels, and alters hepatic IGF-1 gene expression [82]. Intrauterine growth restriction alters the histone code along the length of the gene, and these characteristics persist postnatally. DNA methylation within the gene is also altered in IUGR animals.

Epigenetic changes associated with IUGR are not restricted to the liver. Reports have shown that changes occur in brain, β-cells, and skeletal muscle in this animal model. An elegant study from the Simmons laboratory showed that β-cells exposed to IUGR express lower levels of Pdx1, a transcription factor necessary for β-cell development and function, and this reduction is permanent [81]. They characterized the epigenetic changes in the gene over the life of the animals and showed that silencing of the gene is associated with a progression of repressive chromatin modifications. In the fetal animal the promoter is characterized by the recruitment of the repressive HDAC1 and Sin3A and decreased histone acetylation. After birth the active H3K4me3 marks are removed and replaced by the repressive H3K9me3. Finally, in adulthood, after the onset of diabetes, the promoter is methylated leading to permanent silencing of the gene.

Skeletal muscle in IUGR animals shows a reduction of the GLUT4 glucose transporter gene. A study of the epigenetic changes associated with this decrease in expression found many mechanisms involved in GLUT4 regulation, including histone modification changes, differential recruitment of the repressors HDAC1 and DNMT1, increased H3K9 methylation, and recruitment of the heterochromatin-associated protein HP1α [82]. Hippocampal glucocorticoid receptor mRNA is increased and shows increased H3K4me3 modifications in the promoter in day 0 and day 21 males [83]. In day 0 brains, decreased CpG methylation is seen in IUGR animals, as well as decreased levels of HDAC1, MecP2, and DNMT1. However, an increase in H3K9 and H3K14 acetylation has been reported [84].

Conclusions

A fundamental tenet of modern biology is "the environment shapes the organism." At the species level the process of evolution involves selection of the fittest DNA specimens over time according to the principles outlined by Charles Darwin. The mechanism involved is the inheritance of genetic traits first described by Gregor Mendel and later understood to be attributable to differences in DNA sequence. Since these early days of our understanding that genes and chromosomes function as the backbone of our genetic heredity, our view of heredity has been written in the language of DNA with the assumption that genetic mutations and changes in the nucleotide backbone have driven most descriptions of how phenotypic traits and diseases are handed down from one generation to another.

We now know that this mechanism is only partially correct. The environment shapes the organism through epigenetic mechanisms without effecting changes in DNA sequence. Recent discoveries in the field of epigenetics – the study of heritable changes in gene function that occur without a change in the DNA sequence – have blurred our thinking and are changing the way we as a scientific and clinical community think about heredity. Epigenetic mechanisms such as DNA methylation, histone acetylation, and RNA interference, and their effects in gene activation and inactivation, are increasingly understood to have a profound effect in altering an individual's appearance, transmission of a specific congenital anomaly, and even one's lifetime risk of common diseases such as obesity. Thus we have arrived at the point in our current understanding of "genetics" that while genomic DNA is the template of our heredity, it is the orchestration and regulation of its expression via epigenetic mechanisms in chromatin remodeling, DNA methylation, and miRNA variation that ultimately results in the complexity and diversity among individuals observed in nature.

One of the most exciting attributes of epigenetic inheritance is the pace of change. The environment during development can lead to immediate changes in the phenotype of the organism, which then are passed on to subsequent generations. Epigenetic mechanisms offer great plasticity to the organism's response to environmental challenges. The organism is particularly responsive to environmental challenges during reproduction and development because during gametogenesis epigenetic imprints are erased and re-established. The organism is also vulnerable to untoward environmental influences and toxins that may adversely affect development. The effects are not limited to chemical toxins in the environment, but alterations in maternal nutrition may have effects upon future generations and notably obesity anticipation and prevalence.

In summary, in this chapter we have argued that in accordance with the developmental origins of adult disease hypothesis, perturbations in the in utero environment influence the development of diseases later in life. This was first observed to occur in response to maternal nutritional constraints that resulted in a growth-restricted infant whom later was observed to develop profound changes including obesity, insulin resistance, hypertension, heart disease, and lipid disorders. Working in animal models, multiple and converging lines of evidence have shown that these lifelong disease risks occur through the static reprogramming of gene expression via epigenetic modifications to the regulation of gene expression.

A few comments regarding the potential for the relative contribution of maternal obesity vs. maternal diet are necessary. First, this issue is very difficult to tease apart in human longitudinal cohort studies, but is undoubtedly of necessary importance from a public health standpoint. For example, should it be found that the diet serves as the primary arbitrator, then less emphasis on gestational weight gain and loss and greater emphasis on dietary modifications might be of highest impact. To this end, we emphasize our earlier comments on our data in both a non-human primate mode of maternal high-fat dietary intake [12,13,85–89] as well as maternal smoking [90–92], which suggests that the exposure bears the greater impact in programming both the methylome and histone code. Whether this correlates with long-term benefit in the developing offspring remains to be seen, but is of noted promise.

The field of epigenetic effects on reproduction and development is young but robust. We have discovered a few of the earliest clues in this complex epigenomic code, with many more left to be unraveled. What an exciting time to be at the forefront of biology as we unravel the molecular mechanisms underscoring the developmental origins of disease.

References

1. Bird A. Perceptions of epigenetics. *Nature* 2007;**447**(7143):396–8.

2. Goldberg A D, Allis C D & Bernstein E. Epigenetics: a landscape takes shape. *Cell* 2007;**128**(4):635–8.

3. Roth T L, Roth E D & Sweatt, J D. Epigenetic regulation of genes in learning and memory. *Essays Biochem* 2010;**48**(1):263–74.

4. Feinberg A P. Phenotypic plasticity and the epigenetics of human disease. *Nature* 2007;**447**(7143):433–40.

5. Lillycrop K A & Burdge G C. Epigenetic changes in early life and future risk of obesity. *Int J Obes (Lond)*, 2011;**35**(1):72–83.

6. Luger K, Mader A W, Richmond R K, Sargent D F & Richmond T J. Crystal structure of the nucleosome core particle at 2.8 A resolution. *Nature* 1997;**389**(6648):251–60.

7. Jenuwein T & Allis C D. Translating the histone code. *Science* 2001;**293**(5532):1074–80.

8. Grewal S I & Moazed D. Heterochromatin and epigenetic control of gene expression. *Science* 2003;**301**(5634):798–802.

9. Cedar H & Bergman Y. Linking DNA methylation and histone modification: patterns and paradigms. *Nat Rev Genet* 2009;**10**(5):295–304.

10. Hartil K, Vuguin P M, Kruse M, *et al.* Maternal substrate utilization programs the development of the metabolic syndrome in male mice exposed to high fat in utero. *Pediatr Res* 2009;**66**(4):368–73.

11. McCurdy C E, Bishop J M, Williams S M, *et al.* Maternal high-fat diet triggers lipotoxicity in the fetal livers of nonhuman primates. *J Clin Invest* 2009;**119**(2):323–35.

12. Aagaard-Tillery K M, Grove K, Bishop J, *et al.* Developmental origins of disease and determinants of chromatin structure: maternal diet modifies the primate fetal epigenome. *J Mol Endocrinol* 2008;**41**(2):91–102.

13. Suter M, Bocock P, Showalter L, *et al.* Epigenomics: maternal high-fat diet exposure in utero disrupts peripheral circadian gene expression in nonhuman primates. *FASEB J* 2011;**25**(2):714–26.

14. Jaenisch R & Bird A. Epigenetic regulation of gene expression: how the genome integrates intrinsic and environmental signals. *Nat Genet* 2003;**33**(Suppl):245–54.

15. Ehrlich M. DNA hypomethylation in cancer cells. *Epigenomics* 2009;**1**(2):239–59.

16. Mayer W, Niveleau A, Walter J, Fundele R & Haaf T. Demethylation of the zygotic paternal genome. *Nature* 2000;**403**(6769):501–2.

17. Rougier N, Bourchis D, Gomes D M, *et al.* Chromosome methylation patterns during mammalian preimplantation development. *Genes Dev* 1998;**12**(14):2108–13.

18. Burdge G C & Lillycrop K A. Nutrition, epigenetics, and developmental plasticity: implications for understanding human disease. *Annu Rev Nutr* 2010;**30**:315–39.

19. Delaval K & Feil R. Epigenetic regulation of mammalian genomic imprinting. *Curr Opin Genet Dev* 2004;**14**(2):188–95.

20. Ahmed F. Epigenetics: tales of adversity. *Nature* 2010;**468**(7327):S20.

21. Ruthenburg A J, Allis CD & Wysocka J. Methylation of lysine 4 on histone H3: intricacy of writing and reading a single epigenetic mark. *Mol Cell* 2007;**25**(1):15–30.

22. Wang Z, Schones D E & Zhao K. Characterization of human epigenomes. *Curr Opin Genet Dev* 2009;**19**(2):127–34.

23. MacDonald V E & Howe L J. Histone acetylation: where to go and how to get there. *Epigenetics* 2009;**4**(3):139–43.

24. Ferguson-Smith A C, Cattanach B M, Barton S C, Beechey C V & Surani M A. Embryological and molecular investigations of parental imprinting on mouse chromosome 7. *Nature* 1991;**351**(6328):667–70.

25. Kaneda M. Genomic imprinting in mammals: epigenetic parental memories. *Differentiation* 2011;**82**(2):51–6.

26. da Rocha S T & Ferguson-Smith A C. Genomic imprinting. *Curr Biol* 2004;**14**(16):R646–9.

27. Buiting K. Prader–Willi syndrome and Angelman syndrome. *Am J Med Genet C Semin Med Genet* 2010;**154C**(3):365–76.

28. Glenn C C, Nicholls R D, Robinson W P, *et al.* Modification of 15q11-q13 DNA methylation imprints in unique Angelman and Prader–Willi patients. *Hum Mol Genet* 1993;**2**(9):1377–82.

29. Buiting K, Dittrich B, Robinson W P, *et al.* Detection of aberrant DNA methylation in unique Prader–Willi syndrome patients and its diagnostic implications. *Hum Mol Genet* 1994;**3**(6):893–5.

30. Kelsey G. Imprinting on chromosome 20: tissue-specific imprinting and imprinting mutations in the GNAS locus. *Am J Med Genet C Semin Med Genet* 2010;**154C**(3):377–86.

31. Liu J, Litman D, Rosenberg M J, *et al.* A GNAS1 imprinting defect in pseudohypoparathyroidism type IB. *J Clin Invest* 2000;**106**(9):1167–74.

32. Linglart A, Bastepe M & Juppner H. Similar clinical and laboratory findings in patients with symptomatic autosomal dominant and sporadic pseudohypoparathyroidism type Ib despite different epigenetic changes at the GNAS locus. *Clin Endocrinol (Oxf)* 2007;**67**(6):822–31.

33. Stoger R. Epigenetics and obesity. *Pharmacogenomics* 2008;**9**(12):1851–60.

34. Bernal A J & Jirtle R L. Epigenomic disruption: the effects of early developmental exposures. *Birth Defects Res A Clin Mol Teratol* **88**(10):938–44.

35. Dolinoy D C, Das R, Weidman J R & Jirtle R L. Metastable epialleles, imprinting, and the fetal origins of adult diseases. *Pediatr Res* 2007;**61**(5 Pt 2):30R–7R.

36. Cooney C A, Dave A A & Wolff G L. Maternal methyl supplements in mice affect epigenetic variation and DNA methylation of offspring. *J Nutr* 2002;**132**(8 Suppl):2393S–400S.

37. Waterland R A & Jirtle R L. Transposable elements: targets for early nutritional effects on epigenetic gene regulation. *Mol Cell Biol* 2003;**23**(15):5293–300.

38. Waterland R A, Travisano M, Tahiliani K G, Rached M T & Mirza S. Methyl donor supplementation prevents transgenerational amplification of obesity. *Int J Obes (Lond)* 2008;**32**(9):1373–9.

39. Dolinoy D C, Weidman J R, Waterland R A & Jirtle R L. Maternal genistein alters coat color and protects Avy mouse offspring from obesity by modifying the fetal epigenome. *Environ Health Perspect* 2006;**114**(4):567–72.

40. Dolinoy D C, Weinhouse C, Jones T R, Rozek L S & Jirtle R L. Variable histone modifications at the A(vy) metastable epiallele. *Epigenetics* 2010;**5**(7):637–44.

41. Rubin B S, Murray M K, Damassa D A, King J C & Soto A M. Perinatal exposure to low doses of bisphenol A affects body weight, patterns of estrous cyclicity, and plasma LH levels. *Environ Health Perspect* 2001;**109**(7):675–80.

42. Miyawaki J, Sakayama K, Kato H, Yamamoto H & Masuno H. Perinatal and postnatal exposure to bisphenol a increases adipose tissue mass and serum cholesterol level in mice. *J Atheroscler Thromb* 2007;**14**(5):245–52.

43. Somm E, Schwitzgebel V M, Toulotte A, *et al.* Perinatal exposure to bisphenol a alters early adipogenesis in the rat. *Environ Health Perspect* 2009;**117**(10):1549–55.

44. Dolinoy D C, Huang D & Jirtle R L. Maternal nutrient supplementation counteracts bisphenol A-induced DNA hypomethylation in early development. *Proc Natl Acad Sci U S A* 2007;**104**(32):13056–61.

45. Roseboom T J, van der Meulen J H, Osmond C, *et al.* Coronary heart disease after prenatal exposure to the Dutch famine, 1944–45. *Heart* 2000;**84**(6):595–8.

46. Roseboom T J, van der Meulen J H, Osmond C, *et al.* Plasma lipid profiles in adults after prenatal exposure to the Dutch famine. *Am J Clin Nutr* 2000;**72**(5):1101–6.

47. Hult M, Tornhammar P, Ueda P, *et al.* Hypertension, diabetes and overweight: looming legacies of the Biafran famine. *PLoS One* 2010;**5**(10):e13582.

48. Heijmans B T, Tobi E W, Stein A D, *et al.*, Persistent epigenetic differences associated with prenatal exposure to famine in humans. *Proc Natl Acad Sci U S A* 2008;**105**(44):17046–9.

49. Tobi E W, Lumey L H, Talens R P, *et al.* DNA methylation differences after exposure to prenatal famine are common and timing- and sex-specific. *Hum Mol Genet* 2009;**18**(21):4046–53.

50. Godfrey, K M, Epigenetic gene promoter methylation at birth is associated with child's later adiposity. *Diabetes* 2011;**60**(5):1528–34.

51. Burdge G C, Delange E, Dubois L, *et al.* Effect of reduced maternal protein intake in pregnancy in the rat on the fatty acid composition of brain, liver, plasma, heart and lung phospholipids of the offspring after weaning. *Br J Nutr* 2003;**90**(2):345–52.

52. Bertram C, Trowern A R, Copin N, Jackson A A & Whorwood C B. The maternal diet during pregnancy programs altered expression of the glucocorticoid receptor and type 2 11beta-hydroxysteroid dehydrogenase: potential molecular mechanisms underlying the programming of hypertension in utero. *Endocrinology* 2001;**142**(7):2841–53.

53. Lillycrop K A, Phillips E S, Jackson A A, Hanson M A & Burdge G C. Dietary protein restriction of pregnant rats induces and folic acid supplementation prevents epigenetic modification of hepatic gene expression in the offspring. *J Nutr* 2005;**135**(6):1382–6.

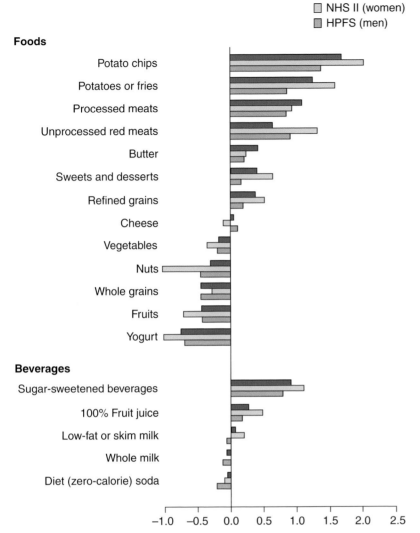

Foods

Potato chips
Potatoes or fries
Processed meats
Unprocessed red meats
Butter
Sweets and desserts
Refined grains
Cheese
Vegetables
Nuts
Whole grains
Fruits
Yogurt

Beverages

Sugar-sweetened beverages
100% Fruit juice
Low-fat or skim milk
Whole milk
Diet (zero-calorie) soda

■ NHS (women)
□ NHS II (women)
▣ HPFS (men)

-1.0   -0.5   0.0   0.5   1.0   1.5   2.0   2.5

Weight change associated with each increased
daily serving, per four-year period (lb)

Figure 2.1. Associations between changes in food and beverage consumption and weight changes every four years, according to study cohort. Study participants included 50 422 women in the Nurses' Health Study (NHS), followed for 20 years (1986 to 2006); 47 898 women in the Nurses' Health Study II (NHS II), followed for 12 years (1991 to 2003); and 22 557 men in the Health Professionals Follow-up Study (HPFS), followed for 20 years (1986 to 2006). Weight changes are reported for each increase in the daily serving of the food or beverage; decreased intake would be associated with the inverse weight changes. There was little evidence of a significant interaction between diet and physical activity (p > 0.10 for the interaction in each cohort). All weight changes were adjusted simultaneously for age, baseline body mass index, sleep duration, and changes in smoking status, physical activity, television watching, alcohol use, and all of the dietary factors shown. The p value is less than 0.001 for all dietary factors with the exception of butter in the NHS II, cheese in the NHS and NHS II, low-fat or skim milk in the NHS and HPFS, diet soda in the NHS, and whole-fat milk in all three cohorts. Reproduced with permission from reference [19], © 2011, *New England Journal of Medicine*.

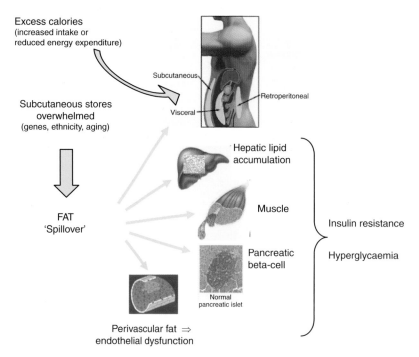

Excess calories
(increased intake or
reduced energy expenditure)

Subcutaneous stores
overwhelmed
(genes, ethnicity, aging)

Subcutaneous

Retroperitoneal

Visceral

FAT
'Spillover'

Hepatic lipid
accumulation

Muscle

Insulin resistance

Pancreatic
beta-cell

Hyperglycaemia

Normal
pancreatic islet

Perivascular fat ⇒
endothelial dysfunction

Figure 5.1. Simple concept of ectopic fat and development of insulin resistance and frank diabetes in non-pregnant individuals. This figure provides a simple conceptual illustration of the development and location of ectopic fat in individuals once they have "overwhelmed" their ability to store safe subcutaneous fat. Certain factors such as gender (females with greater storage capacity), genetics (with family history of diabetes as a broad proxy measure), ethnicity (e.g., South Asians), and aging have relevance to an individual's ability to store fat subcutaneously. Other factors may also be relevant such as smoking but more data are needed to examine this. In temporal terms, liver fat accumulation may be closer to the time of development of diabetes whereas muscle insulin resistance is a more proximal development. Perivascular fat may contribute to vascular dysfunction via a process of adverse vasocrine signaling leading in turn to impaired nutrient blood flow – i.e., vascular insulin resistance. Finally, some recent evidence indicates excess fat may also accumulate in the pancreas to contribute to beta-cell dysfunction, and thus development of diabetes.

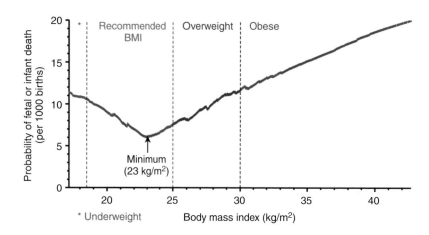

Figure 6.1. Probability of a fetal or infant death with increasing pre-pregnancy body mass index. Reproduced with permission from Tennant *et al.* [17], who constructed the figure using locally weighted scatter plot regression.

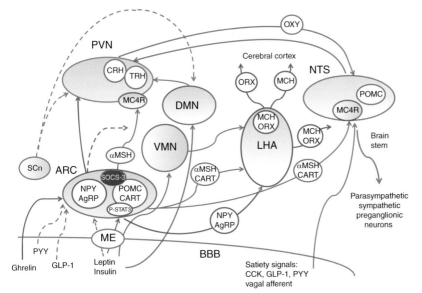

Figure 10.1. Energy balance and hypothalamic regulation. The arcuate nucleus (ARC) is located in the hypothalamus, close to the median eminence (ME) where the blood–brain barrier (BBB) is incomplete allowing blood-borne signals to reach ARC neurons. Leptin, insulin, and ghrelin are the most important hormonal satiety signals and are also actively transported across the BBB where they activate anorexigenic neurons co-expressing alpha melanocyte-stimulating hormone (*a*MSH) and cocaine- and amphetamine-regulated transcript (CART); and inhibit orexigenic neurons co-expressing agouti-related protein and neuropeptide Y (AgRP and NPY). Both populations of neurons project widely throughout the brain. CART is also expressed in the paraventricular hypothalamic nucleus (PVN) and lateral hypothalamic area (LHA). *a*MSH is cleaved from the precusor polypeptide pro-opiomelanocortin (POMC) along with other peptides such as B-endorphin and ACTH. The ARC integrates this information together with inputs from brain stem areas and signals other hypothalamic nuclei such as the ventromedial hypothalamic nucleus (VMN), dorsomedial hypothalamic nucleus (DMH), and PVN, to reduce food intake (pathways shown in red). Signals from the ARC to the PVN and the LHA also increase feeding (shown in green). Divergent projections from the orexin-containing neurons (ORX) and melanin-concentrating hormone (MCH) neurons in the LHA, ascend to the cerebral cortex and descend to the brain stem and spinal cord. Oxytocin-containing neurons (OXY) of the PVN innervate vagal preganglionic parasympathetic neurons involved in gastrointestinal control. Hormones from the gastrointestinal tract including cholecystokinin (CCK) and glucagon-like peptide (GLP-1) modulate these processes through shorter term changes in satiety and hunger. Inputs from the suprachiasmatic nucleus to the PVN and DMN also regulate diurnal feeding patterns. The three possible outputs from the hypothalamus that regulate food intake and energy expenditure are: activation of motor neurons via the brain stem; activation of neuroendocrine neurons in the PVN that secrete corticotrophin-releasing hormone (CRH) and thyrotropin-releasing hormone (TRH) to activate the pituitary axes (e.g., hypothalamic–pituitary–adrenal and hypothalamic–pituitary–thyroid axis activation result in secretion of glucocorticoids and thyroid hormone); autonomic nervous system both sympathetic and parasympathetic, e.g., influencing heart rate and thermogenesis in metabolically active tissues.

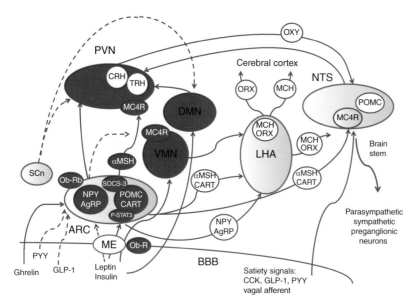

Figure 10.2. Developmental programming of hypothalamic regulation. Areas in red indicate sites susceptible to developmental programming by maternal obesity or neonatal overnutrition. Perhaps not surprisingly those areas most vulnerable to developmental programming lie close to the median eminence (ME) where the blood–brain barrier (BBB) is incomplete allowing blood-borne signals such as leptin to penetrate. Abbreviations as given for Figure 10.1.

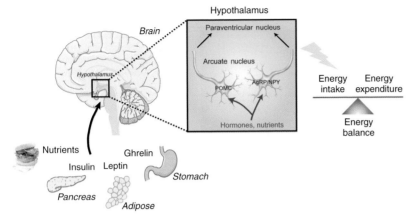

Figure 11.1. Organization of hypothalamic pathways regulating appetite. Highly simplified schematic diagrams to illustrate possible routes and neuronal populations relaying metabolic signals, such as leptin, ghrelin, insulin, and nutrients, from the periphery to the brain. Two distinct populations of neurons in the arcuate nucleus of the hypothalamus – one co-expressing neuropeptide Y (NPY) and Agouti-related protein (AgRP), and the other expressing pro-opiomelanocortin (POMC) – represent major routes for the regulation of body weight by peripheral signals. These neurons send direct projections to discrete populations of neurons, including in the paraventricular nucleus of the hypothalamus, to control energy balance. This figure was created in part using illustrations from "Servier Medical Art" with permission.

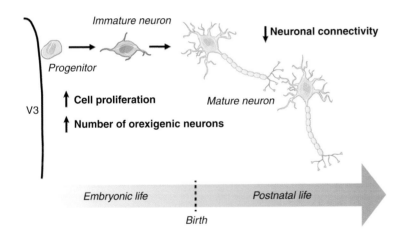

Figure 11.2. Exposure to an obesogenic environment during perinatal life induces marked effects on neuronal wiring in the hypothalamus. The formation of hypothalamic neural circuits occurs in two major phases: one phase (that includes cell proliferation, neuronal migration, and cell fate) during which the numbers of neurons composing the hypothalamus will be established; and another phase during which neuronal connectivity (that includes axon growth and synapse formation) will be established. Exposure to an obesogenic environment (such as maternal obesity and/or postnatal overnutrition) appears to influence each of these developmental events and results in a higher number of orexigenic neurons and disrupted hypothalamic neural projections. This figure was created in part using illustrations from "Servier Medical Art" with permission.

ARH->PVH projections in ob/ob neonates

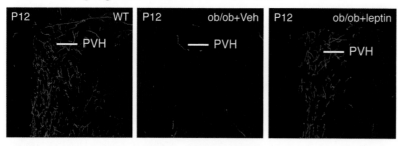

ARH->PVH projections in ob/ob adults

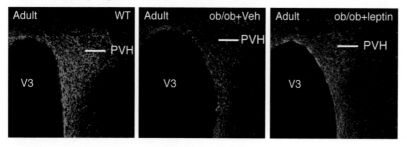

Leptin-induced axon growth

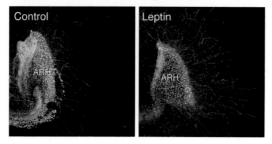

Figure 11.3. Neuroprogramming actions of the adipocyte-derived hormone leptin. In addition to its regulatory role in adults, leptin is an important signal for the development of hypothalamic circuits that control energy homeostasis. Neural projections from the arcuate nucleus (ARH) to the paraventricular nucleus of the hypothalamus (PVH) are disrupted in leptin-deficient (ob/ob) mice. Moreover, leptin appears to act primarily during neonatal critical periods to exert its neurodevelopmental effects. Although daily injections of ob/ob neonates with leptin rescue a normal pattern of innervation by arcuate neurons of the paraventricular nucleus, injections of the hormone in mature animals remain largely ineffective in restoring a normal pattern of arcuate projections. In addition, the application of leptin to isolated explants of the arcuate nucleus induces neurite extension, which suggests that leptin acts directly on arcuate neurons to promote axon growth. Reproduced with permission from [36].

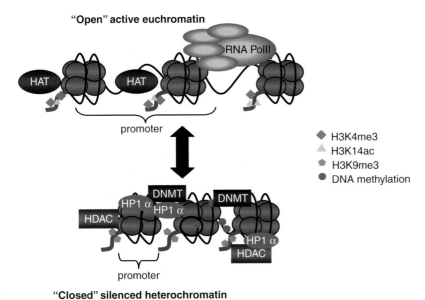

"Open" active euchromatin

HAT

HAT

RNA PolII

promoter

◆ H3K4me3
▲ H3K14ac
⬟ H3K9me3
● DNA methylation

DNMT

HP1 α DNMT
HP1 α

HDAC

HP1 α
HDAC

promoter

"Closed" silenced heterochromatin

Figure 13.1. Characteristics of chromatin structure. Chromatin is organized into euchromatin, which is associated with active gene expression, and tightly compacted heterochromatin, which is associated with gene silencing. Histone modifications such as lysine acetylation (H3K14ac) and H3K4me3 are traditionally associated with euchromatin. Heterochromatin is traditionally enriched for H3K9me3 and DNA methylation as well as other non-histone-associated chromatin proteins such as HP1α.

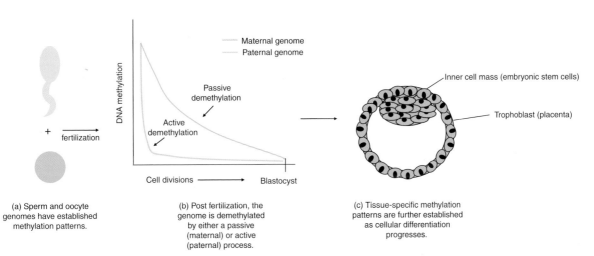

(a) Sperm and oocyte genomes have established methylation patterns.

(b) Post fertilization, the genome is demethylated by either a passive (maternal) or active (paternal) process.

(c) Tissue-specific methylation patterns are further established as cellular differentiation progresses.

Figure 13.2. Establishment of DNA methylation in a fertilized egg. Sperm and egg genomes are methylated before fertilization. After fertilization the genome is demethylated, excluding imprinted genes. The paternal genome is demethylated in an active process, of which the molecular mechanisms remain unknown. The maternal genome is demethylated in a passive manner, through cell-cycle replication without methylation of the newly synthesized strand. Once the embryo reaches the blastocyst stage the methylation patterns of the trophoblast begin to change from that of the inner cell mass. The trophoblast gives rise to the placental tissue and the cells within the inner cell mass will establish distinct methylation patterns as they begin to differentiate.

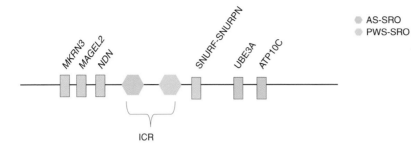

Figure 13.3. The imprinted region on chromosome 15 implicated in Prader–Willi syndrome. On chromosome 15 there is an imprinted region that contains genes that are expressed from either the maternally (pink) or paternally (blue) inherited chromosome. Parent-of-origin expression is controlled by an imprinting control region. Alterations of expression of UBE3A distinctly correlates with Angelman syndrome. Alterations in expression of the four paternally expressed genes has been implicated in the development of Prader–Willi syndrome.

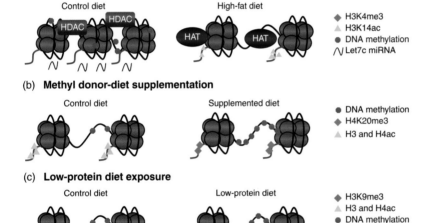

Figure 13.4. Alterations in chromatin structure associated with different in utero constraints. (a) In utero exposure to a high-fat diet is associated with an increase in fetal H3K14ac in non-human primates, as well as a decrease in Let7c miRNA in 15-week-old mice. (b) In utero exposure to a methyl-supplemented maternal diet is associated with an increase in DNA methylation as well as H4K20me3, and decreased histone acetylation in the Agouti mouse model system. (c) Low-protein diet exposure is associated with an increase in histone acetylation as well as DNA methylation and a decrease in H3K9me3 in a rodent model system.

54. Lillycrop K A, Slater-Jefferies J L, Hanson M A, *et al.* Induction of altered epigenetic regulation of the hepatic glucocorticoid receptor in the offspring of rats fed a protein-restricted diet during pregnancy suggests that reduced DNA methyltransferase-1 expression is involved in impaired DNA methylation and changes in histone modifications. *Br J Nutr* 2007;**97**(6):1064–73.

55. Snoeck A, Remacle C, Reusens B & Hoet J J. Effect of a low protein diet during pregnancy on the fetal rat endocrine pancreas. *Biol Neonate* 1990;**57**(2):107–18.

56. Sandovici I, Smith N H, Nitert M D, *et al.* Maternal diet and aging alter the epigenetic control of a promoter-enhancer interaction at the Hnf4a gene in rat pancreatic islets. *Proc Natl Acad Sci U S A* **108**(13):5449–54.

57. Torrens C, Brawley L, Anthony F W, *et al.* Folate supplementation during pregnancy improves offspring cardiovascular dysfunction induced by protein restriction. *Hypertension* 2006;**47**(5):982–7.

58. Burdge G C, Lillycrop K A, Phillips E S, *et al.* Folic acid supplementation during the juvenile-pubertal period in rats modifies the phenotype and epigenotype induced by prenatal nutrition. *J Nutr* 2009;**139**(6):1054–60.

59. Zheng S, Rollet M & Pan Y X. Maternal protein restriction during pregnancy induces CCAAT/ enhancer-binding protein (C/EBPbeta) expression through the regulation of histone modification at its promoter region in female offspring rat skeletal muscle. *Epigenetics* 2011;**6**(2):161–70.

60. Bogdarina I, Welham S, King P J, Burns S P & Clark A J. Epigenetic modification of the renin-angiotensin system in the fetal programming of hypertension. *Circ Res* 2007;**100**(4):520–6.

61. Bogdarina I, Murphy H C, Burns S P & Clark A J. Investigation of the role of epigenetic modification of the rat glucokinase gene in fetal programming. *Life Sci* 2004;**74**(11):1407–15.

62. Benyshek D C, Johnston C S & Martin J F. Glucose metabolism is altered in the adequately-nourished grand-offspring (F3 generation) of rats malnourished during gestation and perinatal life. *Diabetologia* 2006;**49**(5):1117–19.

63. Zambrano E, Martinez-Samayoa P M, Bautista C J, *et al.* Sex differences in transgenerational alterations of growth and metabolism in progeny (F2) of female offspring (F1) of rats fed a low protein diet during pregnancy and lactation. *J Physiol* 2005;**566**(Pt 1):225–36.

64. Martin J F, Johnston C S, Han C T & Benyshek D C. Nutritional origins of insulin resistance: a rat model for diabetes-prone human populations. *J Nutr* 2000;**130**(4):741–4.

65. Oben J A, Mouralidarane A, Samuelsson A M, *et al.* Maternal obesity during pregnancy and lactation programs the development of offspring non-alcoholic fatty liver disease in mice. *J Hepatol* 2010;**52**(6):913–20.

66. Shankar K, Harrell A, Liu X, *et al.* Maternal obesity at conception programs obesity in the offspring. *Am J Physiol Regul Integr Comp Physiol* 2008;**294**(2):R528–38.

67. Gniuli D, Calcagno A, Caristo M E, *et al.* Effects of high-fat diet exposure during fetal life on type 2 diabetes development in the progeny. *J Lipid Res* 2008;**49**(9):1936–45.

68. Ferezou-Viala J, Roy A F, Serougne C, *et al.* Long-term consequences of maternal high-fat feeding on hypothalamic leptin sensitivity and diet-induced obesity in the offspring. *Am J Physiol Regul Integr Comp Physiol* 2007;**293**(3):R1056–62.

69. Chang G Q, Gaysinskaya V, Karatayev O & Leibowitz S F. Maternal high-fat diet and fetal programming: increased proliferation of hypothalamic peptide-producing neurons that increase risk for overeating and obesity. *J Neurosci* 2008;**28**(46):12107–19.

70. Mitra A, Alvers K M, Crump E M & Rowland N E. Effect of high-fat diet during gestation, lactation, or postweaning on physiological and behavioral indexes in borderline hypertensive rats. *Am J Physiol Regul Integr Comp Physiol* 2009;**296**(1):R20–8.

71. Zvonic S, Ptitsyn A A, Conrad S A, *et al.* Characterization of peripheral circadian clocks in adipose tissues. *Diabetes* 2006;**55**(4):962–70.

72. Turek F W, Joshu C, Kohsaka A, *et al.* Obesity and metabolic syndrome in circadian Clock mutant mice. *Science* 2005;**308**(5724):1043–5.

73. Vucetic Z, Kimmel J, Totoki K, Hollenbeck E & Reyes T M. Maternal high-fat diet alters methylation and gene expression of dopamine and opioid-related genes. *Endocrinology* 2010;**151**(10):4756–64.

74. Kaati, G, Bygren L O, and Edvinsson S. Cardiovascular and diabetes mortality determined by nutrition during parents' and grandparents' slow growth period. *Eur J Hum Genet* 2002;**10**(11):682–8.

75. Carone B R, Fauquier L, Habib N, *et al.* Paternally induced transgenerational environmental reprogramming of metabolic gene expression in mammals. *Cell* 2010;**143**(7):1084–96.

76. Joss-Moore L A & Lane R H. The developmental origins of adult disease. *Curr Opin Pediatr* 2009;**21**(2):230–4.

77. Cottrell E C & Ozanne S E. Early life programming of obesity and metabolic disease. *Physiol Behav* 2008;**94**(1):17–28.

78. Fu Q, McKnight R A, Yu X, *et al*. Uteroplacental insufficiency induces site-specific changes in histone H3 covalent modifications and affects DNA-histone H3 positioning in day 0 IUGR rat liver. *Physiol Genomics* 2004;**20**(1):108–16.

79. Lane R H, Kelley D E, Gruetzmacher E M & Devaskar S U. Uteroplacental insufficiency alters hepatic fatty acid-metabolizing enzymes in juvenile and adult rats. *Am J Physiol Regul Integr Comp Physiol* 2001;**280**(1):R183–90.

80. Lane R H, MacLennan N K, Hsu J L, Janke S M & Pham T D. Increased hepatic peroxisome proliferator-activated receptor-gamma coactivator-1 gene expression in a rat model of intrauterine growth retardation and subsequent insulin resistance. *Endocrinology* 2002;**143**(7):2486–90.

81. Park J H, Stoffers D A, Nicholls R D & Simmons R A. Development of type 2 diabetes following intrauterine growth retardation in rats is associated with progressive epigenetic silencing of Pdx1. *J Clin Invest* 2008;**118**(6):2316–24.

82. Raychaudhuri N, Raychaudhuri S, Thamotharan M & Devaskar S U. Histone code modifications repress glucose transporter 4 expression in the intrauterine growth-restricted offspring. *J Biol Chem* 2008;**283**(20):13611–26.

83. Ke X, Schober M E, McKnight R A, *et al*. Intrauterine growth retardation affects expression and epigenetic characteristics of the rat hippocampal glucocorticoid receptor gene. *Physiol Genomics* 2010;**42**(2):177–89.

84. Ke X, Lei Q, James S J, *et al*. Uteroplacental insufficiency affects epigenetic determinants of chromatin structure in brains of neonatal and juvenile IUGR rats. *Physiol Genomics* 2006;**25**(1):16–28.

85. Cox J, Williams S, Grove K, Lane R H & Aagaard-Tillery K M. A maternal high fat diet is accompanied by alterations in the fetal primate metabolome. *Am J Obstet Gynecol* 2009;**201**:281

86. McCurdy C E, Bishop J M, Williams S M, *et al*. Maternal high-fat diet triggers lipotoxicity in the fetal livers of nonhuman primates. *J Clin Invest* 2009;**119**:323–35.

87. Suter M A & Aagaard-Tillery K M. Environmental influences on epigenetic profiles. *Semin Reprod Med* 2009;**27**:380–90.

88. Bocock P N & Aagaard-Tillery K M. Animal models of epigenetic inheritance. *Semin Reprod Med* 2009;**27**:369–79.

89. Segars J H & Aagaard-Tillery K M. Epigenetics in reproduction. *Semin Reprod Med* 2009;**27**:349–50.

90. Aagaard-Tillery K M, Spong C, Thom E, *et al*. Pharmacogenomics of maternal tobacco use: metabolic gene polymorphisms modify risk of adverse pregnancy outcomes. *Obstet Gynecol* 2009;**115**:568–77.

91. Suter M A, Abramovici A, Hu M, *et al. In utero* tobacco exposure epigenetically modifies placental metabolic gene expression. *Metabolism* 2010;**59**:1481–90.

92. Aagaard-Tillery K M, Porter T F, Lane R, Varner M W & LaCoursier D Y. *In utero* tobacco exposure is associated with modified affects of maternal factors on fetal growth. *Am J Obstet Gynecol* 2008;**198**:66–79.

Intervention strategies to improve outcome in obese pregnancies: focus on gestational weight gain

Emily Oken and Matthew W. Gillman

Introduction

Excessive gestational weight gain (GWG) is common and on the rise. While mean weight gains tend to be lower among women entering pregnancy at higher pre-pregnancy weights, weight gain ranges associated with optimal outcomes are also lower for heavier women [1,2]. Thus overweight and obese women are substantially more likely to gain more weight than recommended ("excessive weight gain"), compared with women who were normal weight or underweight entering pregnancy [1].

As summarized in Chapter 4, a large number of observational studies have demonstrated increased risks for adverse short- and long-term pregnancy outcomes associated with excessive GWG [1,3]. For the mother, these adverse outcomes include gestational glucose intolerance, cesarean or complicated vaginal delivery, failure to initiate or maintain breastfeeding, and postpartum weight retention [3,4]. For the child, they include large for gestational age, birth trauma, and infant mortality, as well as increased risk for later obesity [2,3,5–7]. Observational data further suggest that risks for many adverse outcomes associated with greater GWG are similar or greater among obese women than among women of normal pre-pregnancy weight. In studies of birth outcomes among obese women, higher gains appear to raise the risk of large for gestational age more strongly than they reduce the risk of small for gestational age birth [5,8–13]. These findings suggest that reducing GWG among obese women may have beneficial effects without causing undue risk.

The optimal weight gain for obese women is still controversial. As reviewed in Chapter 19, in 2009 the IOM Committee to Reexamine the Weight Gain Guidelines replaced previously vague advice with the recommendation that obese women gain 5 to 9 kg (11 to 20 lbs) in a full-term pregnancy [1]. The recommended range is less than for overweight (7 to 11.5 kg/15.4 to 25.4 lbs) and normal weight (11.5 to 16 kg/25.4 to 35.3 lbs). While 5 to 9 kg (11 to 20 lbs) gain allows for products of conception without any gain in maternal tissue, some observational evidence among obese women suggests that gaining even less than 5 kg (11 lbs), or potentially even losing weight in very obese women, may be optimal for maternal and child outcomes [1,2,8,10], although the balance of risk and benefit likely varies according to the degree of obesity [14]. Observational studies, however, are subject to confounding, which only randomized controlled trials (RCTs) can overcome.

Accordingly, a number of intervention studies to reduce excessive GWG in normal weight as well as overweight and obese women have been planned or conducted in recent years. In this chapter, we discuss published intervention studies that include GWG as a primary or intermediate outcome, focusing especially among overweight or obese women.

We identified six systematic reviews published in English from January 2010 through May 2011 that evaluated intervention studies of the effects of lifestyle interventions, diet, and/or physical activity on GWG (Table 14.1) [15–20]. These papers reviewed multiple databases to identify RCTs or non-randomized interventions. One (Dodd *et al.* [15]) was limited to overweight and obese women. All of the reviews commented on the poor to low quality of the available literature, heterogeneity of interventions, and inconsistent results especially across subgroups (e.g., income, weight category), although publication bias was not a problem. Two of the reviews provided no summary

Table 14.1 Systematic reviews of the literature related to diet, physical activity, or lifestyle interventions during pregnancy published 2010–2011

Reference	Topic	Search	Results	Comments/conclusions
Dodd et al., BJOG 2010 [15]	Systematic review (Cochrane) of RCTs to influence diet and/or lifestyle among overweight/obese pregnant women	PubMed, CENTRAL, clinical trial registers Any language Through 1/2010	9 RCTs 743 women Dietary interventions: GWG 4 studies: mean diff −5.37 kg (95% CI: −6.61 to −4.13) fixed effects −3.10 kg (95% CI: −8.32–2.13) random effects Exercise interventions: no relevant data Other outcomes also included: LGA 3 studies, (RR 2.02, 95% CI: 0.84–4.86) No differences in preterm, pre-eclampsia, GDM, induction, c-section, hemorrhage, infection, birthweight, low birthweight, high birthweight, Apgar <7	7 studies: diet vs. standard care 2 studies: exercise 3 included women with GDM For overweight/obese women, antenatal dietary interventions are of uncertain benefit to limit GWG Quality of studies poor to fair
Gardner et al., Obes Rev 2011 [16]	Systematic review of published controlled trials of interventions that aimed to reduce GWG through changes in diet or physical activity among pregnant women aged 18+ Exclusion: intervention included information only, or non-psychological intervention (e.g., medical/nutritional)	PsycINFO, Medline, EMBASE, AMED, HMIC, CENTRAL English only 1990–February 2010	10 papers including 12 interventions (7 RCTs) 1656 women Weighted mean difference: −1.19 kg (95% CI: −1.74 to −0.65) −2.26 kg (95% CI: −3.28 to −1.24) in overweight-only samples −0.77 kg (95% CI: −1.42 to −0.13) in mixed-weight samples	Moderate heterogeneity No publication bias No moderating effect of pre-pregnancy BMI More weight loss if intervention initiated <12 weeks gestation No clear pattern of which behavior change techniques promoted greater loss (same techniques used in successful and unsuccessful interventions)

Study	Aim	Databases searched	Findings	Comments
Ronnberg & Nilsson, BJOG 2010 [17]	Systematic review of RCTs and non-randomized controlled interventions to reduce excessive GWG Studies evaluated using GRADE criteria	PubMed, Cochrane library, CINAHL, Pedro English/ Scandinavian language Through 8/15/2009	8 studies (4 RCTs) Overall quality "very low" "Because of the heterogeneity in population characteristics, interventions offered, definitions of outcome measures, and durations of intervention, it was not considered appropriate to perform a meta-analysis"	No evidence for publication bias "Results of published intervention trials are of insufficient quality to enable evidence-based recommendations for clinical practice"
Skouteris et al., Obes Rev 2010 [18]	Systematic review of GWG interventions	CINAHL, Global Health, Medline, PsycINFO, Academic Search Premier Published in English 1/2000–4/2010	10 studies 1852 women (No pooled estimates) 6 studies showed significantly less GWG 3 studies showed intervention women more likely to gain within guidelines	Results inconsistent across different groups (income, weight category) Inconsistent in relation to what factors need to be targeted in interventions
Streuling et al., BJOG 2010 [19]	Meta-analysis of RCTs of physical activity during pregnancy with information on GWG	Medline, EMBASE, CENTRAL, ISI Web of Science, BIOSIS Previews, Current Contents, Connect, Journal Citation Reports Through 10/2010	12 RCTs 1073 women Mean difference: −0.61 kg (95% CI: −1.17 to −0.06)	No publication bias Varying quality of studies GWG not primary focus of most studies
Streuling et al., AJCN 2010 [19]	Systematic review of randomized and non-randomized interventions to reduce GWG by modulating diet and physical activity	Medline, EMBASE, CENTRAL, Web of Science English/German Through 1/2010	9 studies (4 RCTs, 3 overweight/obese women only) 1549 women 3 studies significantly lower GWG, 3 studies non-significantly lower GWG in intervention vs. control group Standardized mean difference: −0.22 units (95% CI: −0.38 to −0.05) (about 1.2 kg) Among women with BMI >25: −0.30 (95% CI: −0.54 to −0.06)	"Validity of trials heterogenous" Interventions based on PA and diet counseling, usually combined with weight monitoring, appear to be successful in reducing GWG The standardized mean difference is calculated by dividing the difference of sample means of the two groups by the pooled SD of outcome measurements in the two groups

estimates because they found substantial heterogeneity of populations, interventions, and outcomes [17,18]. The remaining reviews all reported that lifestyle interventions during pregnancy resulted in lower gestational weight gain, with estimates ranging from –0.6 to –5.4 kg compared to the non-intervention group (Table 14.1). Streuling *et al.*[19] included 12 RCTs of physical activity interventions only, and found a mean difference of –0.61 kg (95% CI: –1.17 to –0.06), whereas Dodd *et al.* [15] identified two trials of exercise interventions among obese women, and did not provide a summary estimate because the aims and methods were dissimilar. One [24] was a small (n = 32) RCT of diet v. diet + resistance exercise training in women with diagnosed GDM, showing some metabolic benefits. The other [44] was an RCT of aerobic training among 132 overweight non-diabetic pregnant women, showing improved fitness.

In the remainder of this chapter, we review and summarize the primary literature on GWG interventions, including both RCTs and non-randomized interventions. We include both categories of studies because many of the earliest and/or commonly cited interventions to limit excessive GWG were not RCTs. We include all of the studies addressed in the recent systematic reviews, as well as additional or newer studies we identified on review of references and supplementary literature review using the search terms "gestation or pregnancy," "weight gain," and "intervention or trial or randomized" (1 January 2010 to 31 May 2011). We excluded one study of an inpatient dietary intervention among women with gestational diabetes that lasted only two weeks and did not report GWG or other birth outcomes [21]. We also excluded a study of a physical activity intervention published in Portuguese [22]. Using this approach, we identified 28 separate RCTs published since 2000, of which 17 were published since 2009 (Table 14.2) [22–50]. The largest study analyzed data from 399 women [37], the smallest included only 12 [39]. Studies were conducted in the United States [11], Australia/New Zealand [5], Scandinavia [4], Brazil [3], Canada [2], Western Europe [2], and Iran [2]. We identified an additional seven non-RCT interventions published since 2000 (Table 14.3), which included up to 179 women in the interventions and were conducted in the United States, Canada, and Scandinavia. We expect more results to appear in the literature in the coming years, as ClinicalTrials.gov reveals several ongoing RCTs and the US National Institutes of Health recently invited applications for lifestyle interventions among overweight and obese pregnant women.

We discuss these studies based on the following criteria: (1) efficacy vs. effectiveness; (2) level(s) of the socioecological model; (3) participant characteristics, (4) behavioral targets; (5) intervention delivery; (6) timing of intervention; and (7) outcomes. We conclude with imperatives for future research.

Efficacy vs. effectiveness

To be clinically meaningful, results of interventions must be relevant to specific patient populations in specific settings. Multiple factors determine the external validity, i.e., generalizability or applicability, of interventions, including patient characteristics, treatment settings, and compliance. We often distinguish between the *efficacy* and the *effectiveness* of an intervention to understand its generalizability. Efficacy trials (explanatory trials) determine whether an intervention produces the expected result under ideal circumstances, whereas effectiveness trials (pragmatic trials) measure the degree of beneficial effect under "real world" settings [51]. Using the approach proposed by the US Agency for Healthcare Research and Quality [52], we classified studies according to their concordance with seven criteria for effectiveness trials: primary care population, less stringent eligibility criteria, appropriate health outcomes, sufficiently long study duration, clinically relevant treatment modalities, assessment of adverse events, adequate sample size, and intention-to-treat analysis.

Using the six out of seven criteria as a threshold [52], we identified 12 RCTs as effectiveness studies [23,24,31,33–37,40,41,47,48]. Three quarters (8/12) of the effectiveness RCTs were successful in reducing GWG overall (n = 3) or somewhat, i.e., borderline significance or within a subset (n = 5), whereas one quarter (4/17) of the efficacy RCTs achieved differences in GWG. This finding contrasts with the usual expectation that efficacy studies should be more likely to show an effect, as study populations and settings are often more restricted. However, as all but one of the effectiveness studies were published since 2009, this difference may derive from the relative recency of the interventions rather than reflect any actual superiority of the effectiveness approaches. Three of the non-randomized studies were effectiveness studies. None of the efficacy studies was followed by a subsequently reported effectiveness study. However, one non-randomized effectiveness study [53], which resulted in improved behaviors but no difference in GWG, informed the design of a larger

Table 14.2 Randomized controlled trials (RCTs) of interventions before or during pregnancy that evaluated effects on GWG and related outcomes

Features:

1. Efficacy or effectiveness
2. Level of socioecological model
3. Characteristics of women: weight categories, GDM, low socioeconomic status
4. Behavioral targets: diet, physical activity
5. Intervention delivery
6. Timing of intervention: pre-pregnancy, 1st, 2nd, 3rd trimester
7. Outcomes: GWG only, GWG + other birth outcomes, GWG + distal outcomes

Author	Setting	Population	Intervention	Outcomes	Quality	Reviewed in	Features
Asbee et al. 2009 [23]	USA North Carolina, residents' clinic October 2005–April 2007	Inclusion: 16–26 wks of gestation; 18- to 49-yrs old; singleton; all BMI categories Exclusion: multiple pregnancy; pre-existing diabetes, hypertension, or thyroid disease; pregnancy ending in preterm birth at <37 wks of gestation; less than four antenatal visits Sample size: 144 randomized; 100 analyzed; 40 overweight or obese	Women were randomized to: (1) routine antenatal care, or (2) a lifestyle intervention including a single visit with a dietician for dietary, PA, and GWG advice and GWG tracking and feedback at each visit	Adherence to IOM weight gain recommendations Lower GWG (29 vs. 36 lb, p = 0.01), fewer cesarean sections due to failure to progress (25% vs. 58%, p = 0.02) No effect on other outcomes (operative vaginal delivery, neonatal weight, incidence of pre-eclampsia, GDM, lacerations, shoulder dystocia)	Randomization: computer-generated sequence Allocation concealment: sealed opaque envelopes Blinding: not stated	Dodd *BJOG* [15] Gardner *Obes Rev* [16] Ronnberg *BJOG* [17] Skouteris *Obes Rev* [18] Streuling *AJCN* [20]	1. Effectiveness ("We specifically chose an inexpensive intervention that could be introduced easily into any obstetric practice.") 2. Individual, practice 3. All 4. Diet, PA, GWG advice 5. In-person, dietician 6. 2nd and 3rd trimester 7. GWG + other birth outcomes
Barakat et al. 2009, 2008 [24,66]	Spain January 2000–March 2002	Inclusion: Caucasian, Spanish, "low–middle class", age 25–35 yrs, sedentary, singleton gestation, not at high risk for preterm	Women were randomized to: (1) control group told to maintain level of exercise	Birthweight, length, HC, GA	Randomization: "Randomly assigned"	Streuling *BJOG* [19]	1. Effectiveness 2. Individual 3. Sedentary 4. PA 5. In-person, fitness specialist

155

Table 14.2 (cont.)

Author	Setting	Population	Intervention	Outcomes	Quality	Reviewed in	Features
		Exclusion: medical condition prohibiting exercise in pregnancy, BMI >40 Sample size: 160 randomized, 142 analyzed	(2) group exercise training three times per wk, 35–40 min for 26 wks	All null but trends toward lower GWG (11.5 vs. 12.4 kg) and lower birthweight, less macrosomia (1.4 vs. 10%)	Allocation concealment: concealed Blinding: RAs abstracting data were blinded		6. 2nd and 3rd trimester 7. GWG, birth outcomes
Brankston et al. 2004 [25]	Canada Enrollment period not reported	Inclusion: maternal age 20–40 yrs; 26–32 wks of gestation; BMI <40; diagnosis of gestational diabetes mellitus; not involved in a regular exercise program Sample size: 38 randomized; 32 analyzed	Women were randomized to: (1) standard diabetic diet, asked not to begin structured exercise program, or (2) diet plus circuit-type resistance training three times per wk	No "significant" difference in GWG, gestational age, cesarean sections, or birthweight No difference in incidence of insulin use, but Lower post-meal glucose, less insulin required (0.22 vs. 0.48 u/kg, p < 0.05), and longer time to insulin treatment	Randomization: random number table Allocation concealment: opaque envelopes Blinding: not stated Losses to follow-up: 15%	Dodd *BJOG* [15]	1. Efficacy 2. Individual 3. GDM 4. PA (diet for all) 5. Experienced instructor, in-person, and at home 6. 3rd trimester 7. Glycemic control, birth outcomes
Baciuk et al. 2008 [67]; Cavalcante et al. 2009 [26]	Brazil March 2002– November 2004	Inclusion: low-risk, sedentary women 16–20wks gestation, Exclusion: ≥2 prior cesarean sections, condition prohibiting physical activity Sample size: 71 randomized; 70 analyzed	Women were randomized to: (1) no physical exercise (2) "regular and moderate practice of water aerobics" 50 min three times per wk	Body fat %, FFM, BMI, cardiorespiratory capacity, duration and type of delivery, birthweight, fetal growth No difference in any outcome (slightly higher body fat, lower FFM, p = 0.05)	Randomization: computer-generated list Allocation concealment: opaque envelope Blinding: not reported	Streuling *BJOG* [19]	1. Efficacy 2. Individual 3. Sedentary 4. PA 5. In person 6. 2nd and 3rd trimester 7. Birth outcomes
Clapp et al. 2000 [27]	USA Cleveland, Ohio	Inclusion: no regular exercise, enrolled prior to pregnancy	Women were randomized to: (1) no exercise, or	GWG, cardiorespiratory measures, infant size	Randomization: "randomly assigned"	Streuling *BJOG* [19]	1. Efficacy 2. Individual 3. Sedentary

	Inclusion / Exclusion / Sample	Intervention	Results	Randomization / Allocation / Blinding	Reference	
Enrollment period not reported	Exclusion: substance abuse Sample size: 50 randomized, 46 analyzed Note: women who did not maintain the specified exercise regimen throughout pregnancy or whose antenatal course was abnormal were excluded from data analysis (n = 4)	(2) weight-bearing exercise (treadmill, stair stepper, or step aerobics, 20 min, 3–5 times per wk, beginning at 8 wks and continuing throughout pregnancy	GWG 15.7 vs. 16.3 kg (non-significant) Offspring of intervention women heavier and longer (both lean and fat mass higher), no difference in % body fat, HC, PI Placentae larger	Allocation concealment: "envelope draw" Blinding: not reported		4. PA 5. In person 6. 1st, 2nd, and 3rd trimester 7. GWG, birth outcomes
Garshabi & Faghih Zadeh 2005 [28] Iran April 2003–January 2004	Inclusion: primips, age 20–28 yrs, 17–22 wks gestation, housewives, ≥ high school Exclusion: contraindication to exercise, exercise before pregnancy Sample size: 266 randomized; 212 analyzed (54 intervention women excluded, no controls excluded)	Women were randomized to: (1) control, or (2) exercise three times per wk for 12 wks	GWG 14.1 kg intervention vs. 13.8 kg control (p = 0.63) No difference in gestation length, or birthweight Less LBP, improved spine flexibility	Randomization: "randomized" Allocation concealment: sealed envelopes Blinding: not reported		1. Efficacy 2. Individual 3. Sedentary 4. PA 5. In-person 6. 3rd trimester 7. GWG, birth outcomes, maternal fitness
Guelinckx et al. 2010 [29] Belgium March 2006–January 2008	Inclusion: 15 weeks of gestation, BMI >29 Exclusion: multiple pregnancy, pre-existing diabetes, renal disease, **preterm birth <37 wks (excluded from analysis)** Sample size: 130 randomized; 85 analyzed	Women were randomized to: (1) routine antenatal care (control), or (2) brochure-only (passive), or (3) brochure plus nutritionist lifestyle education in three group sessions (active)	Gestational weight gain, diet, PA, birth outcomes Lower fat intake and higher protein intake in both intervention groups; no difference in GWG (9.8 kg control vs. 10.9 passive and 10.6 active),	Randomization: not stated Allocation concealment: not stated	Gardner *Obes Rev* [16] Dodd *BJOG* [15]	1. Efficacy (groups)/ Effectiveness (brochure) 2. Individual 3. Obese

Table 14.2 (cont.)

Author	Setting	Population	Intervention	Outcomes	Quality	Reviewed in	Features
				% of women gaining within IOM recommendations (23.3% control, (27.0% passive and 26.2% active, p = 0.981), or other birth outcomes	Blinding: not stated Losses to follow-up: 35% excluded after randomization	Skouteris *Obes Rev* [18] Streuling *AJCN* [20]	4. Diet, PA 5. Trained nutritionist, group sessions 6. 2nd and 3rd trimester 7. GWG, diet, PA, birth outcomes
Haakstad & Bø 2011 [30]	Norway September 2007–March 2008.	Inclusion: sedentary nulliparous women, Norwegian speaking, <24 wks gestation Exclusion: >2 miscarriages, severe heart disease, persistent bleeding, multiple pregnancy, illness Sample size: 105 randomized, 79 analyzed	Women were randomized to: (1) supervised aerobic dance 60 min, twice per wk for at least 12 wks + 30 min moderate home exercise five times per wk, or (2) advice not to change usual physical activity level	No difference in GWG (13.0 vs. 13.8 kg, p = 0.38), skinfold thicknesses, or PPWR at 7–8 wks	Randomization: computerized program by independent person Allocation concealment: not reported Blinding: assessor blinded	None	1. Efficacy 2. Individual 3. Sedentary 4. PA only 5. In-person and at home 6. 2nd trimester on, at least 12 wks 7. GWG and PPWR at 7–8 wks
Hopkins *et al.* 2010 [31]	New Zealand December 2004–May 2007	Inclusion: healthy nulliparous women aged 20–40, singleton, gestational age <20 wks Exclusion: substance abuse, condition precluding exercise, personal or family history of type 2 diabetes mellitus Sample size: 98 randomized, 84 analyzed	Women randomized to: (1) home stationary cycling max five times, 40 min per wk, moderate intensity, or (2) continue usual daily activity	No difference in GWG, insulin sensitivity Offspring with lower birthweight, BMI, and cord IGF-I and IGF-2	Randomization: "randomly assigned" Allocation concealment: not reported Blinding: not reported	Streuling *BJOG* [19]	1. Effectiveness 2. Individual 3. All 4. PA only 5. Home 6. 2nd and 3rd trimester 7. GWG, birth outcomes

Study	Population	Intervention	Results	Methods quality	References	Details
Hui et al. 2006 [32]	Canada July–December 2004	Inclusion: <26 wks gestation, no pre-existing diabetes Exclusion: disorder contraindicating exercise Sample size: 52 women, 47 analyzed (26 intervention, 21 controls)	Women were randomized to: (1) usual care, or (2) one weekly group exercise and 3–5 times per wk home exercise DVDs, personalized diet plan with RD	Feasibility, safety, adherence (pilot study) No difference in GWG (14.2 vs. 14.2 kg), newborn weight, GA Higher PA in intervention group	Randomization: not reported Allocation concealment: not reported Blinding: not reported	Gardner *Obes Rev* [16] Skouteris *Obes Rev* [18] Streuling *AJCN* [20]	1. Pilot efficacy 2. Individual, embedded in community prenatal program 3. All 4. PA and diet 5. In-person and home 6. 2nd and 3rd trimester 7. GWG, birth outcomes, PA
Jackson et al. 2011 [33]	USA San Francisco Low-income, ethnically diverse June 2006– December 2007	Inclusion: English-speaking, age ≥18, <26 weeks gestation Exclusion: smoking, alcohol, drug use, or intimate partner violence Sample size: 327 randomized, 321 analyzed	Women were randomized to: (1) a computerized, multimedia, interactive Video Doctor teaching and counseling session about nutrition, exercise, and weight gain, followed by cueing sheet for provider and educational worksheet for patient, with a booster at 4 wks, or (2) usual care	No difference in GWG (intervention 33.4 lb, control 33.6 lb, p = 0.95). Improved knowledge of diet and IOM guidelines, more frequent conversations with providers about diet and physical activity	Randomization: by computer Allocation concealment: not reported Blinding: not reported	None	1. Effectiveness "Our goal was to devise an easy-to-use, brief intervention that could be implemented into clinical practice." 2. Individual, practice 3. All 4. PA, diet, GWG advice 5. Computer-based 6. 2nd trimester (two sessions) 7. GWG, birth outcomes, behaviors

Table 14.2 (cont.)

Author	Setting	Population	Intervention	Outcomes	Quality	Reviewed in	Features
Jeffries et al. 2009 [34]	Australia July 2007–May 2008	Inclusion: ≤14 wks gestation Exclusion: age <18 or >45 yrs, type 1 or type 2 diabetes mellitus, multiple pregnancy, or non-English speaking Sample size: 286 randomized, 236 analyzed	Women were randomized to: (1) receive optimal GWG range for BMI and record weight on graph or table, or (2) standard care	No difference in GWG (0.44 kg/wk vs. 0.46 kg/wk) overall, but lower GWG in overweight women (mean difference 0.12 (95% CI: 0.03–0.22) kg/wk) No difference in adherence to IOM guidelines, birth outcomes	Randomization: no information Allocation concealment: no information Blinding: women blinded to goals of study	Skouteris Obes Rev [18]	1. Effectiveness 2. Individual 3. All 4. GWG advice 5. Unclear 6. 2nd trimester to 36 wks 7. GWG, birth outcomes
Korpi-Hyövälti et al. 2011 [35]	Finland April 2005–May 2006	Inclusion: women living in two rural municipalities, at risk for GDM (BMI >25 kg/m², previous history of GDM or birth of child >4.5 kg, age >40 yrs, family history of diabetes, fasting plasma glucose 4.8–5.5 mmol/l) Exclusion: 1st trimester 2 hr OGTT ≥7.8 mmol/l Sample size: 60 randomized, 54 analyzed	Women were randomized to: (1) early intensive lifestyle intervention including dietary advice at six nutritionist visits and physical activity advice at six physiotherapy visits, or (2) a single-session lifestyle advice combined with a close follow-up	Somewhat lower GWG (11.4 ± 6.0 kg vs. 13.9 ± 5.1 kg, p = 0.062, adjusted by pre-pregnancy weight) No difference in 26–28 wk OGTT results No difference in pre-eclampsia, induction of labor, lacerations, cesarean deliveries, macrosomia, jaundice, gestational length, NICU, higher birthweight	Randomization: computer-generated list Allocation concealment: nurses did not have access to list Blinding: not reported	None	1. Effectiveness "Feasibility study" 2. Individual 3. Rural, high risk for GDM 4. Diet, PA 5. Nutritionist, physiotherapist 6. 2nd trimester 7. At birth

160

Study	Country/Dates	Inclusion/Sample	Intervention	Results	Methods		Outcomes
Laitinen et al. 2009 [36]; Piirainen et al. 2006 [68]	Finland April 2002– November 2005	Inclusion: <17 wks gestation, no metabolic or chronic disease Sample size: 256 women randomized to three arms, 208 analyzed	Women were randomized to: (1) diet (fat, fiber), also given food products/ probiotic, or (2) diet (fat, fiber, products)/ placebo, or (3) control/placebo	Diet + probiotics with improved glucose metabolism (lower glucose, insulin, HOMA) at 3rd trimester and 1, 6, 12 mo postpartum Energy and macronutrient intakes from food diaries No difference in GWG (14.9 kg overall)	Randomization: computer-generated blocks Allocation concealment: sealed envelopes Blinding: probiotics double-blinded in intervention group, single-blinded in control group Diet: not stated Losses to follow-up: 19%	None	1. Effectiveness 2. Individual 3. All 4. Diet 5. In-person, nutritionist 6. 2nd trimester through postpartum 7. Glycemia, diet, birth outcomes, follow-up to 12 mo
Luoto et al. 2011 [37]	Finland October 2007– December 2008	Inclusion: 8–12 wks gestation, at least one GDM RF: pre-pregnancy BMI ≥25, GDM or macrosomia in prior pregnancy, type 2 or type 2 DM in first degree relative, age >40	Women were randomized to: (1) Nurses at intervention sites provided GWG guidelines and graph, physical activity counseling (five sessions), and diet counseling (four sessions), or	At 26–28 weeks no difference in GDM, GWG, gestation length	Randomization: cluster RCT of 14 municipalities matched then randomized by computer	None	1. Effectiveness (follow-up of pilot study) 2. Individual, practice 3. GDM risk

Table 14.2 (cont.)

Author	Setting	Population	Intervention	Outcomes	Quality	Reviewed in	Features
		Exclusion: >1 abnormal value on baseline OGTT, age <18, not Finnish speaking, multiple gestation, substance abuse, condition preventing exercise, mental illness. Sample size: 442 interested and eligible, 399 analyzed	(2) nurses at control sites provided usual care	Less LGA (12% vs. 20%, p = 0.04) and lower birthweight (133 g, p = 0.008) and birthweight for gestational age. Better diet (higher fiber, PUFA; lower saccharose, saturated fat)	Allocation concealment: none. Blinding: not blinded		4. Diet, PA 5. Prenatal nurses 6. 2nd trimester through delivery 7. GWG, birth outcomes
Marquez-Sterling et al. 2000 [38]	USA Florida Recruitment period not reported	Inclusion: "low-risk", sedentary with no exercise for 1 yr prior to pregnancy. Sample size: 20 randomized, 15 analyzed	Women were randomized to: (1) exercise 1 h 3 times per wk for 15 wks, or (2) control (got postpartum exercise prescription)	No difference in GWG (16.2 kg intervention vs. 15.7 kg control), skinfold thicknesses, Apgar scores, or birthweight. Intervention mothers with better fitness	Randomization: "randomly assigned". Allocation concealment: not reported. Blinding: not reported	Streuling BJOG [19]	1. Efficacy 2. Individual 3. Sedentary 4. PA 5. In-person, certified personnel 6. 2nd trimester 7. GWG, birth outcomes, fitness
Ong et al. 2009 [39]	Australia Recruitment period not reported	Inclusion: obese, sedentary, singleton, normal 18 wk ultrasound, no CVD or diabetes. Exclusion: Sample size: 12 randomized	Women were randomized to: (1) 10 wks of home-based supervised cycling three times per wk, wks 18–28, or (2) controls continued usual exercise	No significant lower gain in weight (3.7 vs. 5.2 kg, p = 0.15). Trend to lower 1 h and 2 h glucose at 28-wk OGTT	Randomization: "randomly allocated". Allocation concealment: not reported. Blinding: not reported	Streuling BJOG [19]	1. Efficacy 2. Individual 3. Sedentary, obese 4. PA 5. At home 6. 2nd to 3rd trimester 7. Outcomes at 28 wks

Study	Location	Inclusion/Exclusion	Intervention	Results	Methods	Related reviews	Characteristics
Phelan et al. 2011 [40]	USA Rhode Island 2006–2008	Inclusion: 10–16 wks gestation, BMI 19.8–40, age >18, non-smoking, English speaking, access to telephone Exclusion: >3 miscarriages, major medical or psychiatric disease, weight loss during pregnancy Sample size: 401 randomized, 358 analyzed	Women were randomized to: (1) behavioral intervention based on Polley et al. [41] including one visit with interventionist, weekly postcards, mailed GWG graph with feedback, self-monitoring tools, dietician phone calls, or (2) usual care plus single intervention visit and bimonthly newsletters not focused on weight	Lower risk of excessive GWG in normal weight women (40.2% vs. 52.1%, OR: 0.38; 95% CI: 0.20–0.87; p = 0.003) but not overweight/obese women (OR: 1.4; 95% CI: 0.70–2.7; p = 0.33)	Randomizaton: computer-generated (by study statistician) in randomly varying block sizes and stratified by clinic and BMI category Allocation concealment: opaque envelopes Blinding: physicians and clinic staff blinded	None	1. Effectiveness 2. Individual 3. Normal and overweight/obese 4. Diet, PA, daily self-monitoring 5. Mail/in-person/phone 6. 2nd trimester on 7. Birth outcomes and 6-mo postpartum maternal weight
Polley et al. 2002 [41]	USA Pittsburgh	Inclusion: women at <20 wks of gestation; all BMI categories Exclusion: age <18 yrs, drug abuse, previous pregnancy complication, multiple pregnancy	Women were randomized to: (1) standard antenatal care, or (2) intensive intervention (access to research dietician or psychologist at each antenatal visit), written and	Fewer normal weight women >IOM guidelines (33% vs. 58%, p < 0.05) but more overweight women >IOM (59% vs. 32%, p = 0.09)	Randomization: unclear, "women were randomly assigned" Allocation concealment: not stated	Dodd BJOG [15] Gardner Obes Rev [16] Ronnberg BJOG [17]	1. Effectiveness 2. Individual 3. Normal weight and overweight/obese 4. Diet, PA, GWG

Table 14.2 (cont.)

Author	Setting	Population	Intervention	Outcomes	Quality	Reviewed in	Features
	Recruitment period not reported	Sample size: 120 randomized, 110 followed to delivery	oral information given on (a) appropriate weight gain during pregnancy; (b) exercise during pregnancy; and (c) healthful eating during pregnancy	No differences in physical activity, pre-eclampsia, hypertension, GDM, preterm birth, cesarean section, infant birthweight	Blinding: not stated Losses to follow-up: unable to assess	Skouteris *Obes Rev* [18] Streuling *AJCN* [20]	5. In-person and mail 6. 2nd trimester through delivery 7. GWG and birth outcomes
Quinlivan et al. 2011 [42]	Australia Socioeconomically disadvantaged Recruitment period not reported	Inclusion: no known fetal anomalies, English speaking, plans to keep infant, able to attend antenatal care, BMI ≥25 Sample size: 132 randomized, 124 analyzed	Women were randomized to: (1) 4-step multidisciplinary approach, (i) continuity of provider, (ii) weighing on arrival, (iii) brief dietary intervention by food technologist at each visit, (iv) psychological assessment and intervention if needed or, (2) routine antenatal care	Less GDM: 6% vs. 29%, OR 0.17 (95% CI: 0.03–0.95, p = 0.04) Lower GWG 7.0 vs. 13.8 kg, (−6.7 kg, 95% CI: 4.3–9.1, p < 0.0001) Also increased intake of water, fruit and vegetables, and home-cooked meals, lower intake of SSB, fast foods	Randomization: computer-generated stratified by overweight vs. obese Allocation concealment: sealed opaque envelopes Blinding: not reported	None	1. Efficacy 2. Individual practice 3. Low SES, overweight/obese 4. Diet, GWG 5. In-person (clinical) 6. ?throughout pregnancy 7. Outcomes at 28 wks, birth
Rae et al. 2000 [43]	Australia February 1992–June 1995	Inclusion: women with a diagnosis of gestational diabetes mellitus, <36 weeks of gestation, BMI >110% ideal	Women were randomized to: (1) standard diabetic diet, or	Diet, weight gain, frequency of insulin use, macrosomia	Randomization: "random draw" Allocation concealment: opaque envelopes	Dodd *BJOG* [15]	1. Efficacy 2. Individual 3. GDM, overweight 4. Diet only 5. Research dietician

Study	Setting	Inclusion/Sample	Intervention	Results	Methods		Notes
		Sample size: 125 women randomized, losses to follow-up: 6%	(2) calorie-restricted diet (70% standard)	No difference in any outcome (control group ate less carbohydrates than anticipated) Slightly more women in the intervention group failed to gain, or lost, weight from treatment to delivery (54% vs. 40.7%)	Blinding: women and caregivers blinded		6. 3rd trimester 7. Outcomes at birth
Rhodes et al. 2010 [44]	USA Boston January 2007–June 2009	Inclusion: BMI 25–45, age ≥25, 13–28 wks singleton gestation, Exclusion: smoking, alcohol, major health issues or medications that affect weight, plans to deliver outside of the study medical center, high levels of physical activity lactation in the preceding 3 mo, or being a first-degree relative of a participant Sample size: 46 randomized, 44 analyzed	Women were randomized to: (1) low-fat or (2) low-glycemic low-glycemic load diet two 1-hr in-person visits with biweekly maintenance visits Fats and carbohydrates provided	No difference in GWG from baseline to follow-up: 6.4 kg low GL diet vs. 6.9 kg low-fat diet (p = 0.74) Low GL mothers with greater decrease in CRP, lower increase in total cholesterol and triglycerides Low GL with longer gestation length, higher head circumference, slightly longer No difference in birthweight	Randomization: randomly permuted blocks of 2 and 4 Allocation concealment: sealed envelopes Blinding: none	None	1. Efficacy 2. Individual 3. Overweight/obese 4. Diet only 5. In-person, foods provided 6. 2nd and 3rd trimesters 7. GWG, diet, physiology, and infant outcomes at birth

Table 14.2 (cont.)

Author	Setting	Population	Intervention	Outcomes	Quality	Reviewed in	Features
Santos et al. 2005 [45]	Brazil March 2000–March 2002	Inclusion: healthy non-smoking women age >20 yrs, early pregnancy BMI 26–31 kg/m², gestational age <20 wk, compliance with 1-wk run-in period, no DM or hypertension, no contraindications to exercise. Sample size: 92 randomized, 72 analyzed	Women were randomized to: (1) supervised exercise 60 min, three times per wk through delivery, or (2) once-weekly focus group, relaxation training, no exercise advice	Improved cardiorespiratory capacity No difference in GWG, gestation length, birthweight	Randomization: blocked sequence given by statistician Allocation concealment: opaque envelopes Blinding: unblinded	Dodd BJOG [15] Streuling BJOG [19]	1. Efficacy 2. Individual 3. Overweight 4. PA only 5. In-person 6. 2nd and 3rd trimesters 7. Birth outcomes, fitness
Sedaghati et al. 2007 [46]	Iran	Inclusion: healthy sedentary women Exclusions: absolute or relative contraindications to exercise in pregnancy Sample size: 100 randomized, 90 analyzed	Women were randomized to: (1) 30-min cycling exercise three times per wk, moderate intensity, or (2) control	Lower GWG (13.55 kg vs. 15.1 kg, p < 0.001) No increase in lower back pain in intervention women compared with controls GWG strongly correlated with LBP	Randomization: not reported Allocation concealment: not reported Blinding: not reported Intervention: women who did not attend the sessions were excluded	Streuling BJOG [19]	1. Efficacy 2. Individual 3. Sedentary 4. PA only 5. In-person 6. 2nd and 3rd trimesters 7. GWG, LBP
Thornton et al. 2009 [69]	USA Urban NY/NJ June 1998–May 2005	Inclusion: singleton pregnancy, 12–28 wks of gestation, BMI ≥30 Exclusion: pre-existing diabetes, hypertension, or chronic renal disease	Women were randomized to: (1) standard antenatal care, or	Lower GWG (mean 11 lb vs. 31 lb, p < 0.001), lower GH (3% vs. 9%, p = 0.046), lower GDM (10% vs. 16%, p = 0.12), lower 6-wk	Randomization: random number table Allocation concealment: opaque envelopes	Dodd BJOG [15]	1. Effectiveness 2. Individual 3. Urban, obese 4. Diet only 5. In-person by RD

	Sample / Inclusion	Intervention	Results	Methods	Citation	Items
	Sample size: 257 women randomized, 232 analyzed	(2) monitored group (visit to dietician and detailed diet protocol)	postpartum maternal weight (200 vs. 227, p < 0.001), no difference in pre-eclampsia, preterm birth, cesarean section, birthweight	Blinding: not stated; Losses to follow-up: 10%	Streuling AJCN [20]	6. 2nd and 3rd trimesters; 7. Birth outcomes and 6-wk postpartum mother's weight
Weisman et al. 2011 [48]	Pennsylvania	Inclusion: non-pregnant women age 18–35 yrs, capable of becoming pregnant; Exclusion: non-English speaking; Sample size: 692 randomized, 362 with follow-up information at 12 wks, 45 with information on pregnancy outcome at 12 mo post-intervention	Women were randomized 2:1 to: (1) Strong Healthy Women intervention, with six, 2-hr sessions over 12 wks, or (2) no intervention	At 14 wks, intervention women with higher self-efficacy, greater intent for healthy behaviors, and improved behaviors. Among subset with pregnancy (n = 45), lower GWG 23.8 vs. 34.2 lbs, mean difference –10.5 lb (95% CI: –24.3 to 3.4)	Randomization: not reported; Allocation concealment: not reported; Blinding: not reported	None	1. Effectiveness; 2. Individual; 3. Low-income rural; 4. Diet and physical activity; 5. In-person (groups); 6. Pre-pregnancy; 7. Outcomes of intervention GWG on a subset, no other birth outcomes
Wolff et al. 2008 [49]	Denmark; Recruitment period not reported	Inclusion: "early" pregnancy, BMI ≥30, non-diabetic, White; Exclusion: smoking, age <18 or >45 yrs, multiple pregnancy, medical complications; Sample size: 73 women randomized, 23 post-randomization exclusions/loss, 50 women analyzed	Women were randomized to: (1) standard antenatal care, or (2) intensive intervention (ten, 1-hr visits with dietician at each antenatal visit)	Mean GWG, pre-eclampsia, hypertension, gestational diabetes, cesarean section, infant birthweight; Lower energy intake, GWG 6.6 kg vs. 13.3 kg, (6.7 kg; 95% CI: 2.6–10.8 kg, p = 0.002); lower s-insulin and leptin (27 w), lower s-insulin and b-glucose (36 w)	Randomization: computer-generated random number table; Allocation concealment: not stated; Blinding: not stated; Losses to follow-up: 32%	Dodd BJOG [15]; Gardner Int J Obes [49]; Ronnberg BJOG [17]; Skouteris Obes Rev [18]	1. Efficacy; 2. Individual; 3. Obese; 4. Diet only; 5. In-person with dietician; 6. 2nd and 3rd trimesters; 7. GWG and birth outcomes, maternal weight at 4 wks, postpartum

Table 14.2 (cont.)

Author	Setting	Population	Intervention	Outcomes	Quality	Reviewed in	Features
Yeo 2009 [50]	US November 2001–July 2006	Inclusion: gestational age <14 weeks, sedentary, lower than average fitness Exclusion: hypertension, diabetes, contraindication to exercise, recommendation of MD, inability to communicate Sample size: 124 randomized, 81% obese	Women were randomized to: (1) moderate intensity walking, or (2) gentle stretching, each 40 mins, five times per wk, from 18 wks to delivery	No difference in mean GWG (15.4 vs. 15.9 kg, p "ns") but 0% walkers vs. 11% stretchers had adequate GWG Stretchers had lower HR and BP, and were more adherent	Randomization: pre-generated allocation schedule Allocation concealment: sealed envelopes Blinding: not reported	Streuling BJOG [19]	1. Efficacy 2. Individual 3. Sedentary 4. PA only 5. In-person 6. 2nd and 3rd trimesters 7. GWG, fitness measures

BP: blood pressure; CVD: cardiovascular disease; CRP: C-reactive protein ; FFM: fat-free mass; GA: gestational age; GH: gestational hypertension; GDM-RF: gestational diabetes mellitus; GWG: gestational weight gain; HC: head circumference; HOMA: homeostatic model assessment; HR: heart rate; LBP: lower back pain; NICU: neonatal intensive care unit; OGTT: oral glucose tolerance test; PA: physical activity; PI: ponderal index; PPWR: postpartum weight retention; PUFA: polyunsaturated fatty acid; RD: registered dietician; SSB: sugar-sweetened beverages.

Table 14.3 Non-randomized interventions during pregnancy that evaluated effects on GWG and related outcomes

Author	Setting	Population	Intervention	Outcomes	Study design / comparison group	Reviewed in	Features
Artal et al. 2007 [58]	USA St. Louis Recruitment period not reported	Inclusion: GDM, BMI >25, GA <33 wks, ability to maintain moderate exercise Exclusion: unclear Sample size: 96 total, 39 intervention, 57 control	Education on healthy low-fat diet, consistent carbohydrate intake, moderate exercise, GWG goals	More intervention women with weight maintenance or loss to delivery (46% vs. 21%), no difference in infant birthweight, delivery method	Assigned to control if contraindication to or declined exercise: received medical nutrition therapy and GDM management program	None	1. Efficacy 2. Individual 3. Overweight/ obese, GDM 4. PA, diet, GWG goals 5. In-person 6. 3rd trimester 7. GWG and birth outcomes
Claesson et al. 2008 [59] Claesson et al. 2011 [63] Claesson et al. 2010 [71]	Sweden November 2003–December 2005	Inclusion: BMI ≥30 Exclusion: not Swedish speaking, pre-pregnancy diabetes, thyroid disease, or psychiatric disease Sample size: 155 intervention, 193 control 238 at 1 yr, 155 at 2 yrs	Trained midwife delivered motivational interview in early pregnancy, 30-min wkly session, 1–2 times per wk water aerobics	Intervention group with lower GWG (8.7 vs. 11.3 kg), more likely to gain <7 kg (36% vs. 21%) No difference in birthweight, GA, or mode of delivery No difference in anxiety or depressive symptoms At 12 mo PPWR –2.2 kg intervention vs. 0.4 kg control, p = 0.046	All obese pregnant women in two nearby cities, same exclusion criteria, routine care	Gardner *Obes Rev* [16] Skouteris *Obes Rev* [18] Ronnberg *BJOG* [17] Streuling *AJCN* [20]	1. Efficacy 2. Individual and organizational 3. Obese 4. Diet, PA 5. In-person, midwife 6. 2nd trimester through postpartum 7. Birth outcomes, postpartum mother's weight

Table 14.3 (cont.)

Author	Setting	Population	Intervention	Outcomes	Study design / comparison group	Reviewed in	Features
Gray-Donald et al. 2000 [57]	Canada Quebec Control July 1995–March 1996 Intervention April 1996–January 1997	Inclusion: Cree women in one of four communities, <26 wks gestation Exclusion: pre-gestational diabetes Sample size: 219 women (107 control, 112 intervention) Mean BMI: 29.6 control, 30.8 intervention	Research and Cree nutritionists and Cree health workers dietary advice focus on improved dairy, fruit and vegetable intake, and lower intake of energy-dense, nutrient-poor foods; via individual counseling, radio broadcasts, pamphlets, exercise groups, cooking demonstrations	Energy and nutrient intake, at 27 wks GWG GDM and glucose screen results at 28 wks gestation Birthweight, macrosomia, PPWR No effect on any outcomes	Pre-post intervention design ITT analysis	Gardner Obes Rev [16] Ronnberg BJOG [17] Skouteris Obes Rev [18] Streuling AJCN [20]	1. Effectiveness 2. Individual, community 3. Cree 4. Diet 5. In-person (nutritionists and health workers) and public campaign 6. 2nd to 3rd trimesters 7. GDM results, GWG and birth outcomes, 6-wk postpartum weight
Kinnunen et al. 2007 [53]	Finland August 2004–January 2005	Inclusion: women attending one of six maternity clinics, nulliparous, Finnish speaking Exclusion: age <18yrs, type1 or type 2 DM, twin gestation, disability, pregnancy complications, psychiatric illness, substance abuse Sample size: 105 (69 intervention, 63 control)	GWG recommendations (IOM), physical activity counseling session with four boosters, dietary counseling (regular meals with breakfast, ≥5 fruits/vegetables, high-fiber bread, ≤1 high-sugar snack)	GWG per IOM, diet, MET min/wk No effect on GWG (14.6 vs. 14.3 kg, p = 0.77) or PA Lower decrease in high-fiber bread, increase in fruits/ vegetables, increase in fiber, Fewer macrosomic infants (0% vs. 15%, p = 0.006)	Women attending control clinics; received usual care Analysis did not account for clustering	Gardner Obes Rev [16] Ronnberg BJOG [17] Skouteris Obes Rev [18] Streuling AJCN [20]	1. Effectiveness 2. Individual 3. All 4. Diet, PA, GWG advice 5. In-person 6. 1st trimester delivery 7. GWG, birth outcomes

Study	Location, Date	Inclusion/Exclusion/Sample	Intervention	Results	Design	References
Olson et al. 2004 [62]	Upstate NY March 2000–April 2001	Inclusion: BMI 19.8–29.0, prenatal care <3rd trimester, age ≥18 yrs, competent, singleton Exclusion: medical condition affecting body weight Sample size: 560 (179 intervention, 381 controls)	Clinical GWG guidance and monitoring, mailed patient education	Overall no significant difference in mean GWG (14.80 kg control vs. 14.10 kg int, $p = 0.09$) or PPWR (1.31 kg control vs. 0.59 kg int, $p = 0.14$) In low-income (normal and overweight) women 52% vs. 33% adequate GWG	Historical control: women enrolled in a previous observational study 1995–1997	Gardner Obes Rev [16] Ronnberg BJOG [17] Skouteris Obes Rev [18] Streuling AJCN [20]
Shirazian et al. 2010 [60]	USA New York City 2007–2008	Inclusion: singleton, pre-preg BMI ≥30, no underlying medical condition, first trimester Exclusion: chronic medical condition, multiple gestation, preterm delivery Sample size: 28 recruited, 21 intervention, and 20 controls	Lifestyle modification program (LMP), a comprehensive program on nutrition, exercise, and weight control in pregnancy to limit weight gain to 15 lbs. Six structured seminars led by study coordinators, and 1–1, in-person, or phone sessions	Lower GWG (17 vs. 34 lbs, $p = 0.003$), no difference in gestation length, infant birthweight, pre-eclampsia, cesarean delivery, fetal complications, labor complications, postpartum complications	Prospective matched controlled study design; controls were matched by starting BMI, parity, and socioeconomic status during the same study period cared for at the same institution Intervention women excluded if did not attend intervention	Gardner Obes Rev [16] Streuling AJCN [20]

Olson et al. 2004 [62]:
1. Effectiveness
2. Individual and clinic
3. Normal and overweight
4. GWG monitoring, a bit on diet/PA
5. In clinic, via mail
6. 2nd trimester through delivery
7. GWG and 12-mo PPWR

Shirazian et al. 2010 [60]:
1. Efficacy
2. Individual
3. Obese, low-income, Medicaid
4. Diet, PA, GWG advice
5. In-person, phone
6. 2nd trimester through delivery
7. GWG, birth outcomes

effectiveness study with a cluster RCT design that also did not influence GWG, but was associated with lower fetal growth and likelihood of large for gestational age (LGA) [37]. Additionally, one small effectiveness trial (n = 120 randomized), which was successful in reducing excessive GWG among normal weight women only [41], was followed by a larger effectiveness trial (n = 401) randomized, which also found a lower risk of excessive GWG among normal weight but not overweight/obese women [40].

Social ecological model

Increasingly, obesity experts are suggesting that that a transdisciplinary and multilevel approach is essential for understanding and ultimately preventing obesity [54,55]. Behaviors such as dietary intake and physical activity, resulting in an imbalance between energy input and expenditure, are the final common pathway leading to excess weight gain. However, upstream factors, including mood, self-efficacy, and self-image often underlie these behaviors. Furthermore, interpersonal, organizational, community, and policy influence, shape, and constrain individual behaviors. The social ecological model [56] provides a framework for mapping these influences (Figure 14.1).

While all interventions addressed individual-level behaviors, few addressed personal barriers to behavior change, such as self-efficacy, mood, or self-esteem. Only four of the RCTs and two of the non-randomized interventions attempted to influence obstetric care delivery.

Practice level changes included adding extra routine prenatal visits, training clinicians or dieticians to provide counseling in healthy eating and physical activity, having obstetric clinicians chart and provide feedback on GWG, and offering healthy eating or exercise training via individual sessions, classes, or interactive computer. One non-randomized study, performed among the Cree of James Bay, Quebec, Canada, developed an intervention for the entire community [57]. That intervention, which included training of nutritionists and local health workers to deliver messages via local radio broadcasts about healthful eating in pregnancy, supermarket tours, and cooking demonstrations as well as via individual counseling, was not successful in influencing GWG or related outcomes including obesogenic diet, GDM, and infant birthweight, although the investigators did observe a reduction in caffeine intake in pregnancy and an increase in folate intake postpartum. Another study, a small RCT (n = 52), which embedded an individual-level intervention within a community prenatal program, also found no effect on GWG [32]. We did not identify any studies that attempted to influence GWG by acting upon interpersonal relationships, or any that evaluated the effects of governmental policies.

Participant characteristics

Inclusion and exclusion criteria differed among the various studies. In general, studies that included physical activity as the primary intervention limited enrollment to women who had been sedentary. Most of the

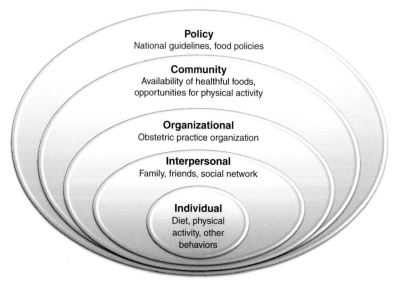

Figure 14.1. Social ecological model: levels of influence on obesity-related pregnancy outcomes.

studies excluded women with a diagnosed history of type 1 or type 2 diabetes before pregnancy. However, some, especially those with a primary outcome of improving glucose metabolism, targeted women with gestational diabetes mellitus (GDM) in the index pregnancy [25,43,58], and two included women at high risk for developing GDM based on having one or more of the following risk factors: pre-pregnancy overweight, age >40 years, GDM or macrosomia in a prior pregnancy, diabetes in a first degree relative, or elevated fasting glucose in early pregnancy [35,37].

Of particular relevance to this book, several studies targeted women who were overweight and/or obese entering pregnancy [29,39,42–45,47,49], including three non-randomized studies [58–60]. Of the exercise-only interventions, one targeted women who were overweight [45], one included women who were both obese and sedentary prior to pregnancy [39], and one included women who were overweight or obese and diagnosed with GDM [58]. While many of these studies were successful in reducing GWG (Table 14.2), the majority of the RCTs among overweight and obese women showed no effect [28,38,42–45]. Furthermore, among the successful interventions, the absolute effect sizes were often small, and generally did not substantially increase the proportion of women who were gaining within recommended ranges.

Additional investigators performed stratified analyses to look for different intervention effects among women across weight categories. Phelan et al.[40] stratified randomization according to normal weight (19.8–26.0 kg/m²) or overweight/obese (26.1–40 kg/m²) pre-pregnancy BMI [61]. They observed that normal weight women randomized to the intervention had a lower risk of excessive GWG (OR 0.38; 95% CI: 0.20–0.87) compared to normal weight women randomized to the control condition, but among overweight/obese women there was no difference by study arm in risk for excessive GWG (OR 1.4; 95% CI: 0.70–2.7). Similarly, Jeffries et al. [34] found no effect of the intervention overall (mean difference, 0.02 kg/week; 95% CI: −0.02–0.07 kg/week), or among underweight, normal, or obese women, but women who were overweight had significantly reduced GWG in the intervention vs. control arm (mean difference, 0.12 kg/week; 95% CI: 0.03–0.22 kg/week). In contrast, however, in the study by Polley et al. [41] the intervention significantly decreased the percentage of normal weight women who exceeded the IOM recommendations

(33% vs. 58%, p < 0.05), but there was no benefit among overweight/obese women, in fact rather there was a non-significant increase in excessive GWG (59% vs. 32%, p = 0.09). In the study by Olson et al. [62], the intervention effected no changes in GWG among either normal weight or overweight women overall, compared with historical controls, but among low-income women there was a significant difference between the control and intervention groups in the proportion exceeding recommended weight gains, with similar effects seen among both normal weight and overweight women. Finally, in the study by Asbee et al. [23], there was no statistically significant difference in adherence across BMI groups between the intensive counseling and routine care groups. Thus, there has been substantial heterogeneity across various studies regarding the sensitivity of women of pre-pregnancy weight status to intervention messages, and many have not shown substantial benefit among overweight and obese women.

Behavioral targets

Behavioral targets of the different interventions included some combination of diet and physical activity, and messages regarding GWG tracking/advice. Eleven RCTs, and none of the non-randomized studies, used physical activity as the primary behavioral target of the intervention. Five RCTs focused on diet and physical activity, five focused on diet only, four included all three targets, and one included diet and GWG advice but not physical activity. One intervention relied entirely on weight gain advice and tracking [34]. In contrast, others emphasized dietary and exercise behavior changes over a focus on weight gain [33]. Among the non-RCT interventions, one targeted diet only; one targeted physical activity and diet; and four targeted diet, physical activity, and GWG advice.

The exact intervention content differed across the studies, especially for diet and physical activity. For example, some dietary interventions included recommendations to follow national dietary guidelines [62]. Some interventions included advice to limit total energy intake (kcal), either with general advice such as 20 kcal/kg body weight [40,43], or individualized to a woman's weight category or other characteristics [23,35]. A number of the interventions focused on the macronutrient composition of the diet, although recommendations varied substantially: e.g., one study recommended 9% to 11% of calories from proteins and 50% to 55% from carbohydrates [29]; whereas another recommended 30% of calories from proteins and 40% from carbohydrates [23]. Several emphasized diets low in fat [35,37,40,41], whereas others focused on the quality of dietary fats [33,36,37]. One study particularly focused on the relative influences of a reduction of dietary fats or a decrease in the glycemic load of the diet [44]. Several interventions focused on foods and food groups rather than nutrients, with various messages aimed at limiting intake of energy-dense foods, fast foods, sugary foods, or snacks containing high levels of sugar and/or fat, and increased intake of fruits, vegetables, whole-grain foods, and low-fat dairy [29,33,37,41]. Different physical activity regimens included general physical activity advice or structured physical activity at home (advice for regular physical activity, stationary cycle use, walking, stretching) or in individual or group exercise classes (aerobic, resistance training, water aerobics, aerobic dance).

In general, the studies included GWG advice that was in line with the 1990 US Institute of Medicine guidelines [61], including the non-US studies, as none of the interventions began after the 2009 guidelines were released [1].

Intervention delivery

Very few studies have explained the theoretical basis of the intensity or mode of delivery [16]. Most of the interventions were delivered in person at a study center or prenatal practice, by trained study staff, dieticians, or obstetric clinicians. Most were delivered in individual one-on-one sessions, though a few included group visits, especially for physical activity. The two community-based interventions were delivered part in community settings; one of these studies was the only one that reported using lay health workers. Some of the physical activity interventions that recommended home exercises included a home visit for training. Two studies included a mailed component – one incorporated biweekly mailed newsletters prompting healthy eating and exercise habits [41], and another mailed five newsletters with messages about GWG, physical activity, and diet during pregnancy that included a postcard on which the women could ask questions [62]. Only one study used electronic technology to deliver intervention messages [33]. This study used the Video Doctor, a computer program delivered on laptop computers in the clinic setting that conducted in-depth

behavioral risk assessments, delivered tailored counseling messages, and produced printed output for both the patient and clinician. However, patients had only a single encounter with the Video Doctor followed by a brief booster Video Doctor visit four weeks later. No studies used newer technologies such as mobile phones, text messaging, or internet platforms to deliver intervention messages or promote tracking of behaviors.

Timing and duration of intervention

Most of the interventions commenced in the second trimester and continued to delivery, although some lasted only into the early third trimester [39]. A notable exception was studies that recruited women after diagnosis of GDM, which generally occurred at around 28 weeks gestation. A few studies began in the first trimester [27,53], and several continued into the postpartum period [30,36,40,47,62,63]. One pre-pregnancy intervention recruited healthy non-pregnant women, who were randomized to attend six group intervention sessions over a 12-week period or usual care. Among the subset of women (45 of 692 randomized) who went on to have a pregnancy within 12 months of completing the intervention, those who had been in the intervention arm had lower GWG [64].

Outcomes

By virtue of our inclusion criteria, all studies included information on GWG. Most included total GWG, i.e., the difference in weight gain from pre-pregnancy to just before delivery. Two studies reported weight gain during the period of intervention delivery [42,58]. Most of the studies also included other birth outcomes, including gestational age, infant birthweight, and related measures, e.g., small or large for gestational age, macrosomia, and route of delivery. Some included complications of pregnancy (pre-eclampsia, GDM) or delivery (birth trauma). Some of the studies, especially those that included a physical activity intervention, included measures of maternal body fat or cardiorespiratory fitness, and a few had detailed measures of glucose homeostasis. One study assessed neonatal body fat [27], and one had cord blood measures of insulin-like growth factors [31]. Some, but not all, of the studies, reported maternal behaviors such as self-reported diet.

While most reviews have not attempted to summarize intervention effects on outcomes other than GWG, the recent meta-analysis by Dodd *et al.* [15] found no reduced risk of GDM, LGA birth, or other birth outcomes [15]. Another systematic review by the UK's National Institute for Health and Clinical Excellence (NICE) found inconsistent or no evidence for a benefit of lifestyle interventions during pregnancy for gestation length, birthweight, or rates of cesarean delivery or macrosomia [65].

Conclusions

On the whole, the literature suggests that interventions to improve diet or physical activity during pregnancy or reduce excessive GWG have been moderately successful in doing so but the degree of restriction, if achieved, is generally modest. Most studies are underpowered for clinical outcomes, but meta-analyses have hitherto not indicated that any clinical benefit has been achieved. The dearth of studies among overweight and obese women, the heterogeneity of study designs and intervention content, the lack of important clinical outcomes, and the relatively low methodologic quality of most studies preclude firm inferences regarding how best to modify GWG.

Our review of published interventions reveals several imperatives for future research:

- Observational studies to further characterize behavioral determinants of GWG, which will serve as foci for behavior change in RCTs.
- RCTs with sample sizes large enough to
  - examine as outcomes not only weight gain but also
    - clinically important outcomes for mother and child, and
    - body composition and metabolic mediators; and
  - examine effect modification (subgroup analysis) according to participant characteristics such as race/ethnicity, weight status, and age.
- RCTs with attention to proven theory and methodologic quality, including method of randomization, masking, high retention rates, valid measures, and appropriate analytic approaches.
- RCTs that include subpopulations at highest risk including obese women, racial/ethnic minorities, and women from lower socioeconomic position.
- RCTs that distinguish whether benefits to maternal–child outcomes operate through

changes in weight gain or via metabolic pathways that do not involve changes in weight.
- RCTs that address efficacy and effectiveness; for effectiveness trials, that invoke several levels of the social ecological model including health systems.
- RCTs that measure and report adverse events and outcomes.
- RCTs that estimate cost-effectiveness.
- RCTs that involve longer term maternal and child follow-up.
- Decision–analytic approaches to evaluating optimal GWG that balance short- and long-term outcomes for both mother and child.

References

1. Institute of Medicine and National Research Council of the National Academies. *Weight Gain During Pregnancy: Reexamining the Guidelines.* (Washington, DC: National Academies Press, 2009).

2. Oken E, Kleinman K P, Belfort M B, Hammitt J K & Gillman M W. Associations of gestational weight gain with short- and longer-term maternal and child health outcomes. *Am J Epidemiol* 2009;**170**:173–80.

3. Siega-Riz A M, Viswanathan M, Moos M K, *et al.* A systematic review of outcomes of maternal weight gain according to the Institute of Medicine recommendations: birthweight, fetal growth, and postpartum weight retention. *Am J Obstet Gynecol* 2009;**201**:339 e1–14.

4. Herring S, Oken E, Rifas-Shiman S, *et al.* Weight gain in pregnancy and risk of maternal hyperglycemia. *Am J Obstet Gynecol* 2009;**201**:61e1–7.

5. Chen A, Feresu S A, Fernandez C & Rogan W J. Maternal obesity and the risk of infant death in the United States. *Epidemiology* 2009;**20**:74–81.

6. Oken E, Taveras E M, Kleinman K P, Rich-Edwards J W & Gillman M W. Gestational weight gain and child adiposity at age 3 years. *Am J Obstet Gynecol* 2007;**196**:322e1–8.

7. Oken E, Rifas-Shiman S L, Field A E, Frazier A L & Gillman M W. Maternal gestational weight gain and offspring weight in adolescence. *Obstet Gynecol* 2008;**112**:999–1006.

8. Cedergren M I. Optimal gestational weight gain for body mass index categories. *Obstet Gynecol* 2007;**110**:759–64.

9. Kiel D W, Dodson E A, Artal R, Boehmer T K & Leet T L. Gestational weight gain and pregnancy outcomes in obese women: how much is enough? *Obstet Gynecol* 2007;**110**:752–8.

10. Nohr E A, Vaeth M, Baker J L, *et al*. Combined associations of prepregnancy body mass index and gestational weight gain with the outcome of pregnancy. *Am J Clin Nutr* 2008;**87**:1750–9.

11. Vesco K K, Dietz P M, Rizzo J, *et al*. Excessive gestational weight gain and postpartum weight retention among obese women. *Obstet Gynecol* 2009;**114**:1069–75.

12. Vesco K K, Sharma A J, Dietz P M, *et al*. Newborn size among obese women with weight gain outside the 2009 Institute of Medicine recommendation. *Obstet Gynecol* 2011;**117**:812–18.

13. Hinkle S N, Sharma A J & Dietz P M. Gestational weight gain in obese mothers and associations with fetal growth. *Am J Clin Nutr* 2010;**92**:644–51.

14. Beyerlein A, Schiessl B, Lack N & von Kries R. Associations of gestational weight loss with birth-related outcome: a retrospective cohort study. *BJOG* 2011;**118**:55–61.

15. Dodd J M, Grivell R M, Crowther C A & Robinson J S. Antenatal interventions for overweight or obese pregnant women: a systematic review of randomised trials. *BJOG* 2010;**117**:1316–26.

16. Gardner B, Wardle J, Poston L & Croker H. Changing diet and physical activity to reduce gestational weight gain: a meta-analysis. *Obes Rev* 2011;**12**(7):e602–20.

17. Ronnberg A K & Nilsson K. Interventions during pregnancy to reduce excessive gestational weight gain: a systematic review assessing current clinical evidence using the Grading of Recommendations, Assessment, Development and Evaluation (GRADE) system. *BJOG* 2010;**117**:1327–34.

18. Skouteris H, Hartley-Clark L, McCabe M, *et al*. Preventing excessive gestational weight gain: a systematic review of interventions. *Obes Rev* 2010;**11**:757–68.

19. Streuling I, Beyerlein A, Rosenfeld E, *et al*. Physical activity and gestational weight gain: a meta-analysis of intervention trials. *BJOG* 2010;**118**:278–84.

20. Streuling I, Beyerlein A & von Kries R. Can gestational weight gain be modified by increasing physical activity and diet counseling? A meta-analysis of interventional trials. *Am J Clin Nutr* 2010;**92**:678–87.

21. Magee M S, Knopp R H & Benedetti T J. Metabolic effects of 1200-kcal diet in obese pregnant women with gestational diabetes. *Diabetes* 1990;**39**:234–40.

22. Prevedel T, Calderon I, De Conti M, Consonni E & Rudge M. Maternal and perinatal effects of hydrotherapy in pregnancy. *Revista Brasileira de Ginecologia e Obstetricia* 2003;**25**:53–9.

23. Asbee S M, Jenkins T R, Butler J R, *et al*. Preventing excessive weight gain during pregnancy through dietary and lifestyle counseling: a randomized controlled trial. *Obstet Gynecol* 2009;**113**:305–12.

24. Barakat R, Lucia A & Ruiz J R. Resistance exercise training during pregnancy and newborn's birth size: a randomised controlled trial. *Int J Obes (Lond)* 2009;**33**:1048–57.

25. Brankston G N, Mitchell B F, Ryan E A & Okun N B. Resistance exercise decreases the need for insulin in overweight women with gestational diabetes mellitus. *Am J Obstet Gynecol* 2004;**190**:188–93.

26. Cavalcante S R, Cecatti J G, Pereira R I, *et al*. Water aerobics II: maternal body composition and perinatal outcomes after a program for low risk pregnant women. *Reprod Health* 2009;**6**:1.

27. Clapp J F, 3rd, Kim H, Burciu B, Lopez B. Beginning regular exercise in early pregnancy: effect on fetoplacental growth. *Am J Obstet Gynecol* 2000;**183**:1484–8.

28. Garshasbi A & Faghih Zadeh S. The effect of exercise on the intensity of low back pain in pregnant women. *Int J Gynaecol Obstet* 2005;**88**:271–5.

29. Guelinckx I, Devlieger R, Mullie P & Vansant G. Effect of lifestyle intervention on dietary habits, physical activity, and gestational weight gain in obese pregnant women: a randomized controlled trial. *Am J Clin Nutr* 2010;**91**:373–80.

30. Haakstad L A & Bø K. Effect of regular exercise on prevention of excessive weight gain in pregnancy: a randomised controlled trial. *Eur J Contracept Reprod Health Care* 2011;**16**:116–25.

31. Hopkins S A, Baldi J C, Cutfield W S, McCowan L & Hofman P L. Exercise training in pregnancy reduces offspring size without changes in maternal insulin sensitivity. *J Clin Endocrinol Metab* 2010;**95**:2080–8.

32. Hui A L, Ludwig S M, Gardiner P, *et al*. Community-based exercise and dietary intervention during pregnancy: a pilot study. *Can J Diabetes* 2006;**30**:169–75.

33. Jackson R A, Stotland N E, Caughey A B & Gerbert B. Improving diet and exercise in pregnancy with Video Doctor counseling: a randomized trial. *Patient Educ Couns* 2011;**83**:203–9.

34. Jeffries K, Shub A, Walker S P, Hiscock R & Permezel M. Reducing excessive weight gain in pregnancy: a randomised controlled trial. *Med J Aust* 2009;**191**:429–33.

35. Korpi-Hyovalti E A, Laaksonen D E, Schwab U S, *et al*. Feasibility of a lifestyle intervention in early pregnancy to prevent deterioration of glucose tolerance. *BMC Public Health* 2011;**11**:179.

36. Laitinen K, Poussa T & Isolauri E. Probiotics and dietary counselling contribute to glucose regulation

during and after pregnancy: a randomised controlled trial. *Br J Nutr* 2009;**101**:1679–87.

37. Luoto R, Kinnunen T I, Aittasalo M, *et al.* Primary prevention of gestational diabetes mellitus and large-for-gestational-age newborns by lifestyle counseling: a cluster-randomized controlled trial. *PLoS Med* 2011;**8**:e1001036.

38. Marquez-Sterling S, Perry A C, Kaplan T A, Halberstein R A & Signorile J F. Physical and psychological changes with vigorous exercise in sedentary primigravidae. *Med Sci Sports Exerc* 2000;**32**:58–62.

39. Ong M J, Guelfi K J, Hunter T, *et al.* Supervised home-based exercise may attenuate the decline of glucose tolerance in obese pregnant women. *Diabetes Metab* 2009;**35**:418–21.

40. Phelan S, Phipps M G, Abrams B, *et al.* Randomized trial of a behavioral intervention to prevent excessive gestational weight gain: the Fit for Delivery Study. *Am J Clin Nutr* 2011;**93**(4):772–9.

41. Polley B A, Wing R R & Sims C J. Randomized controlled trial to prevent excessive weight gain in pregnant women. *Int J Obes Relat Metab Disord* 2002;**26**:1494–502.

42. Quinlivan J A, Lam L T & Fisher J. A randomised trial of a four-step multidisciplinary approach to the antenatal care of obese pregnant women. *Aust N Z J Obstet Gynaecol* 2011;**51**:141–6.

43. Rae A, Bond D, Evans S, *et al.* A randomised controlled trial of dietary energy restriction in the management of obese women with gestational diabetes. *Aust N Z J Obstet Gynaecol* 2000;**40**:416–22.

44. Rhodes E T, Pawlak D B, Takoudes T C, *et al.* Effects of a low-glycemic load diet in overweight and obese pregnant women: a pilot randomized controlled trial. *Am J Clin Nutr* 2010;**92**:1306–15.

45. Santos I A, Stein R, Fuchs S C, *et al.* Aerobic exercise and submaximal functional capacity in overweight pregnant women: a randomized trial. *Obstet Gynecol* 2005;**106**:243–9.

46. Sedaghati P, Zaiee V & Ardjmand A. The effect of an ergometric training program on pregnants weight gain and low back pain. *Gazz Med Ital-Arch Sci Med* 2007;**166**:209–13.

47. Thornton Y S. Preventing excessive weight gain during pregnancy through dietary and lifestyle counseling: a randomized controlled trial. *Obstet Gynecol* 2009;**114**:173; author reply 173–4.

48. Weisman C S, Hillemeier M M, Downs D S, *et al.* Improving women's preconceptional health: long-term effects of the Strong Healthy Women behavior change intervention in the Central Pennsylvania Women's Health Study. *Womens Health Issues* 2011;**21**(4):265–71.

49. Wolff S, Legarth J, Vangsgaard K, Toubro S & Astrup A. A randomized trial of the effects of dietary counseling on gestational weight gain and glucose metabolism in obese pregnant women. *Int J Obes (Lond)* 2008;**32**:495–501.

50. Yeo S. Adherence to walking or stretching, and risk of preeclampsia in sedentary pregnant women. *Res Nurs Health* 2009;**32**:379–90.

51. Godwin M, Ruhland L, Casson I, *et al.* Pragmatic controlled clinical trials in primary care: the struggle between external and internal validity. *BMC Med Res Methodol* 2003;**3**:28.

52. Gartlehner G, Hansen R A, Nissman D, Lohr K N & Carey T S. Criteria for distinguishing effectiveness from efficacy trials in systematic reviews. Technical Review 12. (Prepared by the RTI-International/University of North Carolina Evidence-based Practice Center under Contract No. 290–02–0016.) AHRQ Publication No. 06–0046. (Rockville, MD: Agency for Healthcare Research and Quality, 2006).

53. Kinnunen T I, Pasanen M, Aittasalo M, *et al.* Preventing excessive weight gain during pregnancy – a controlled trial in primary health care. *Eur J Clin Nutr* 2007;**61**:884–91.

54. Rayner G, Gracia M, Young E, *et al.* Why are we fat? Discussions on the socioeconomic dimensions and responses to obesity. *Global Health* 2010;**6**:7.

55. Davison K K & Birch L L. Childhood overweight: a contextual model and recommendations for future research. *Obes Rev* 2001;**2**:159–71.

56. Stokols D, Allen J & Bellingham R L. The social ecology of health promotion: implications for research and practice. *Am J Health Promot* 1996;**10**:247–51.

57. Gray-Donald K, Robinson E, Collier A, *et al.* Intervening to reduce weight gain in pregnancy and gestational diabetes mellitus in Cree communities: an evaluation. *CMAJ* 2000;**163**:1247–51.

58. Artal R, Catanzaro R B, Gavard J A, Mostello D J & Friganza J C. A lifestyle intervention of weight-gain restriction: diet and exercise in obese women with gestational diabetes mellitus. *Appl Physiol Nutr Metab* 2007;**32**:596–601.

59. Claesson I M, Sydsjo G, Brynhildsen J, *et al.* Weight gain restriction for obese pregnant women: a case-control intervention study. *BJOG* 2008;**115**:44–50.

60. Shirazian T, Monteith S, Friedman F & Rebarber A. Lifestyle modification program decreases pregnancy weight gain in obese women. *Am J Perinatol* 2010;**27**:411–14.

61. Institute of Medicine. *Nutrition During Pregnancy.* (Washington, DC: National Academy Press, 1990).

62. Olson C M, Strawderman M S & Reed R G. Efficacy of an intervention to prevent excessive gestational weight gain. *Am J Obstet Gynecol* 2004;**191**:530–6.

63. Claesson I M, Sydsjo G, Brynhildsen J, *et al.* Weight after childbirth: a 2-year follow-up of obese women in a weight-gain restriction program. *Acta Obstet Gynecol Scand* 2011;**90**:103–10.

64. Weisman C S, Hillemeier M M, Downs D S, Chuang C H & Dyer A M. Preconception predictors of weight gain during pregnancy: prospective findings from the Central Pennsylvania Women's Health Study. *Womens Health Issues* 2011;**20**:126–32.

65. Campbell F, Johnson M, Messina J, Guillaume L & Goyder E. Behavioural interventions for weight management in pregnancy: a systematic review of quantitative and qualitative data. *BMC Public Health* 2011; **11**:491.

66. Barakat R, Stirling J R & Lucia A. Does exercise training during pregnancy affect gestational age? A randomised controlled trial. *Br J Sports Med* 2008;**42**:674–8.

67. Baciuk E P, Pereira R I, Cecatti J G, Braga A F & Cavalcante S R. Water aerobics in pregnancy: cardiovascular response, labor and neonatal outcomes. *Reprod Health* 2008;**5**:10.

68. Piirainen T, Isolauri E, Lagstrom H & Laitinen K. Impact of dietary counselling on nutrient intake during pregnancy: a prospective cohort study. *Br J Nutr* 2006;**96**:1095–104.

69. Thornton Y S, Smarkola C, Kopacz S M & Ishoof S B. Perinatal outcomes in nutritionally monitored obese pregnant women: a randomized clinical trial. *J Natl Med Assoc* 2009;**101**:569–77.

70. Bechtel-Blackwell D A. Computer-assisted self-interview and nutrition education in pregnant teens. *Clin Nurs Res* 2002;**11**:450–62.

71. Claesson I M, Josefsson A & Sydsjo G. Prevalence of anxiety and depressive symptoms among obese pregnant and postpartum women: an intervention study. *BMC Public Health* 2010;**10**:766.

15

Interventional strategies to improve outcome in obese pregnancies: insulin resistance and gestational diabetes

Scott M. Nelson and Lucilla Poston

Introduction

In this chapter we address the metabolic sequelae of maternal obesity, and by detailing effects on glucose, lipid, and protein metabolism, parallels with type 2 diabetes are highlighted. These similarities and the success of lifestyle intervention strategies for the prevention of type 2 diabetes may provide a road map for the development of strategies to modify maternal hyperglycemia – a key determinant of pregnancy complications.

Maternal metabolism

Lipid metabolism

Lipid metabolism undergoes major adjustment during pregnancy as although there is no change in either basal carbohydrate oxidation or non-oxidizable carbohydrate metabolism there is a significant 50% to 80% increase in basal fat oxidation during pregnancy and also in response to glucose [1]. There is also a marked hyperlipidemia in pregnancy [2–4]. Specifically very low-density lipoprotein (VLDL) triglyceride concentrations increase three-fold from 14 weeks gestation to term [5], with concomitant decreases in hepatic lipase activity [2]. This increase in plasma triglyceride concentration results may drive in the appearance of small, dense low-density lipoprotein (LDL) particles, particularly in late pregnancy [6]. Plasma cholesterol levels rise to a lesser degree due to an early decrease in LDL followed by a modest continuous rise in high-density lipoprotein (HDL) (particularly the HDL-2 subfraction) by over 40% after 14 weeks gestation [5]. HDL cholesterol exhibits a triphasic profile, rising to a peak at 25 weeks, and then declining to 32 weeks with maintenance at this level until term [7]. These changes

in lipoprotein concentrations are associated with the progressive increases in estradiol, progesterone, and human placental lactogen [7], and estrogens are known to enhance VLDL production and decrease hepatic lipase activity and may play a key role in the accumulation of triglycerides in lipoproteins of higher density than VLDL [8].

In obese pregnant women this hyperlipidemia is exaggerated. Total and VLDL triglycerides are increased further and plasma HDL are even lower; in contrast, LDL is unaltered [9–11]. The relative inability of insulin to suppress whole-body lipolysis leads to a marked increase in plasma free fatty acids in obese patients [12], thereby further amplifying the already higher concentrations associated with obesity [13]. The increases in fat oxidation are also maintained even in the absence of changes to carbohydrate metabolism, with an inverse correlation between endogenous glucose production and fat oxidation from pre-pregnancy to early gestation [1]. Lastly the susceptibility of LDL to oxidation, a classic associate of endothelial dysfunction, atherosclerosis, and cell toxicity is exacerbated by maternal obesity [14]. Collectively the pattern of dyslipidemia observed in obese pregnancy is therefore similar to those observed in non-pregnant obese individuals [15].

This dyslipidemia may also contribute to obesity-related vascular complications including pre-eclampsia – with maternal hypertriglyceridemia being a characteristic of women destined to develop pre-eclampsia [16–23]. The observed changes in triglycerides in pre-eclampsia are accompanied by an almost three-fold higher VLDL1, a two-fold increase in VLDL2 concentration [20,22], marked increases in free fatty acids, and a three-fold increase in small dense

Maternal Obesity, ed. Matthew W. Gillman and Lucilla Poston. Published by Cambridge University Press. © Cambridge University Press 2012.

LDL, with a reduction in large buoyant LDL subfractions [6,20,24,25]. It is these small dense LDL particles, which are increased in both pre-eclampsia and obesity, that are highly atherogenic and capable of promoting foam cell formation and endothelial dysfunction [26], with further impairment of endothelial function by elevated free fatty acids. Collectively this pattern suggests that obese women or women with excessive gestational weight gain may have sufficient pre-existing or newly acquired dyslipidemia to facilitate the acute development of placental bed atherosis and pre-eclampsia. Furthermore this association in conjunction with increased inflammation, would provide a potential explanation for the strong epidemiological associations of pre-eclampsia with pre-pregnancy BMI and excessive gestational weight gain [20,27,28].

Amino acid metabolism

In pregnancy the mother uses the majority of amino acids for protein synthesis, with a reduction in the amount oxidized by approximately 10% [29]. Although counter-intuitively there is no increase in measured protein synthesis in the first trimester, there is an increase in the second and third trimester of 15% and 25% respectively [30–33]. These are greater than can simply be accounted for by highly active protein synthesis in the fetus and placenta, implying an overall increase in protein synthesis in maternal tissues including the liver, breasts, and uterus. The impact of maternal protein turnover on the fetus is striking, with a greater maternal protein synthesis in the second trimester being associated with an increase in birth length and accounting for 26% of its overall variance [34]. The proportion of maternal amino acid metabolism that is directed toward fetal protein synthesis rather than oxidation, can also modify birthweight, with 34% of the variance of birthweight related to this shift, presumably due more to fat-free mass than to fat mass [29].

At present the impact of obesity on maternal and fetal amino acid metabolism is unknown. However, in non-pregnant obese women protein synthesis is stimulated less in a hyperinsulinemic state in comparison with lean women, with no difference in protein oxidation [35]. Obesity is also associated with a greater supply of gluconeogenic amino acids to the liver with preference of their use over glycogen for glucose production [36]. Lastly, visceral lean mass is positively correlated with maternal protein turnover [34]. Collectively these data would suggest that the anabolic response to pregnancy

may be impaired in obese women, raising the possibility that mechanisms may exist to limit what would otherwise be greater fetal growth in a hyperinsulinemic and glucose-rich environment.

Glucose metabolism and insulin resistance

In normal pregnancy, dynamic changes in maternal glucose homeostasis and insulin sensitivity accompany the alterations in lipid and protein metabolism. In early pregnancy, maternal fasting glucose decreases by 2 mg/dl very early in gestation (weeks 6 to 10), with little further decrease by the third trimester [37]. Basal hepatic glucose production increases with advancing gestation (16%–30%), as does total gluconeogenesis to meet the increasing needs of the placenta and fetus [38–41]. Postprandial glucose concentrations are also elevated and the glucose peak is prolonged during pregnancy [42]. These increases in glucose production occur despite rises in fasting insulin concentrations [38], and are also relative to maternal body weight, such that glucose production per kilogram body weight does not change throughout pregnancy [41]. Commensurate with the increased rate of glucose production, there is an increased contribution of carbohydrate to oxidative metabolism in late pregnancy, with an adjusted rate of carbohydrate oxidation of 282 g/d at 37 weeks gestation, which then falls to 210g/d by three months postpartum [43].

Facilitating these alterations in glucose homeostasis are marked changes in insulin secretion and sensitivity. During early pregnancy, glucose tolerance is normal or slightly improved and peripheral (muscle) sensitivity to insulin and hepatic basal glucose production is normal [38,44,45]. This increased peripheral insulin sensitivity is accompanied by a greater than normal sensitivity to the blood glucose-lowering effect of exogenously administered insulin in the first trimester, which disappears in the second and third trimesters. Longitudinal studies of glucose tolerance during gestation demonstrate an increased insulin response to oral glucose in the first trimester relative to pre-pregnancy values [44], with a subsequent progressive increase in nutrient-stimulated insulin responses despite only a minor deterioration in glucose tolerance, consistent with progressive insulin resistance [44]. Notably there is also an independent effect of pregnancy on β-cell function independent of the observed changes in insulin; however, the etiology of this effect is at present unknown although may include the incretins GIP and GLP-1 [46,47]. Overall the insulin sensitivity of late normal pregnancy is reduced by 50% to 70% compared to normal, non-pregnant women [38,44,45,48], with increases in basal insulin and the response to glucose with concomitant decreases in insulin clearance [44,49,50]. Consequently, by the third trimester basal and 24-h mean insulin concentrations may double and the first and second phases of insulin release are 3- to 3.5-fold greater in late pregnancy [44].

Maternal obesity and glucose homeostasis

The impact of obesity on these changes is substantial, in particular the decline in fasting glucose in early gestation is reduced, and glucose is not reduced at all in severely obese women [37]. In late gestation the normal reduction in peripheral insulin sensitivity of 50% [44] is reduced further by 15% in obese women as determined by the Quantitative Insulin Sensitivity Check Index (QUICKI) [51] – a validate surrogate for direct measurement of insulin sensitivity using the euglycemic–hyperinsulinemic clamp [52]. In addition there is marked peripheral and hepatic insulin resistance, which manifests as reduced insulin-mediated glucose disposal, a large reduction in insulin-stimulated carbohydrate oxidation, and a reduction in insulin suppression of endogenous glucose production, all of which are reversed in the postpartum period [53]. Importantly the overall effects of this impaired insulin resistance are not limited to glucose. In the postprandial state, this obesity-related insulin resistance exaggerates the normal circulatory increases in metabolic fuels, i.e., glucose, lipids, and amino acids. In fact the fasting, postprandial, and integrated 24-hour plasma concentrations of all three macronutrients are affected by enhanced insulin resistance in obese women. Consequently the impaired glucose uptake exposes the fetus to hyperglycemia; the inability to suppress whole body lipolysis leads to an increase in free fatty acids available for placental transfer; and the decreased ability of insulin to suppress amino acid turnover causes an elevation in maternal concentrations of branched-chain amino acids, facilitating transfer of excess protein substrate to the fetus. These alternative nutrient pathways may independently contribute to macrosomia as higher maternal serum triglycerides and amino acid profiles (serine, threonine, lysine, proline, ornithine, and arginine) have been associated with higher offspring birthweight independent of maternal glucose or pre-pregnancy BMI, which have strong independent associations with a birthweight greater than the 90th percentile [54–58].

Although the precise mechanisms regulating insulin sensitivity are uncertain, it would appear that preconceptual fat mass is a major determinant. Pre-pregnancy lean women exhibit an inverse correlation between changes in insulin sensitivity and fat mass, which is not seen in obese women [1,59]. Obese women do, however, exhibit a negative relationship between the decrease in insulin sensitivity and accretion of fat mass during pregnancy [1]. Additionally although changes in insulin sensitivity related to later pregnancy are primarily mediated at the peripheral level and secondarily at the hepatic level, elevated levels of non-esterified free fatty acids in later pregnancy may also contribute to peripheral and hepatic insulin resistance [60,61], with adipose-derived estrogen facilitating further increases in lipids. The peripheral resistance may be mediated by reduced adipose tissue insulin receptor substrate-1 protein levels, which are 43% lower in obese women with gestational diabetes than they are in obese women without gestational diabetes [13]. Circulating concentrations of peroxisome proliferator-activated receptor-γ (PPARγ) mRNA and protein are also less than normal [13], and given that PPARγ acts as an important regulator of adipose lipid storage and as a regulator of insulin sensitivity, this reduction may contribute to the insulin-mediated suppression of lipolysis in obese pregnancy.

The consequences of maternal insulin resistance

Gestational diabetes

Pre-existing diabetes and poor maternal glycemic control have classically been associated with adverse pregnancy outcome. However, over the last decade several studies have led to the universal recognition that pre-existing diabetes reflects the tip of the iceberg. First, treatment of women with an abnormal glucose challenge test but normal oral glucose tolerance test reduced the risk of macrosomia [16]. This finding raised the possibilities that maternal hyperglycemia below the traditional thresholds for overt diabetes increases the risk of adverse maternal and fetal outcomes, and that treating such women improves perinatal outcomes. In recent years, three major studies sought to further address these central questions in gestational diabetes diagnosis and treatment. The Australian

Carbohydrate Intolerance Study in Pregnant Women Trial Group (ACHOIS) published a randomized controlled trial treating mild hyperglycemia in pregnant women who did not reach diagnostic criteria for gestational diabetes, but had 75 g OGTT results between 140 and 199 mg/dl, consistent with glucose intolerance [62]. The investigators found a reduction in the composite endpoint of perinatal death, shoulder dystocia, bone fracture, and nerve palsy in the treatment group compared with the group receiving routine care. Subsequently, a randomized controlled trial by Landon *et al.* similarly included women who did not reach diagnostic thresholds for gestational diabetes but in whom a 100g OGTT was not entirely normal [63]. This trial similarly demonstrated a reduction in macrosomia, shoulder dystocia, cesarean delivery, and hypertensive disorders with treatment. In 2008, the Hyperglycemia and Adverse Pregnancy Outcome (HAPO) study, a prospective, blinded, multinational observational study, including almost 25 000 pregnant women, published its main findings [64]. Unlike the two randomized controlled trials, HAPO was not designed to evaluate the efficacy of treating maternal hyperglycemia, but to provide data elucidating the relationship between maternal glucose concentrations and adverse perinatal outcomes. Many hoped HAPO would provide a maternal glycemic threshold for such outcomes and thereby lead to consensus on firm diagnostic criteria and treatment goals for gestational diabetes. Instead, validating previous findings HAPO showed a continuous association between rising maternal glucose concentrations and large for gestational age, pre-eclampsia, and primary cesarean section. The HAPO study also showed a positive association between maternal hyperglycemia and neonatal hypoglycemia, cord blood serum c-peptide, premature delivery, intensive neonatal care, and hyperbilirubinemia. Due to the continuous nature of the associations found, there was no clear threshold above which adverse events occurred, which might have easily guided precise values at which gestational diabetes should be diagnosed.

With the publication of these studies, the International Association of the Diabetes and Pregnancy Study Groups (IADPSG), an international group consisting of representatives from regional and national groups with a focus on gestational diabetes, established a new set of guidelines [65]. Key differences exist between these new guidelines and previous versions (Table 15.1, [66]). First, to address the rising prevalence of pre-existing diabetes in pregnancy properly,

the IADPSG recommends screening high-risk women at the initial visit with use of random plasma glucose, fasting plasma glucose, or glycosylated hemoglobin paired with diagnostic thresholds in accordance with guidelines for the diagnosis of non-gestational diabetes. In addition, the diagnosis of gestational diabetes can be made at the initial visit with a fasting plasma glucose between 5.1 mmol/l (92 mg/dl) and 7 mmol/l (126 mg/dl), thus including most women who would not have been considered to have gestational diabetes under most previous national guidelines. In agreement with the majority of previous guidelines, they recommend all women not yet diagnosed with gestational diabetes to be screened at 24 to 28 weeks gestation with the fasting 75 g OGTT. However, the interpretation of the OGTT represents a significant change. Unlike the WHO criteria, under the IADPSG guidelines not only can an abnormal fasting or two-hour plasma glucose be used for diagnosis, the IADPSG also recommends an abnormal one-hour plasma glucose is sufficient for diagnosis. Moreover any one of these three time-points can be abnormal for the diagnosis of gestational diabetes.

Translation of the continuous association between maternal glycemia and adverse perinatal outcomes seen in HAPO into diagnostic thresholds required the panel to reach consensus. Mean concentrations for fasting, one-hour, and two-hour OGTT plasma glucose concentrations for the entire study cohort were used. The selected thresholds represent an odds ratio of 1.75 for birthweight, cord c-peptide, and fetal percent body weight being greater than the 90th percentile, relative to the odds of those outcomes at mean glucose values (Table 15.1).

If the IADPSG recommendations are widely adopted, the timely diagnosis of pre-gestational type 2 diabetes and of gestational diabetes will likely improve, but they will also greatly increase the numbers of women identified with these conditions. Notably application of this system of testing and criteria is predicted to result in a per pregnancy incidence of gestational diabetes of over 16% – a major change in terms of UK obstetric practice from current levels of 3.5%. This rate appears unacceptably high to many clinicians and would represent a radical redefinition of the diagnosis in many countries. An alternative approach rather than the OR threshold of 1.75, would be to base thresholds on the cost-effectiveness of screening and treatment of GDM based on a woman's hypothetical individual risk of disease [67]. The relevance of such an approach

Table 15.1 Published criteria for the screening and diagnosis of hyperglycemia in pregnancy (1998–2010)

Organization	Screening	Diagnosis
ADIPS (1998) The Australasian Diabetes in Pregnancy Society	Universal screening recommended except in areas where resources are limited or incidence of GDM[a] is low, then selective screening based on risk factors may be appropriate. Screen at 26–30 wks. Screen with a 50 g non-fasting GCT[b]; positive if 1 h ≥ 7.8 mmol/l (140 mg/dl). Confirm with 75 g OGTT[cd]	75 g OGTT positive if **one or more abnormal values:** Fasting ≥ 5.5 mmol/l (99 mg/dl) 2 h ≥ 8.0 mmol/l (145 mg/dl) (9.0 mmol/l or 162 mg/dl in New Zealand)
WHO (1999) World Health Organization	Risk assessment in first trimester. If high risk, screen in first trimester. All others, screen at 24–28 wks. Screen/diagnose with 75 g OGTT.	75 g OGTT positive for GDM if **one or more abnormal values:** Fasting ≥ 7.0 mmol/l (126 mg/dl) 2 h ≥ 11.1 mmol/l (200 mg/dl) Positive for impaired glucose tolerance if fasting < 7.0 mmol/l (126 mg/dl) and 2 h ≥ 7.8 mmol/l (140 mg/dl) Women classified as either diabetes mellitus or impaired fasting glucose by WHO criteria should be diagnosed with gestational diabetes mellitus
ACOG (2001) American College of Obstetricians and Gynecologists	Risk assessment or perform universal screening at 24–28 wks. Low-risk[e] patients may be excluded from screening. Screen with 50 g 1 h GCT. Positive if 1 h > 7.2 mmol/l (130 mg/dl) or 7.8 mmol/l (140 mg/dl). Diagnose with 100 g OGTT.	Positive 100 g 3 h OGTT requires **two abnormal values** from either of two sets of criteria: Carpenter/Coustan: Fasting ≥ 5.3 mmol/l (95 mg/dl) 1 h ≥ 10.0 mmol/l (180 mg/dl) 2 h ≥ 8.6 mmol/l (155 mg/dl) 3 h ≥ 7.8 mmol/l (140 mg/dl) National Diabetes Data Group: Fasting ≥ 5.8 mmol/l (105 mg/dl) 1 h ≥ 10.5 mmol/l (190 mg/dl) 2 h ≥ 9.2 mmol/l (165 mg/dl)
SOGC (2002) Society of Obstetricians and Gynaecologists of Canada	Each of the following approaches is acceptable: Routine screening at 24–28 wks with 50 g GCT, using threshold of 7.8 mmol/l (140 mg/dl) except in low-risk patients.[f] Non-screening is also acceptable. Consider the recommendations given by the Fourth International Workshop-Conference for screening women at high risk for GDM early in pregnancy and again at 24–28 wks if initial results are negative.	100 g OGTT as recommended by ACOG (2001) or the 75 g OGTT as recommended by the ADA (2002) Specifically do not recommend use of the WHO criteria for diagnosis
Japan (2002) The Committee of the Japan Diabetes Society	Screen all patients at the first visit using a random plasma glucose. If value is 5.5 mmol/l (99 mg/dl) or higher, perform a 75 g OGTT at that time with use of a 1 h plasma glucose level. Screen all at 24–28 wks. Screen using the 75 g OGTT.	75 g OGTT positive if **two abnormal values**: Fasting ≥ 5.3 mmol/l (95 mg/dl) 1 h ≥ 10.0 mmol/l (180 mg/dl) 2 h ≥ 8.6 mmol/l (155 mg/dl)

Table 15.1 (cont.)

Organization	Screening	Diagnosis
Austrian (2004)	Screen high-risk groups in the first trimester. Screen all at 24–28 wks. Screen using 75 g OGTT.	75 g OGTT positive if **one or more abnormal values:** Fasting ≥ 5.3 mmol/l (95 mg/dl) 1 h ≥ 10.0 mmol/l (180 mg/dl) 2 h ≥ 8.6 mmol/l (155 mg/dl)
Joslin Diabetes Center (2005)	Perform risk assessment at first prenatal visit.[g] Screen average-risk women at 24–28 wks. Screen using a 50 g OGTT. Abnormal if 1 hr ≥ 7.8 mmol/l (140 mg/dl). If abnormal, diagnose with 100 g OGTT.	100 g OGTT: Positive 100 g 3 h OGTT requires **two abnormal values:** Fasting ≥ 5.8 mmol/l (105 mg/dl) 1 h ≥ 10.6 mmol/l (190 mg/dl) 2 h ≥ 9.2 mmol/l (165 mg/dl) 3 h ≥ 8.0 mmol/l (145 mg/dl)
AACE (2007) American Association of Clinical Endocrinologists	Screen all pregnant women for diabetes. Screen low-risk women at 24–28 wks. Screen high-risk women at 20 wks.[h] Screen using a 75 g OGTT with addition of a 1 h plasma glucose level.	75 g OGTT positive if **two** abnormal values met: Fasting ≥ 5.3 mmol/l (95 mg/dl) 1 h ≥ 10.0 mmol/l (180 mg/dl) 2 h ≥ 8.6 mmol/l (155 mg/dl)
5th International Workshop-Conference on Gestational Diabetes Mellitus (2007)	Risk assessment should be performed at the first prenatal visit.[i] Low-risk women do not require any routine testing. High-risk women should undergo screening as soon as possible (as below). All other women should have screening at 24–28 wks. Screening can be done as 50 g GCT followed by diagnostic OGTT if abnormal. Abnormal if 1 h ≥ 7.8 mmol/l (140 mg/dl). Or proceed directly to a diagnostic OGTT.	Diagnostic testing can be done with either the 75 g OGTT or the 100 g OGTT 100 g OGTT positive for GDM if **two or more** are true: Carpenter/Coustan: Fasting ≥ 5.3 mmol/l (95 mg/dl) 1 h ≥ 10.0 mmol/l (180 mg/dl) 2 h ≥ 8.6 mmol/l (155 mg/dl) 3 h ≥ 7.8 mmol/l (140 mg/dl) 75 mg OGTT positive for GDM if two or more are true: Fasting ≥ 5.3 mmol/l (95 mg/dl) 1 h ≥ 10.0 mmol/l (180 mg/dl) 2 h ≥ 8.6 mmol/l (155 mg/dl)
Brazilian Society of Endocrinology and Metabolism (2008)	Screen for risk factors and obtain a fasting glucose at the first antenatal visit. Any fasting glucose > 5.6 mmol/l (100 mg/dl) is abnormal and should prompt further testing. After the 24th week of pregnancy, any fasting glucose above 4.7 mmol/l (85 mg/dl) is a positive screen and should lead to further testing. Screen all women at 24–28 wks using the 50 g GCT. Positive if 1 h > 7.2 mmol/l (130 mg/dl) or 7.8 mmol/l (140 mg/dl). Use the 75 g OGTT for confirmation.	A fasting glucose > 6.1 mmol/l (110 mg/dl) at any week confirms GDM 75 g OGTT positive as per WHO criteria GDM if **one or more abnormal values:** Fasting ≥ 7.0 mmol/l (126 mg/dl) 2 h ≥ 11.1 mmol/l (200 mg/dl) Impaired glucose tolerance if: Fasting < 7.0 mmol/l (126 mg/dl) and 2 h ≥ 7.8 mmol/l (140 mg/dl) Women classified as either diabetes mellitus or impaired fasting glucose by WHO criteria should be diagnosed with gestational diabetes mellitus

Organization	Screening	Diagnosis
HKCOG (2008) Hong Kong College of Obstetricians and Gynaecologists	Perform risk assessment at first antenatal visit.[j] Screen all women at 24–30 wks using the 50 g OGTT or a fasting plasma glucose. In an urgent situation such as late presentation of obstetric complications that could be related to GDM, a random glucose > 200 is diagnostic. 50 g GCT results abnormal if > 7.8 mmol/l (140 mg/dl) in the international population or > 7.0 mmol/l (126 mg/dl) in the local population. Women with risk factors should proceed directly to the 75 g OGTT after initial visit. If initial testing is normal, repeat at 28–30 wks. Follow abnormal screen with diagnostic 75 g OGTT.	75 g OGTT positive as per WHO criteria. GDM if **one or more abnormal values:** Fasting ≥ 7.0 mmol/l (126 mg/dl) 2 h ≥ 11.1 mmol/l (200 mg/dl) Impaired glucose tolerance if: fasting < 7.0 mmol/l (126 mg/dl) and 2 h ≥ 7.8 mmol/l (140 mg/dl) Women classified as either diabetes mellitus or impaired fasting glucose by WHO criteria should be diagnosed with gestational diabetes mellitus
USPSTF (2008) US Preventive Services Task Force	No recommendation made for routine screening due to insufficient evidence. Until there is better evidence, clinicians should discuss screening with patients and make case-by-base decisions. If a decision is made to screen for gestational diabetes, they cite most screening is done between 24 and 28 wks and the 50 g GCT is the most common test used in the US followed by the 100 g OGTT for confirmation.	100 g OGTT positive when there are **two or more** abnormal values Diagnostic threshold values are not provided
NICE UK (2008) National Institute for Health and Clinical Excellence, United Kingdom	Perform risk assessment at the initial visit. Women with any risk factors should be **offered testing** for GDM.[k] If a woman has had GDM in a prior pregnancy, she should be offered SMBG at 16–18 wks and repeat OGTT at 28 wks if initial testing is normal. Women without risk factors should be **offered an OGTT** at 24–28 wks. Screen using the 75 g OGTT.	75 g OGTT positive as per WHO criteria GDM if **one or more abnormal values**: Fasting ≥ 7.0 mmol/l (126 mg/dl) 2 h ≥ 11.1 mmol/l (200 mg/dl) Impaired glucose tolerance if: Fasting < 7.0 mmol/l (126 mg/dl) and 2 h ≥ 7.8 mmol/l (140 mg/dl) Women classified as either diabetes mellitus or impaired fasting glucose by WHO criteria should be diagnosed with gestational diabetes mellitus
ADA (2010) American Diabetes Association	Risk assessment should take place at the first prenatal visit. Do not screen low-risk women.[l] Screen high-risk women at the initial visit to identify pre-gestational diabetes.[m] If negative at first visit, high-risk women should be retested at 24 **and** 28 wks. Women of average risk should be universally screened between 24 and 28 wks. Initial screening: Hemoglobin A1c by NGSP-certified, standardized method, fasting plasma glucose, 1-step 75 g OGTT with 2-h glucose level, **or** random plasma glucose in a patient with classic symptoms of hyperglycemia	

Table 15.1 (*cont.*)

Organization	Screening	Diagnosis
	2-step approach: Perform a 50 g glucose challenge test and if 1 h plasma or serum glucose >130 mg/dL or >140 mg/dl,[n] move on to either the 100 g OGTT or the 75 g OGTT for diagnosis. 1-step approach: 75 g OGTT; this approach may be cost-effective in high-risk populations.	
IADPSG (2010) International Association of Diabetes and Pregnancy Study Groups	First prenatal visit: Measure FPG, A1C, or random plasma glucose on all or only high-risk women. If results indicate overt diabetes, treatment and follow-up as for pre-existing diabetes. If results not diagnostic of overt diabetes, and fasting plasma glucose ≥5.1 mmol/l (92 mg/dl) but <7.0 mmol/l (126 mg/dl), diagnose as GDM, and fasting plasma glucose <5.1 mmol/l (92 mg/dl), test for GDM from 24–28 weeks gestation with a 75 g OGTT. 24–28 weeks gestation: diagnosis of GDM: 2 h 75 g OGTT: perform after overnight fast on all women not previously found to have overt diabetes or GDM during testing earlier in this pregnancy. Overt diabetes if fasting plasma glucose ≥7.0 mmol/l (126 mg/dl). GDM if one or more values equals or exceeds thresholds indicated. Normal if all values on OGTT less than thresholds indicated.	**One or more** of these values from a 75 g OGTT must be equaled or exceeded for the diagnosis of GDM: Fasting ≥ 5.1 mmol/l (92 mg/dl) 1 h ≥ 10.0 mmol/l (180 mg/dl) 2 h ≥ 8.5 mmol/l (153 mg/dl) To diagnose overt diabetes in pregnancy: FBG ≥ 7.0 mmol/l (126 mg/dl) A1C ≥ 6.5% (DCCT/UKPDS standardized) Random plasma glucose ≥ 11.1 mmol/l (200mg/dl) plus confirmation by FBG or A1C

[a] Gestational diabetes mellitus.

[b] Glucose challenge test.

[c] Oral glucose tolerance test (OGTT).

[d] All OGTTs listed are assumed to be performed after an overnight fast of 8–14 hrs and after at least three days of an unrestricted diet (≥150 g carbohydrate per day) and unlimited physical activity.

[e] Low risk defined as age < 25 years, BMI < 25, not member of a high-risk racial or ethnic group, no previous history of abnormal glucose tolerance, no previous history of adverse obstetric outcomes usually associated with GDM, no known diabetes in a first-degree relative.

[f] Low risk defined as maternal age < 25, Caucasian or member of other ethnic group with low prevalence of diabetes, no previous history of GDM or glucose intolerance, pregnant body mass index < 27, no family history of diabetes in first-degree relative, no history of GDM-associated adverse pregnancy outcomes.

[g] Low risk defined as white race age < 25 weight normal before pregnancy no history of abnormal glucose metabolism, no history of poor obstetric outcome. High risk defined as member of high-risk ethnic group (Black or African American, Hispanic/Latina, American Indian or Alaskan Native, Asian (South or East Asian), Native Hawaiian or other Pacific Islander, Inidgenous Australian), or obese (>20% above ideal body weight), or previous history of gestational diabetes, or glycosuria, or strong family history of diabetes, or impaired OGTT or impaired fasting flucose, or previous baby > 9lbs birthweight.

[h] Risk factors for gestational diabetes mellitus includes age >25 years, overweight or obese state, family history of diabetes mellitus (i.e., in a first-degree relative), history of abnormal glucose metabolism, history of poor obstetric outcome, history of delivery of an infant with a birthweight >9 lbs, history of polycystic ovary syndrome, Latino/Hispanic, non-Hispanic Black, Asian American, Native American, or Pacific Islander ethnicity, fasting (no energy intake for at least 8 hours) plasma glucose concentration >85 mg/dl or 2 hour postprandial glucose concentration > 140 mg/dl (indicates need to perform a 75 g OGTT).

[i] Low risk if all the following present: member of an ethnic group with a low prevalence of GDM, no known diabetes in first-degree relatives, age < 25 years, weight normal before pregnancy, weight normal at birth, no history of abnormal glucose metabolism, no history of poor obstetric outcome. High risk defined as severe obesity, strong family history of type 2 diabetes, or previous history of GDM, impaired glucose metabolism, or glucosuria.

[j] Risk factors for Asian/Chinese women include maternal age ≥ 35, BMI ≥ 25 before pregnancy or at booking in the first trimester, family history of diabetes (especially in parents), carrier of the α-thallasemia trail, carrier of HBsAg, history of: GDM, macrosomic infant, unexplained stillbirth, congenital malformations compatible with diabetic embryopathy, pre-eclampsia/eclampsia, current pregnancy: conceived after ART/IVF especially if for conditions such as PCOS, multiple pregnancy, hemoglobin > 13 g/dl in first

Table 15.1 *(cont.)*

trimester, polyhydramnios, fetal size > date, recurrent and significant glycosuria, currently on medications such as steroid or other immunosuppressants, unexplained fetal demise, or unexplained macrosomic infant.

[k] Risk factors include BMI > 30 kg/m², previous infant weighing ≥ 4500 g, previous GDM, first-degree relative with diabetes, family origin with a high prevalence of diabetes (specifically women whose country of family origin is Saudi Arabia, United Arab Emirates, Iraq, Jordan, Syria, Oman, Qatar, Kuwait, Lebanon, or Egypt).

[l] Low-risk group defined as age <25 years, normal body weight, no family history of diabetes, no history of abnormal glucose metabolism, no history of poor obstetric outcome, not a member of an ethnic/racial group with a high prevalence of diabetes (e.g., Hispanic America, Native American, Asian American, African American, Pacific Islander).

[m] High-risk group defined as those with marked obesity, personal history of GDM, glycosuria, or a strong family history of diabetes.

[n] ADA guidelines allow either threshold, noting that at the >130 mg/dl cut-off, the yield is increased to 90% from 80% for the higher threshold.

(Modified from Leary *et al.* 2010 [66])

is strengthened by recent studies that attempt to estimate the risks of GDM based on patient characteristics and medical history [68,69]. However, national socioeconomic status and health care policies would result in persistence of different national guidelines, with a major attraction of the IADPSG approach being a unified approach to GDM. Randomized controlled trials of treating women identified by the new criteria may be the best way of determining the effectiveness and cost-effectiveness of revised guidelines.

Intervention strategies

Given the continuous associations of maternal glycemia with perinatal complications, a shift toward early prevention of gestational diabetes appears logical but is largely untested. Obese women are an easily identified group at increased risk with the other short- and long-term complications for the mother and child providing the stimulus for rapid development of an intervention to improve outcomes. To date, none has been validated for clinical use. Undoubtedly, the most successful intervention will be that which prevents development of obesity before the reproductive years. However, the high rates of obesity among adolescent girls and the upward trends of obesity among pregnant women suggests that this is not immediately attainable. As reviewed above, we have a good understanding of the changes in metabolism accompanying obesity in pregnancy and central to these is the development of insulin resistance and its metabolic sequelae. Since there are strong similarities between the risk profile for type 2 diabetes and the hyperglycemia, hyperinsulinemia, and dyslipidemia that characterize maternal obesity, the extensive literature addressing interventions in type 2 diabetes and gestational diabetes may provide guidance.

Lifestyle modification as a preventative strategy for type 2 diabetes mellitus

Lifestyle intervention is now a critical component of the treatment strategy for diabetes, hypertension, cardiovascular disease, and obesity in non-pregnant patients [70,71]. Importantly, effective lifestyle intervention strategies can prevent or at least delay the progression to type 2 diabetes in high-risk individuals (summarized in Table 15.2; [72–76]). Notably the Finnish Diabetes Prevention Study (DPS), in addition to a 58% reduction in the incidence of diabetes incidence, also achieved within one year, a reduction in weight, BMI, waist circumference, fasting plasma glucose, two-hour plasma glucose, serum triglycerides, and serum total cholesterol:HDL cholesterol ratio in the intervention group [72]. In the US Diabetes Prevention Program (DPP), attainment of 7% weight loss was achieved by 50% of participants at 24 weeks and 74% had achieved the physical activity targets, importantly this was also accompanied by reductions in plasma glucose [76]. These studies raise the exciting possibility that lifestyle modification in a similar form could be applied to pregnancy to prevent the onset of metabolic and obesity-related complications.

Safety of exercise in pregnancy

In theory there are potential risks to the fetus during maternal exercise, including stimulation of uterine contractility [77], decreased uteroplacental flow due to preferential shunting to skeletal muscles [78], potentially fetal hypoglycemia secondary to increased glucose used by skeletal muscles, and reductions in circulating maternal glucose [79] and hyperthermia from exercise. In reality although exercise and particularly high-impact exercise in early pregnancy has

Table 15.2 Summary of the four lifestyle intervention studies that aimed at preventing type 2 diabetes in non-pregnant subjects with impaired glucose tolerance

Study	Cohort size	Intervention	Mean BMI (kg/m²)	Duration (years)	RRR (%)	ARR (%)	NNT
Malmö	217	Dietary and/or increased physical activity or training.	26.6	5	63	18	28
DPS	523	Aim for ≥5% reduction in bodyweight respectively through diet and physical activity. *Diet:* a reduction in dietary fat to <30 proportion of total energy (E%) and saturated fat to <10%E, while increasing fiber to ≥15 g/1000 kcal. Achieved by face-to-face consultation sessions (from 30 min to 1 h) with the study nutritionist at weeks 0, 1–2, and 5–6 and at months 3, 4, 6, and 9, i.e., altogether seven sessions during the first year and every three months thereafter. *Physical activity:* Aim of moderate physical activity of ≥30mins/day achieved through progressive, individually tailored circuit type moderate intensity resistance training sessions, exercise competitions, voluntary group walking, and hiking.	31.0	3	58	12	22
DPP	2161[a]	Aim for ≥7% reduction in bodyweight respectively through diet and physical activity. *Diet:* a healthy low-calorie, low-fat diet. *Physical activity:* moderate intensity, such as brisk walking, for at least 150 minutes per week.	34.0	3	58	15	21
Da Qing	500	Exercise, diet or exercise + diet	25.8	6	46	27	25
IDDP-1	531	Physical activity target of moderate physical activity of >30mins/day and dietary advice including reduction in total calories, refined carbohydrates and fats, avoidance of sugar, and inclusion of fiber-rich foods.	25.7	3	28	15	19

RRR = relative risk reduction
ARR = absolute risk reduction/1000 person-years
NNT = numbers needed to treat to prevent one case of diabetes over 12 months
[a] Combined numbers for placebo and diet and exercise groups

been associated with an increased risk of miscarriage, once beyond 18 weeks, physical activity has not been associated with adverse obstetric complications [80], and with respect to preterm birth may even be protective [81–84]. Furthermore maternal hypoglycemia even in type 1 diabetes has not been consistently associated with adverse neurodevelopment in the offspring, although in these patients maternal plasma β-hydroxyburate, an index of ketosis and potentially the necessity for alternative fuel use, has been negatively associated with psychomotor and intellectual development [85,86].

Given that physical activity may improve insulin resistance, thereby reducing circulating glucose levels and decreasing the amount of glucose available for the fetus, there is the potential for a benefit on fetal adiposity. To date three different meta-analyses have demonstrated that leisure time physical activity (LTPA) is not associated with birthweight [87–89]. However, vigorous endurance exercise during the third trimester was associated with a 200 to 500 g lower birthweight [90,91]. Should birthweight be similarly reduced across the whole range this might be detrimental as the incidence of small for gestational age babies would be increased. However, if this reduction in birthweight was restricted to women who are at risk of delivering LGA infants, this could be beneficial and may reduce birth complications and the need for operative delivery. In support of this assertion, in one study moderate or vigorous physical activity for at least two hours per week was associated with a reduced risk of delivering a large for gestational age infant (OR 0.3; 95% CI: 0.2–0.7), but was not accompanied by an increase in small for gestational age infants [92]. Nonetheless, reduction of birthweight among offspring of mothers with gestational diabetes has been accompanied by improvement in significant perinatal and neonatal metabolic sequelae [62,63,93]. In a recent study of children at the age of four to five years from a subgroup of women who took part in one of these trials [62] Gillman *et al.* reported that there was no difference in BMI between the control and intervention groups. This finding could argue against a "programmed" risk of obesity by maternal hyperglycemia [94].

Lifestyle modification as a strategy for improving glycemic control in gestational diabetes mellitus

Given the positive impact of lifestyle modification on type 2 diabetes, a similar approach has been applied to GDM. Initial management of affected women now consists of glucose monitoring and lifestyle modification including dietary counseling and a diet that restricts carbohydrates to 35% to 40% of daily calories [95,96]. This type of counseling is based on data demonstrating that carbohydrate restriction decreases maternal glucose concentrations and improves maternal and fetal outcomes [97]. Furthermore in obese women with diabetes, a 30% to 33% calorie restriction (to ~25 kcal/kg actual weight per day) reduced hyperglycemia and plasma triglycerides with no increase in ketonuria [98]. However, despite diet being a core component of management, dietary advice alone is insufficient for many GDM patients [99], and outcomes are improved if it is combined with pharmacological therapy including metformin [62,100,101]. Although metformin may seem an attractive therapeutic option in obese pregnancy, in one small RCT of 40 women with polycystic ovarian syndrome it did not reduce the incidence of GDM [102]. Furthermore metformin is not as effective as lifestyle intervention in preventing type 2 diabetes in women with a history of gestational diabetes [103]. Two randomized controlled trials in the UK are currently addressing the potential benefit of metformin in obese pregnant women; the EMPOWaR study (ISRCTN 5127984) and the MOP trial (NCT01273584).

Regular physical activity has repeatedly been shown to improve glycemic control in women with GDM [104–107], primarily due to the physiological pregnancy-related increases in insulin resistance being reduced by moderate-intensity daily physical activity [108,109]. However, most of these trials studied the effects of a short-term exercise program (i.e., a single bout or only several weeks). Studies on longer lasting exercise programs, especially those continuing into the third trimester of pregnancy, are currently lacking. Further most studies have concerned the treatment and not the prevention of GDM, but given the positive impact on type 2 diabetes studies of prophylactic lifestyle modification are needed.

Lifestyle modification as a strategy for preventing gestational diabetes mellitus

Epidemiological studies have suggested that physical activity prior to and during pregnancy may significantly reduce the risk of gestational diabetes [110]. Not surprisingly, the highest reduction is seen in women engaged in leisure time physical activity during both time periods (RR 0.31; 95% CI: 0.12–0.79 for development of gestational diabetes) [111]. To date, however, there is a paucity of trial data examining the role of lifestyle modification for the prevention of gestational diabetes [112]. A pilot study examining controlled energy intake during pregnancy (8350 kJ/d, 200 g/d carbohydrate) combined with exercise at 30% $VO_{2\,peak}$, demonstrated that this combination was better than mild exercise alone at controlling blood glucose concentrations as indicated by a fasting oral glucose tolerance test in late pregnancy [112]. However, subsequent application of this combined exercise and lifestyle program was only to a small cohort of women at risk of GDM (n = 23), and although GDM was prevented, the small numbers prevent any firm conclusion [112]. Larger, purely physical activity-based, studies are currently being undertaken, but they are still modest in size [113] and appear limited relative to the non-pregnant diabetes prevention studies, which aimed for a combination of modification of diet, exercise, and also attainment of weight loss.

With respect to diet, the aim is to reduce postprandial glucose levels and thereby excessive fetal growth [114]. Low-glycemic index diets are frequently used to reduce postprandial glucose peaks as well as fasting glucose levels [115]. Unfortunately, assessment of a role in the prevention of insulin resistance in pregnancy is limited. Moses demonstrated that a low-GI diet (n = 32) compared to a high-GI diet (n = 30) was associated with a reduction in fasting glucose and a reduction in birthweight and incidence of large for gestational age [116]. Fraser established that a high-fiber diet (n = 13) as compared to a normal pregnancy diet (n = 12) significantly attenuated postprandial insulin secretion [117]. Clapp combined these principles with an exercise program and demonstrated in a randomized controlled trial of 20 women that the combination of a low-glycemic diet and exercise significantly reduced birthweight, ponderal index, and maternal fasting blood glucose [118].

Together, these lifestyle modification trials are still too small to provide definitive conclusions [119], but suggest that diets that are characterized by low GI and high fiber content combined with exercise would be appropriate for obesity [120].

Interventions for maternal obesity

Among obese pregnant women, the primary outcome of any intervention study requires careful choice. As detailed in Chapter 14, the majority of those underway, or the preliminary studies already published, focus on prevention of excessive gestational weight gain as defined by the Institute of Medicine (IOM). Observational studies show that women whose GWG falls within the 1990 IOM guidelines experience a better pregnancy outcome, and the new IOM 2009 guidelines provide new and more evidence-based targets for each category and, for the first time a specific weight gain range for obese women (5–9 kg) [121] (Table 15.3). However, as described above, excessive GWG is only weakly associated with several of the primary abnormalities linked to obesity including GDM and pre-eclampsia. Nevertheless, if observational studies are translatable to effects of intervention, prevention of excessive GWG among pregnant women could reduce the risk of LGA, cesarean section, postpartum weight gain, and, potentially, childhood obesity.

In contrast, in view of the close association between obesity and insulin resistance as outlined above, and the proposed role that this plays in GDM, pre-eclampsia, and macrosomia, maternal insulin resistance may be an alternative primary outcome in intervention studies. As discussed above, dietary and exercise regimes for treatment of gestational diabetes have shown some promise with respect to improvement of adverse outcomes. These interventional strategies in GDM do provide a template for trials in obesity. In practical terms, the lifestyle interventions that are offered to obese women to limit weight gain and to prevent insulin resistance, namely increased physical activity and dietary advice and individual counseling, may differ only slightly from those used to treat GDM, although they may start earlier in pregnancy.

As described above, physical activity is a modifiable factor that may reduce insulin resistance during pregnancy, and is likely to reduce GWG. In a recent study from the Project Viva cohort, mid-pregnancy walking (OR 0.92; 95% CI: 0.83–1.01, per 30 minutes per day) and vigorous physical activity (OR 0.76; 95% CI: 0.60–0.97, per 30 minutes per day) were inversely associated with excessive GWG [122]. Dietary advice, whether to reduce insulin resistance or calories, involves avoidance of simple sugars and saturated fats with adherence to a "healthy diet," but the emphasis will slightly differ. Dietary energy density is also a modifiable factor, which may assist pregnant women to manage weight gain, but this remains to be proven in adequately powered trials [122–125]. Although in some studies dietary glycemic load has not been found to be associated with GWG [125], one study suggested that low-glycemic index diet does reduce GWG [118]. Focusing on prevention of weight gain, if misinterpreted by the pregnant women, has the disadvantage that it may increase the risk of inappropriate fasting or excessive caloric restriction leading to excessive ketonuria and ketonemia, and the potential to adversely impact upon neurocognitive and motor skill development of the offspring [85,126]. A focus on dietary quality may have beneficial effects without such risks. Certainly altering diet composition in obese women is feasible, but whether these changes are adequate to have an impact on clinical outcomes is the subject of several ongoing clinical trials.

Perhaps the greatest challenge for obese women, however, is to achieve any behavioral changes in diet or physical activity. Most of the studies published to date do not report the theory upon which interventions are based [127]. Understanding barriers to behavioral

Table 15.3 Summary of ongoing lifestyle intervention studies in relation to weight gain and/or obesity

Ongoing studies

Althuizen *et al.* (New Life study)	Randomized controlled trial	Healthy nulliparous women (7 months pregnant) n = 300 (The Netherlands).	Tailored advice on physical activity and diet.	Gestational weight gain in relation to IOM guidelines, BMI, and skinfold thickness.
Brand-Miller (the CHOPP study)	Randomized controlled trial	Pregnant women n = 1650 (Sydney, Australia).	Low-glycemic index diet from 12–16 weeks until delivery.	Large for gestational age delivery; childhood obesity.
Chasan-Taber *et al.* (the BABY study)	Randomized controlled trial	Pregnant sedentary women with GDM in a prior pregnancy n = 364 (Western Massachusetts, USA).	Tailored advice on physical activity.	Incidence of gestational diabetes, physical activity levels, and circulating concentrations of glucose, insulin, leptin, TNF-α, resistin, CRP, adiponectin.
Dodd *et al.* (the LIMIT trial)	Randomized controlled trial	Overweight and obese pregnant women n = 2500 (Australia).	Dietary package and lifestyle advice.	Gestational weight gain.
Hauner *et al.*	Randomized controlled trial	Pregnant and lactating women n = 210 (Munich, Germany).	n-3 fatty acids from 15 weeks gestation until 4 months postpartum.	Body mass of newborn with follow-up until age 5.
Ko *et al.*	Randomized uncontrolled	Pregnant women receiving prenatal care (Washington, USA).	Vigorous physical activity.	Central adiposity 6–8 weeks postpartum.
Krummel *et al.*	Randomized controlled trial	Obese pregnant women (Cincinnati, USA).	Dietary docosahexanoic acid (DHA) supplements from 24–28 weeks gestation until term.	Maternal insulin sensitivity.
Louto *et al*	Cluster randomized controlled trial	Women at risk of gestational diabetes (overweight, age 40 years or older, earlier macrosomic child, diabetic first-degree relatives) (Finland).	Tailored diet and physical activity counseling, five visits to public health nurse. Monthly group session with physiotherapist.	Primary: gestational diabetes, birthweight. Secondary: maternal weight gain, childhood weight at one year; requirement for insulin treatment in pregnancy.
Ludwig *et al*	Randomized controlled trial	Overweight and obese (BMI >25, <45) pregnant women (Boston, USA).	Low glycemic load.	Birthweight z-score.
Nagle *et al.*	Randomized controlled trial	214 women with BMI ≥ 30 who are less than 17 weeks gestation.	Intervention arm will consist of care in a midwifery continuity of care model and receive an informational leaflet on managing weight gain in pregnancy.	Proportion of women with a gestational weight gain within IOM guidelines.
Parat *et al.*	Randomized controlled trial	Overweight or obese women (Paris, France).	Counseling on healthy eating and modest exercise.	30% reduction in rapid infancy weight gain at two years.
Oostdam *et al.* (Fit for 2 study)	Randomized controlled trial	Dutch women obese (BMI > 30) or overweight with history of macrosomia or abnormal glucose tolerance in previous pregnancy or first-grade relative with type 2 GDM. Two groups of 64 subjects.	Intensive exercise program (two days per week, 60 min each day).	Maternal fasting plasma glucose and relative insulin resistance. Primary neonatal outcome birthweight, QUALY.

Table 15.3 (cont.)

Ongoing studies

Poston et al. (the UPBEAT Study)	Pilot trial followed by randomized controlled trial	1560 obese pregnant women (UK).	Tailored advice on physical activity and diet. Group sessions.	Pilot study: change in dietary and physical activity behaviors, QUALY, and barriers to behavioral change. RCT: maternal insulin resistance. Primary neonatal outcome: birthweight, QUALY.
Shaheta et al	(1) Observational study (2) Randomized controlled trial	(1) All pregnant women delivering in District General Hospital. (2) Women with a BMI > 40.	Measurement of waist circumference at booking and 20/40 weeks. Metformin plus exercise vs. metformin.	Macrosomia, pre-eclampsia, and GDM.
Shen et al.	Randomized controlled trial	All BMI pregnant women (Manitoba, USA).	Community-based lifestyle intervention package (diet and exercise) during and after pregnancy.	Excessive gestational weight gain.
Walsh et al.	Randomized controlled trial	720 secundigravid women whose first baby was macrosomic, defined as a birthweight greater than 4000 g, will be recruited at their first antenatal visit.	Low-glycemic index carbohydrate diet vs. no dietary intervention.	Mean birthweight centiles and ponderal indices.
Vintner et al.	Randomized controlled trial	Obese (BMI > 30) pregnant women n = 360 (Odense, Denmark).	Individualized counseling on diet and physical activity.	Multiple obesity-related adverse pregnancy outcomes.

change using validated instruments in obese pregnant women is a prerequisite in development of a successful intervention. Obese women are likely to have low self-esteem, and as pre-pregnancy weight increases, so do psychosocial measures of perceived stress, trait anxiety, and depressive symptoms [128]. Furthermore women who gain excess weight in pregnancy relative to the IOM 1990 guidelines are more likely to demonstrate symptoms of depression [129]. The barriers to physical activity are also substantial, with 85% of women identifying lack of time, tiredness, and the inherent physical constraints of pregnancy [130]. Socioeconomic factors are also important as pregnant women who are younger, less educated, with a higher BMI, and who have more children are more likely to eat a poor quality and energy-dense diet [131]. Pilot trials of complex interventions are an essential preliminary step [132], with objective measurement of dietary and physical activity before and after the intervention, to prove efficacy of the intervention prior to embarking on large randomized controlled trials. These feasibility studies also offer insight into the practical issues that underpin success or failure [133].

The future: early identification and treatment of those at greatest risk

Although initially intervention studies have focused on targeting all obese women, clearly accurate targeting of interventions to those at greatest risk will be more cost-effective. In contrast to the wealth of studies and validated risk scores for the prediction of type 2 diabetes, the literature on the first trimester prediction of gestational diabetes and pregnancy complications is still limited. Some preliminary evidence suggests that combining simple maternal demographic and clinical characteristics will allow detection rates similar to those for type II diabetes (Figure 15.1), but external validation is still required [68]. Progress has recently been made with prediction algorithms for pre-eclampsia, and a composite algorithm with GDM as an outcome should be feasible due to the similarity of risk factors [134].

Conclusions

The maternal obesity "epidemic" has stimulated the need for development of effective interventions to improve pregnancy outcome. The rationale for new interventions should incorporate a detailed understanding of the maternal metabolic environment and its consequences for the health of the mother and the child.

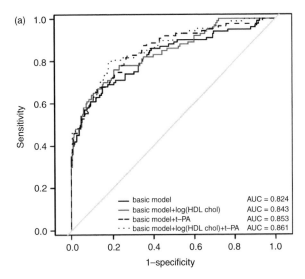

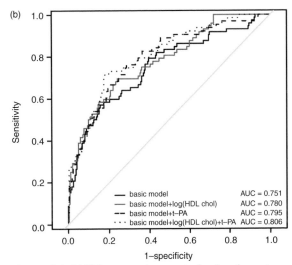

Figure 15.1. (a) ROC curves and summaries for all mothers using a basic model (including age, gestational age at sampling, BMI, ethnicity, family history of diabetes, and prior GDM) and with addition of independent predictors (HDL cholesterol and t-PA). AUC, area under ROC curve. (b) ROC curves and summaries for women with no prior GDM using a basic model (including age, gestational age at sampling, BMI, ethnicity, and family history of diabetes) and with addition of independent predictors (HDL cholesterol and t-PA). Reproduced with permission from Savvidou *et al.* 2010 [68].

Several randomized controlled trials are planned or underway, and using slightly different strategies should inform the best approach to effective intervention.

References

1. Okereke N C, Huston-Presley L, Amini S B, Kalhan S & Catalano P M. (2004) Longitudinal changes in energy

expenditure and body composition in obese women with normal and impaired glucose tolerance. *Am J Physiol Endocrinol Metab*;**287**:e472–9.

2. Alvarez J J, Montelongo A, Iglesias A, Lasuncion M A & Herrera, E. Longitudinal study on lipoprotein profile, high density lipoprotein subclass, and postheparin lipases during gestation in women. *J Lipid Res* 1996;**37**:299–308.

3. Knopp R H, Warth M R & Carrol C J. Lipid metabolism in pregnancy. I. Changes in lipoprotein triglyceride and cholesterol in normal pregnancy and the effects of diabetes mellitus. *J Reprod Med* 1973;**10**:95–101.

4. Warth M R, Arky R A & Knopp R H. Lipid metabolism in pregnancy. III. Altered lipid composition in intermediate, very low, low, and high-density lipoprotein fractions. *J Clin Endocrinol Metab* 1975;**41**:649–55.

5. Fahraeus L, Larsson-Cohn U & Wallentin L. Plasma lipoproteins including high density lipoprotein subfractions during normal pregnancy. *Obstet Gynecol* 1985;**66**:468–72.

6. Sattar N, Greer I A, Louden J, et al. Lipoprotein subfraction changes in normal pregnancy: threshold effect of plasma triglyceride on appearance of small, dense low density lipoprotein. *J Clin Endocrinol Metab* 1997;**82**:2483–91.

7. Desoye G, Schweditsch M O, Pfeiffer K P, Zechner R & Kostner G M. Correlation of hormones with lipid and lipoprotein levels during normal pregnancy and postpartum. *J Clin Endocrinol Metab* 1987;**64**:704–12.

8. Sacks F M & Walsh B W. Sex hormones and lipoprotein metabolism. *Curr Opin Lipidol* 1994;**5**:236–40.

9. Merzouk H, Meghelli-Bouchenak M, el-Korso N, Belleville J & Prost J. Low birth weight at term impairs cord serum lipoprotein compositions and concentrations. *Eur J Pediatr* 1998;**157**:321–6.

10. Ramsay J E, Ferrell W R, Crawford L, et al. Maternal obesity is associated with dysregulation of metabolic, vascular, and inflammatory pathways. *J Clin Endocrinol Metab* 2002;**87**:4231–7.

11. Rajasingam D, Seed P T, Briley A L, Shennan A H & Poston L. A prospective study of pregnancy outcome and biomarkers of oxidative stress in nulliparous obese women. *Am J Obstet Gynecol* 2009;**200**:395e391–9.

12. Sivan E, Homko C J, Chen X, Reece E A & Boden G. Effect of insulin on fat metabolism during and after normal pregnancy. *Diabetes* 1999;**48**:834–8.

13. Catalano P M, Nizielski S E, Shao J, et al. Downregulated IRS-1 and PPARgamma in obese women with gestational diabetes: relationship to FFA during pregnancy. *Am J Physiol Endocrinol Metab* 2002;**282**:e522–33.

14. Sanchez-Vera I, Bonet B, Viana M, et al. Changes in plasma lipids and increased low-density lipoprotein susceptibility to oxidation in pregnancies complicated by gestational diabetes: consequences of obesity. *Metabolism* 2007;**56**:1527–33.

15. Sattar N, Tan C E, Han T S, et al. Associations of indices of adiposity with atherogenic lipoprotein subfractions. *Int J Obes Relat Metab Disord* 1998;**22**:432–9.

16. Bevier W C, Fischer R & Jovanovic L. Treatment of women with an abnormal glucose challenge test (but a normal oral glucose tolerance test) decreases the prevalence of macrosomia. *Am J Perinatol* 1999;**16**:269–75.

17. Enquobahrie D A, Williams M A, Butler C L, et al. Maternal plasma lipid concentrations in early pregnancy and risk of preeclampsia. *Am J Hypertens* 2004;**17**(7):574–81.

18. Lorentzen B, Drevon C A, Endresen M J & Henriksen T. Fatty acid pattern of esterified and free fatty acids in sera of women with normal and pre-eclamptic pregnancy. *Br J Obstet Gynaecol* 1995;**102**(7):530–7.

19. Potter J M & Nestel P J. The hyperlipidemia of pregnancy in normal and complicated pregnancies. *Am J Obstet Gynecol* 1979;**133**(2):165–70.

20. Ramsay J E, Ferrell W R, Crawford L, et al. Divergent metabolic and vascular phenotypes in pre-eclampsia and intrauterine growth restriction: relevance of adiposity. *J Hypertens* 2004;**22**(11):2177–83.

21. Rajasingam D, Seed P T, Briley A L, Shennan A H & Poston L. A prospective study of pregnancy outcome and biomarkers of oxidative stress in nulliparous obese women. *Am J Obstet Gynecol* 2009;**200**(4):395e391–9.

22. Sattar N, Greer I A, Louden J, et al. Lipoprotein subfraction changes in normal pregnancy: threshold effect of plasma triglyceride on appearance of small, dense low density lipoprotein. *J Clin Endocrinol Metab* 1997;**82**:2483–91.

23. Vadachkoria S, Woelk G B, Mahomed K, et al. Elevated soluble vascular cell adhesion molecule-1, elevated homocyst(e)inemia, and hypertriglyceridemia in relation to preeclampsia risk. *Am J Hypertens* 2006;**19**(3):235–42.

24. Hubel C A, Shakir Y, Gallaher M J, McLaughlin M K & Roberts J M. Low-density lipoprotein particle size decreases during normal pregnancy in association with triglyceride increases. *J Soc Gynecol Investig* 1998;**5**(5):244–50.

25. Llurba E, Casals E, Domínguez C, et al. Atherogenic lipoprotein subfraction profile in preeclamptic women with and without high triglycerides: different pathophysiologic subsets in preeclampsia. *Metabolism* 2005;**54**(11):1504–9.

26. Griffin B A, Freeman D J, Tait G W, *et al.* Role of plasma triglyceride in the regulation of plasma low density lipoprotein (LDL) subfractions: relative contribution of small, dense LDL to coronary heart disease risk. *Atherosclerosis* 1994;**106**(2):241–53.

27. Institute of Medicine, National Research Council. *Weight Gain During Pregnancy: Reexamining the Guidelines.* (Washington, DC: The National Academies Press, 2009).

28. Sebire N J, Jolly M, Harris J P, *et al.* Maternal obesity and pregnancy outcome: a study of 287,213 pregnancies in London. *Int J Obes Relat Metab Disord* 2001;**25**(8):1175–82.

29. Duggleby S L & Jackson A A. Higher weight at birth is related to decreased maternal amino acid oxidation during pregnancy. *Am J ClinNutr* 2002;**76**:852–7.

30. deBenoist B, Jackson A A, Hall J S & Persaud C. Whole-body protein turnover in Jamaican women during normal pregnancy. *Hum Nutr Clin Nutr* 1985;**39**:167–79.

31. Jackson A A. Measurement of protein turnover during pregnancy. *Hum Nutr Clin Nutr* 1987;**41**:497–8.

32. Thompson G N & Halliday D. Protein turnover in pregnancy. *Eur J Clin Nutr* 1992;**46**:411–17.

33. Willommet L, Schutz Y, Whitehead R, Jequier E & Fern E B. Whole body protein metabolism and resting energy expenditure in pregnant Gambian women. *Am J Physiol Endocrinol Metab* 1992;**263**:e624–31.

34. Duggleby S L & Jackson A A. Relationship of maternal protein turnover and lean body mass during pregnancy and birth length. *Clin Sci (Lond)* 2001;**101**:65–72.

35. Chevalier S, Marliss E B, Morais J A, Lamarche M & Gougeon R. Whole-body protein anabolic response is resistant to the action of insulin in obese women. *Am J Clin Nutr* 2005;**82**:355–65.

36. Chevalier S P, Burgess S C, Malloy C R *et al.* The greater contribution of gluconeogenesis to glucose production in obesity is related to increased whole-body protein catabolism. *Diabetes* 2006;**55**:675–81.

37. Mills J L, Jovanovic L, Knopp R, *et al.* Physiological reduction in fasting plasma glucose concentration in the first trimester of normal pregnancy: the diabetes in early pregnancy study. *Metabolism*1998;**47**:1140–4.

38. Catalano P M, Tyzbir E D, Wolfe R R, *et al.* Longitudinal changes in basal hepatic glucose production and suppression during insulin infusion in normal pregnant women. *Am J Obstet Gynecol* 1992;**167**:913–19.

39. Kalhan S C, D'Angelo L J, Savin S M & Adam P A. Glucose production in pregnant women at term gestation. Sources of glucose for human fetus. *J Clin Invest* 1979;**63**:388–94.

40. Assel B, Rossi K & Kalhan S. Glucose metabolism during fasting through human pregnancy: comparison of tracer method with respiratory calorimetry. *Am J Physiol Endocrinol Metab* 1993;**265**:e351–6.

41. Kalhan S, Rossi K, Gruca L, Burkett E & O'Brien A. Glucose turnover and gluconeogenesis in human pregnancy. *J Clin Invest* 1997;**100**:1775–81.

42. Cousins L, Rigg L, Hollingsworth D, *et al.* The 24-hour excursion and diurnal rhythm of glucose, insulin, and C-peptide in normal pregnancy. *Am J Obstet Gynecol* 1980;**136**:483–8.

43. Butte N F, Hopkinson J M, Mehta N, Moon J K & Smith E O B. Adjustments in energy expenditure and substrate utilization during late pregnancy and lactation. *Am J Clin Nutr* 1999;**69**:299–307.

44. Catalano P M, Tyzbir E D, Roman N M, Amini S B & Sims E A. Longitudinal changes in insulin release and insulin resistance in nonobese pregnant women. *Am J Obstet Gynecol* 1991;**165**:1667–72.

45. Catalano P M, Tyzbir E D, Wolfe R R, *et al.* Carbohydrate metabolism during pregnancy in control subjects and women with gestational diabetes. *Am J Physiol Endocrinol Metab* 1993;**264**:e60–7.

46. Meier J J, Gallwitz B, Askenas M, *et al.* Secretion of incretin hormones and the insulinotropic effect of gastricinhibitory polypeptide in women with a history of gestational diabetes. *Diabetologia* 2005;**48**(9):1872–81.

47. Cypryk K, Vilsbøll T, Nadel I, *et al.* Normal secretion of the incretin hormones glucose-dependent insulinotropic polypeptide and glucagon-like peptide-1 during gestational diabetes mellitus. *Gynecol Endocrinol* 2007;**23**(1):58–62.

48. Ryan E A, O'Sullivan M J & Skyler J S. Insulin action during pregnancy. Studies with the euglycemic clamp technique. *Diabetes* 1985;**34**:380–9.

49. Catalano P M, Drago N M & Amini S B. Longitudinal changes in pancreatic beta-cell function and metabolic clearance rate of insulin in pregnant women with normal and abnormal glucose tolerance. *Diabetes Care* 1998;**21**:403–8.

50. Agardh C D, Aberg A & Norden N E. Glucose levels and insulin secretion during a 75 g glucose challenge test in normal pregnancy. *J Intern Med* 1996;**240**:303–9.

51. Endo S, Maeda K, Suto M, *et al.* Differences in insulin sensitivity in pregnant women with overweight and gestational diabetes mellitus. *Gynecol Endocrinol* 2006;**22**(6):343–9.

52. Kirwan J P, Huston-Presley L, Kalhan S C & Catalano P M. Clinically useful estimates of insulin sensitivity during pregnancy: validation studies in women with normal glucose tolerance and gestational diabetes mellitus. *Diabetes Care* 2001;**24**(9):1602–7.

53. Sivan E, Chen X, Homko C J, Reece E A & Boden G. Longitudinal study of carbohydrate metabolism in healthy obese pregnant women. *Diabetes Care* 1997;**20**:1470–5.

54. Di Cianni G, Miccoli R, Volpe L, *et al.* Maternal triglyceride levels and newborn weight in pregnant women with normal glucose tolerance. *Diabet Med* 2005;**22**:21–5.

55. Kalkhoff R K, Kandaraki E, Morrow P G, *et al.* Relationship between neonatal birth weight and maternal plasma amino acid profiles in lean and obese nondiabetic women and in type I diabetic pregnant women. *Metabolism*1988;**37**:234–9.

56. Nolan C J, Riley S F, Sheedy M T, Walstab J E & Beischer N A. Maternal serum triglyceride, glucose tolerance, and neonatal birth weight ratio in pregnancy. *Diabetes Care* 1995;**18**:1550–6.

57. Schaefer-Graf U M, Graf K, Kulbacka I, *et al.* Maternal lipids as strong determinants of fetal environment and growth in pregnancies with gestational diabetes mellitus. *Diabetes Care* 2008;**31**:1858–63.

58. HAPO Study Cooperative Research Group. Hyperglycemia and Adverse Pregnancy Outcome (HAPO) Study: associations with maternal body mass index. *BJOG* 2010;**117**:575–84.

59. Catalano P M, Roman-Drago N M, Amini S B & Sims E A. Longitudinal changes in body composition and energy balance in lean women with normal and abnormal glucose tolerance during pregnancy. *Am J Obstet Gynecol* 1998;**179**:156–65.

60. Sivan E, Homko C J, Whittaker P G, *et al.* Free fatty acids and insulin resistance during pregnancy. *J Clin Endocrinol Metab* 1998;**83**:2338–42.

61. Homko C J, Cheung P & Boden G. Effects of free fatty acids on glucose uptake and utilization in healthy women. *Diabetes* 2003;**52**:487–91.

62. Crowther C A, Hiller J E, Moss J R, *et al.* Effect of treatment of gestational diabetes mellitus on pregnancy outcomes. *N Engl J Med* 2005;**352**:2477–86.

63. Landon M B, Spong C Y, Thom E, *et al.* (2009) A multicenter, randomized trial of treatment for mild gestational diabetes. *N Engl J Med*;**361**:1339–48.

64. Metzger B E, Lowe L P, Dyer A R, *et al.* Hyperglycemia and adverse pregnancy outcomes. *N Engl J Med* 2008;**358**:1991–2002.

65. International Association of Diabetes and Pregnancy Study Groups Consensus Panel. International association of diabetes and pregnancy study groups recommendations on the diagnosis and classification of hyperglycemia in pregnancy. *Diabetes Care* 2010;**33**:676–82.

66. Leary J, Pettitt D J & Jovanovic L. Gestational diabetes guidelines in a HAPO world. *Best Pract Res Clin Endocrinol Metab* 2010;**24**(4):673–85.

67. Round J A, Jacklin P, Fraser R B, *et al.* Screening for gestational diabetes mellitus: cost-utility of different screening strategies based on a woman's individual risk of disease. *Diabetologia* 2011; **54**: 256–63.

68. Savvidou M, Nelson S M, Makgoba M, *et al.* First-trimester prediction of gestational diabetes mellitus: examining the potential of combining maternal characteristics and laboratory measures. *Diabetes* 2010;**59**:3017–22.

69. Nanda S, Savvidou M, Syngelaki A, Akolekar R & Nicolaides K H. Prediction of gestational diabetes mellitus by maternal factors and biomarkers at 11 to 13 weeks. *Prenat Diagn.* 2011;**31**:135–41.

70. Graham I, Atar D, Borch-Johnsen K, *et al.* European guidelines on cardiovascular disease prevention in clinical practice: executive summary. *Eur Heart J* 2007;**28**:2375–414.

71. Rydén L, Standl, E, Bartnik, M *et al.* Guidelines on diabetes, pre-diabetes, and cardiovascular diseases: executive summary. The Task Force on Diabetes and Cardiovascular Diseases of the European Society of Cardiology (ESC) and of the European Association for the Study of Diabetes (EASD). *Eur Heart J* 2007;**28**:88–136.

72. Lindstrom J, Louheranta A, Mannelin M, *et al.* The Finnish Diabetes Prevention Study (DPS): lifestyle intervention and 3-year results on diet and physical activity. *Diabetes Care* 2003;**26**:3230–36.

73. Eriksson K F & Lindgarde F. Prevention of type 2 (non-insulin-dependent) diabetes mellitus by diet and physical exercise. The 6-year Malmo feasibility study. *Diabetologia* 1991;**34**:891–8.

74. Pan X R, Li G W, Hu Y H, *et al.* Effects of diet and exercise in preventing NIDDM in people with impaired glucose tolerance. The Da Qing IGT and Diabetes Study. *Diabetes Care* 1997;**20**:537–44.

75. Ramachandran A, Snehalatha C, Mary S, *et al.* The Indian Diabetes Prevention Programme shows that lifestyle modification and metformin prevent type 2 diabetes in Asian Indian subjects with impaired glucose tolerance (IDPP-1). *Diabetologia* 2006;**49**:289–97.

76. Diabetes Prevention Program Research Group. Reduction in the incidence of type 2 diabetes with lifestyle intervention or metformin. *N Engl J Med* 2002;**346**:393–403.

77. Spinnewijn W E, Lotgering F K, Struijk P C & Wallenburg H C. Fetal heart rate and uterine contractility during maternal exercise at term. *Am J Obstet Gynecol* 1996;**174**:43–8.

78. Kennelly M M, Geary M, McCaffrey N, *et al.* Exercise-related changes in umbilical and uterine artery waveforms as assessed by Doppler ultrasound scans. *Am J Obstet Gynecol* 2002;**187**:661–6.

79. Bonen A, Campagna P, Gilchrist L, Young D C & Beresford P. Substrate and endocrine responses during exercise at selected stages of pregnancy. *J Appl Physiol* 1992;**73**:134–42.

80. Madsen M, Jorgensen T, Jensen M L, *et al.* Leisure time physical exercise during pregnancy and the risk of miscarriage: a study within the Danish National Birth Cohort. *BJOG* 2007;**114**:1419–26.

81. Misra D P, Strobino D M, Stashinko E E, Nagey D A & Nanda J. Effects of physical activity on preterm birth. *Am J Epidemiol* 1998;**147**:628–35.

82. Berkowitz G S, Kelsey J L, Holford T R & Berkowitz R L. Physical activity and the risk of spontaneous preterm delivery. *J Reprod Med* 1983;**28**:581–8.

83. Evenson K R, Siega-Riz A M, Savitz D A, Leiferman J A & Thorp J M, Jr. Vigorous leisure activity and pregnancy outcome. *Epidemiology* 2002;**13**:653–9.

84. Hatch M, Levin B, Shu X O & Susser M. Maternal leisure-time exercise and timely delivery. *Am J Public Health* 1998;**88**:1528–33.

85. Rizzo T, Metzger B E, Burns W J & Burns K. Correlations between antepartum maternal metabolism and child intelligence. *N Engl J Med* 1991;**325**:911–16.

86. Rizzo T A, Dooley S L, Metzger B E, *et al.* Prenatal and perinatal influences on long-term psychomotor development in offspring of diabetic mothers. *Am J Obstet Gynecol* 1995;**173**(6):1753–8.

87. Lokey E A, Tran Z V, Wells C L, Myers B C & Tran A C. Effects of physical exercise on pregnancy outcomes: a meta-analytic review. *Med Sci Sports Exerc* 1991;**23**:1234–9.

88. Kramer M S & McDonald S W. Aerobic exercise for women during pregnancy. *Cochrane Database Syst Rev* 2006;**3**:CD000180.

89. Leet T & Flick L. Effect of exercise on birthweight. *Clin Obstet Gynecol* 2003;**46**:423–31.

90. Bell R J, Palma S M & Lumley J M. The effect of vigorous exercise during pregnancy on birth-weight. *Aust N Z J Obstet Gynaecol* 1995; **35**:46–51.

91. Clapp J F, 3rd & Dickstein S. Endurance exercise and pregnancy outcome. *Med Sci Sports Exerc* 1984;**16**:556–62.

92. Alderman B W, Zhao H, Holt V L, Watts D H & Beresford S A. Maternal physical activity in pregnancy and infant size for gestational age. *Ann Epidemiol* 1998;**8**:513–19.

93. Langer O, Yogev Y, Most O & Xenakis E M. Gestational diabetes: the consequences of not treating. *Am J Obstet Gynecol* 2005;**192**(4):989–97.

94. Gillman M W, Oakey H, Baghurst P A *et al.* Effect of treatment of gestational diabetes mellitus on obesity in the next generation. *Diabetes Care* 2010;**33**:964–8.

95. Reece EA, Leguizamón G & Wiznitzer A. Gestational diabetes: the need for a common ground. *Lancet* 2009;**373**:1789–97.

96. American Diabetes Association. Gestational diabetes mellitus. *Diabetes Care* 2003;**26**:s103–s5.

97. Major C A, Henry M J, De Veciana M & Morgan M A. The effects of carbohydrate restriction in patients with diet-controlled gestational diabetes. *Obstet Gynecol* 1998;**91**:600–4.

98. Franz M J, Horton E S, Sr., Bantle J P, *et al.* Nutrition principles for the management of diabetes and related complications. *Diabetes Care* 1994;**17**:490–518.

99. Moses R G, Barker M, Winter M, Petocz P & Brand-Miller J C. Can a low glycemic index diet reduce the need for insulin in gestational diabetes mellitus? *Diabetes Care* 2009;**32**:996–1000.

100. Tuffnell D J, West J & Walkinshaw S A. Treatments for gestational diabetes and impaired glucose tolerance in pregnancy. *Cochrane Database Syst Rev* 2003;**3**:CD003395.

101. Rowan J A, Hague W M, Gao W, Battin M R & Moore M P. Metformin versus insulin for the treatment of gestational diabetes. *N Engl J Med* 2008;**358**:2003–15.

102. Fougner K J, Vanky E & Carlsen S M. Metformin has no major effects on glucose homeostasis in pregnant women with PCOS: results of a randomized double-blind study. *Scand J Clin Lab Invest* 2008;**68**:771–6.

103. Ratner R E, Christophi C A, Metzger B E, *et al.* Prevention of diabetes in women with a history of gestational diabetes: effects of metformin and lifestyle interventions. *J Clin Endocrinol Metab* 2008;**93**:4774–9.

104. Jovanovic-Peterson L, Durak E P & Peterson C M. Randomized trial of diet versus diet plus cardiovascular conditioning on glucose levels in gestational diabetes. *Am J Obstet Gynecol* 1989;**161**:415–19.

105. Avery M D & Walker A J. Acute effect of exercise on blood glucose and insulin levels in women with gestational diabetes. *J Matern Fetal Med* 2001;**10**:52–8.

106. Brankston G N, Mitchell B F, Ryan E A & Okun N B. Resistance exercise decreases the need for insulin in overweight women with gestational diabetes mellitus. *Am J Obstet Gynecol* 2004;**190**:188–93.

107. Garcia-Patterson A, Martin E, Ubeda J, *et al.* Evaluation of light exercise in the treatment of gestational diabetes. *Diabetes Care* 2001;**24**:2006–7.

108. Clapp J F, 3rd, Rokey R, Treadway J L, *et al.* Exercise in pregnancy. *Med Sci Sports Exerc* 1992;**24**:s294–300.

109. Clapp J F, 3rd & Capeless E L. The changing glycemic response to exercise during pregnancy. *Am J Obstet Gynecol* 1991;**165**:1678–83.

110. Dempsey J C, Butler C L, Sorensen T K, *et al.* A case-control study of maternal recreational physical activity and risk of gestational diabetes mellitus. *Diabetes Res Clin Pract* 2004;**66**:203–15.

111. Dempsey J C, Sorensen T K, Williams M A, *et al.* Prospective study of gestational diabetes mellitus risk in relation to maternal recreational physical activity before and during pregnancy. *Am J Epidemiol* 2004;**159**:663–70.

112. Weissgerber T L, Wolfe L A, Davies G A & Mottola M F. Exercise in the prevention and treatment of maternal-fetal disease: a review of the literature. *Appl Physiol Nutr Metab* 2006;**31**:661–74.

113. Oostdam N, van Poppel M N, Eekhoff E M, Wouters M G & van Mechelen W. Design of FitFor2 study: the effects of an exercise program on insulin sensitivity and plasma glucose levels in pregnant women at high risk for gestational diabetes. *BMC Pregnancy Childbirth* 2009;**9**:1.

114. Dornhorst A & Frost G. The principles of dietary management of gestational diabetes: reflection on current evidence. *J Hum Nutr Diet* 2002;**15**:145–56; quiz 57–9.

115. Thomas D & Elliott E J. Low glycaemic index, or low glycaemic load, diets for diabetes mellitus. *Cochrane Database Syst Rev* 2009;**1**:CD006296.

116. Moses R G, Luebcke M, Davis W S, *et al.* Effect of a low-glycemic-index diet during pregnancy on obstetric outcomes. *Am J Clin Nutr* 2006;**84**:807–12.

117. Fraser R B, Ford F A & Milner R D. A controlled trial of a high dietary fibre intake in pregnancy – effects on plasma glucose and insulin levels. *Diabetologia* 1983;**25**:238–41.

118. Clapp J F, 3rd. Maternal carbohydrate intake and pregnancy outcome. *Proc Nutr Soc* 2002;**61**:45–50.

119. Tieu J, Crowther C A & Middleton P. Dietary advice in pregnancy for preventing gestational diabetes mellitus. *Cochrane Database Syst Rev* 2008;**2**:CD006674.

120. Thomas D E, Elliott E J & Baur L. Low glycaemic index or low glycaemic load diets for overweight and obesity. *Cochrane Database Syst Rev* 2007;**3**:CD005105.

121. Rasmussen K M, Yaktine A L. (eds) Institute of Medicine & National Research Council Committee to Reexamine IOM Pregnancy Weight Guidelines. *Weight Gain During Pregnancy: Reexamining the Guidelines.* (Washington DC: National Academies Press, 2009).

122. Stuebe A M, Oken E & Gillman M W. Associations of diet and physical activity during pregnancy with risk for excessive gestational weight gain. *Am J Obstet Gynecol* 2009;**201**:58e1–8.

123. Kramer M S & Kakuma R. Energy and protein intake in pregnancy. *Cochrane Database Syst Rev* 2003;**4**:CD000032.

124. Olafsdottir A S, Skuladottir G V, Thorsdottir I, Hauksson A & Steingrimsdottir L. Maternal diet in early and late pregnancy in relation to weight gain. *Int J Obes (Lond)* 2006;**30**:492–9.

125. Deierlein A L, Siega-Riz A M & Herring A. Dietary energy density but not glycemic load is associated with gestational weight gain. *Am J Clin Nutr* 2008;**88**:693–9.

126. Stehbens J A, Baker G L & Kitchell M. Outcome at ages 1, 3, and 5 years of children born to diabetic women. *Am J Obstet Gynecol* 1977;**127**:408–13.

127. Gardner B, Wardle J, Poston L & Croker H. Changing diet and physical activity to reduce gestational weight gain: a meta-analysis. *Obesity Rev* 2011;**12**:e602–20.

128. Laraia B A, Siega-Riz A M, Dole N & London E. Pregravid weight is associated with prior dietary restraint and psychosocial factors during pregnancy. *Obesity (Silver Spring)* 2009;**17**:550–8.

129. Webb J B, Siega-Riz A M & Dole N. Psychosocial determinants of adequacy of gestational weight gain. *Obesity (Silver Spring)* 2009;**17**:300–9.

130. Evenson K R, Moos M K, Carrier K & Siega-Riz A M. Perceived barriers to physical activity among pregnant women. *Matern Child Health J* 2008;**13**:364–75.

131. Rifas-Shiman S L, Rich-Edwards J W, Kleinman K P, Oken E & Gillman M W. Dietary quality during pregnancy varies by maternal characteristics in Project Viva: a US cohort. *J Am Diet Assoc* 2009;**109**:1004–11.

132. Craig P, Dieppe P, Macintyre S, *et al.* Developing and evaluating complex interventions: the new Medical Research Council guidance. *BMJ* 2008;**337**:a1655.

133. Kinnunen T I, Aittasalo M, Koponen P, *et al.* Feasibility of a controlled trial aiming to prevent excessive pregnancy-related weight gain in primary health care. *BMC Pregnancy Childbirth* 2008;**8**:37.

134. North R A, McCowan L M, Dekker G A, *et al.* Clinical risk prediction for pre-eclampsia in nulliparous women: development of model in international prospective cohort. *BMJ* 2011;**342**:d1875.

Chapter

16

Intervention strategies to improve outcome in obese pregnancies: micronutrients and dietary supplements

Lisa M. Bodnar and Meredith S. Parrott

Introduction

A vast body of literature supports strong associations between maternal obesity and risk of a wide range of birth and pregnancy outcomes (see Chapters 4 and 6). Notably, these health risks increase as obesity becomes more severe. With the rising rates of severe obesity among women of childbearing age, we are in urgent need of effective interventions that will improve the outcome in obese pregnancy.

Intervening to improve maternal micronutrient status may be one means by which poor outcomes may be prevented. Many of the poor outcomes prevalent among obese pregnant women, including some congenital malformations, gestational diabetes, hypertensive disorders of pregnancy, and stillbirth have been linked with maternal micronutrient deficiencies [1]. Moreover, although obesity is considered a state of overnutrition, micronutrient deficiencies may be more common among obese women than their leaner counterparts.

In the current chapter, we review data highlighting the vulnerability of obese women to multiple micronutrient deficiencies and discuss potential mechanisms explaining this poorer overall micronutrient status in obesity. We then summarize evidence supporting the effectiveness of nutrition interventions at preventing key birth outcomes among obese pregnant women. Finally, we provide recommendations for research needed to fill major knowledge gaps in this important area.

Obese pregnant women are vulnerable to multiple nutrient deficiencies

In this section, we explore notable nutrient deficiencies observed in obesity, with a focus on reproductive-aged and pregnant women, if available (Table 16.1). For a recent, detailed review of micronutrient deficiencies in general obese populations, see Garcia *et al.* [2].

Folate

Adequate folate in the periconceptional period has been shown to prevent neural tube defects (NTD). Evidence suggests that folate status is compromised by being overweight/obese and also indicates that obese women of childbearing age are at high risk for folate deficiency. Using the National Health and Nutrition Examination Survey (NHANES) III and NHANES 1999–2000 data including a total of 8369 non-pregnant women aged 17 to 49 years, Mojtabai *et al.* [3] demonstrated that obese women of childbearing age in the United States consumed significantly less folate than leaner women, with a significant inverse relationship between folate intake and body mass index (BMI). In addition, these authors also reported that increased BMI was associated with a lower serum folate concentration, even after controlling for differences in folate intake from diet and supplements. Specifically, multiple regression analyses adjusting for age, race/ethnicity, and folate intake illustrated that each $10 \, \text{kg/m}^2$ increase in BMI was associated with a 0.92 ng/ml or 1.91 ng/ml decline in serum folate in NHANES III and NHANES 1999–2000, respectively. Interestingly, while authors of another analysis of premenopausal women in NHANES III observed a similar increased risk of poor serum folate in obese compared with normal weight women, there was no difference in red blood cell (RBC) concentrations of folate, a longer term marker of folate status (OR 0.84; 95% CI: 0.55–1.29)[4].

In a study of 67 Spanish women aged 20 to 35 years, Ortega *et al.* [5] reported that obese women were at a

Maternal Obesity, ed. Matthew W. Gillman and Lucilla Poston. Published by Cambridge University Press. © Cambridge University Press 2012.

Table 16.1 Observed relationships between obesity and micronutrient status in women by pregnancy status[a]

Micronutrient	Obese non-pregnant women	Obese pregnant women
Folate	Some studies report significantly less folate consumption[b] An inverse relationship exists between folate intake and BMI Elevated BMI is associated with lower serum folate, controlling for folate intake Obese women may be at greater risk of folate deficiency[b]	In the latter half of pregnancy, serum folate concentrations are significantly less in women with pre-pregnancy obesity[b]
Antioxidants	Obese women have a higher likelihood of selenium deficiency and marginal vitamin C status[b] The odds of low vitamin E, α- and β-carotene, and other carotenoids are greater among obese women[b]	BMI does not appear to be associated with mid-trimester ascorbic acid or retinol concentrations Ascorbic acid concentrations are significantly lower in women who subsequently deliver SGA[c] infants compared with those who deliver AGA[d] infants
Vitamin D	Obese women have lower serum 25(OH)D concentrations and are at higher risk of deficiency[b]	Pregravid BMI is associated with lower 25(OH)D concentrations and higher prevalence of vitamin D deficiency at <21 weeks gestation Neonates of overweight and obese women are about twice as likely to be vitamin D deficient compared to those of lean women
Trace minerals	An inverse relationship between adiposity and serum iron concentrations may exist Adiposity predicts decreased iron absorption	Obesity may be associated with high hemoglobin and reduced prevalence of antepartum iron-deficient anemia Pre-pregnancy obesity predicts postpartum anemia High pregravid BMI is correlated with lower plasma zinc concentrations in early pregnancy[b]
Calcium	Higher calcium intake is associated with lower odds of adiposity Supplementation in women with low intake may result in decreased body weight and fat mass	The relationship between calcium and adiposity in pregnancy is unclear

[a] Refer to text for specific references.
[b] Compared with non-obese women or those of normal weight.
[c] Small for gestational age, defined as <10%.
[d] Appropriate for gestational age.

significantly greater risk than leaner women of having serum folate concentrations <14.9 nmol/l, which is considered at risk for deficiency (OR 6.2; 95% CI: 1.9–20.3). Notably, they observed no difference in dietary intake of folate between obese and leaner women. Like the results by Mojtabai, these results suggest that rather than differences in intake, biologic mechanisms are at play in obese women that may reduce blood folate concentrations.

We are aware of only one study that has addressed the association between adiposity and folate in pregnant women. In a cross-sectional analysis of 608 pregnant Korean women, mean serum folate concentrations in the latter half of pregnancy were significantly lower in those women with pre-pregnancy obesity compared with women who were underweight before pregnancy [6]. However, the results were not adjusted for confounders.

Antioxidants

Low concentrations of antioxidants have consistently been reported among obese individuals in the published literature [2]. In an analysis of 4327 non-pregnant premenopausal women from NHANES III, Kimmons et al. observed that compared with normal weight women (BMI 18.5–24.9 kg/m²), obese (BMI ≥30 kg/m²) women were more likely to have low concentrations of multiple antioxidants after adjustment for age and race/ethnicity [4]. Specifically, obese women had a greater likelihood of selenium deficiency (<100 μg/l; OR 1.6; 95% CI: 1.0–2.5) and marginal vitamin C status (<0.4 mg/dl; OR 2.5; 95% CI: 1.8–3.5). They also reported that obesity was associated with greater odds of low concentrations of vitamin E, α-carotene, ß-carotene, and other carotenoids (ß-cryptoxanthin, lutein/zeaxanthin, and lycopene), but not vitamin A.

Evidence relating obesity and antioxidant status during pregnancy is limited. In a cohort of 208 obese primiparous women enrolled in the placebo arm of the randomized controlled Vitamins in Pre-eclampsia (VIP) trial [7], BMI was not associated with second-trimester plasma ascorbic acid (vitamin C) or retinol concentrations [8]. However, the authors did find that concentrations of ascorbic acid were 10.2 μmol/l (95% CI: 1.2–19.0 μmol/l) lower in obese women who subsequently delivered small for gestational age (SGA) <10th percentile neonates compared with obese women who delivered appropriate for gestational age infants. Interestingly, they also observed a significant association between maternal BMI and elevation in the ratio of second-trimester plasma α-tocopherol: γ-tocopherol. This ratio may be a marker of a poor quality diet [9].

Vitamin D

The association between obesity and vitamin D status has been well described in many populations [2]. Compared with leaner women, obese women have significantly lower serum concentrations of 25--hydroxyvitamin D (25(OH)D, the indicator of vitamin D nutritional status) [10] and are at higher risk of vitamin D deficiency [4]. Vitamin D insufficiency and deficiency are common among pregnant women, and the relationship between adiposity and vitamin D has been explored in pregnancy. In a US cohort of Black and White nulliparas, pregravid obesity was associated with significantly lower adjusted 25(OH)D concentrations (56.5 vs. 62.7 nmol/l) as well as a higher prevalence of vitamin D deficiency (61% vs. 36%) at <21 weeks gestation, which remained statistically significant after confounder adjustment [11]. In addition, overweight

and obese women were approximately twice as likely as lean women to deliver neonates with vitamin D deficiency as measured by levels in cord blood at delivery.

Trace minerals

Iron

An inverse relationship between adiposity (measured by BMI, waist circumference, and fat mass) and serum iron concentration has been described in American Hispanic women [12]. In addition, other authors have demonstrated that adiposity predicts lower iron absorption in reproductive-age women [13]. In pregnant women, obesity may be associated with higher concentrations of hemoglobin and reduced prevalence of anemia [14, 15] compared with those of normal weight, while in the postpartum period, maternal pre-pregnancy obesity predicts postpartum anemia [16].

Zinc

There appears to be a relationship between zinc status and obesity in both children and adults [2]. Moreover, high pre-pregnancy BMI has been significantly correlated with lower plasma zinc concentrations in early pregnancy. In a cross-sectional study of 1474 women at <14 weeks gestation, researchers reported that those women in the highest quartile of BMI (mean BMI 36 kg/m²) had significantly lower plasma zinc concentrations than those individuals in lower BMI quartiles [17].

Calcium

In observational studies, low calcium intake has been shown to be correlated with greater fat mass, as well as greater risk of future weight and fat mass gain [18]. Zemel and colleagues further supported this relationship in the NHANES III dataset [19]. They demonstrated that the odds of being in the highest body fat quartile was significantly reduced among non-pregnant women in the highest quartile of calcium and dairy product intake compared to women in the lowest quartile of intake (OR 0.16; 95% CI: 0.03–0.88). In addition, some data also suggest that calcium or dairy food supplementation may assist in fat and weight loss among individuals with poor calcium intake [18]. For instance, Major et al. randomized 63 overweight/obese women to calcium plus vitamin D supplementation vs. placebo for 15 weeks and demonstrated that in women with very low baseline calcium intake, supplementation was associated with a significant decrease in body weight and fat mass [20]. To our knowledge, the relationship between calcium and adiposity in pregnancy has not yet been elucidated.

Synopsis of micronutrient deficiencies in obese pregnant women

As summarized above, data demonstrate that obese women of childbearing potential are at increased risk for multiple micronutrient deficiencies, but evidence in pregnant populations is scarce. Increased BMI in non-pregnant women is associated with decreased serum folate, 25(OH)D, ascorbic acid, vitamin E, total carotenoids, and selenium in a variety of populations. Among pregnant women, greater pre-pregnancy adiposity is associated with significantly lower serum folate and 25(OH)D concentrations compared with leaner counterparts [21] but the relationship between adiposity and other important micronutrients in the prenatal period remains unclear. Because pregnancy is a time of tremendous physiologic change, it is uncertain if conclusions that we draw regarding poor micronutrient status in obesity among non-pregnant women are generalizable to pregnant women. We are currently conducting a study of pregnant women to evaluate the association between pre-pregnancy obesity and nutritional status, defined using a wide range of nutritional biomarkers assayed in mid-pregnancy. We hope that these data help to fill knowledge gaps relating micronutrient status and adiposity in pregnancy.

Proposed mechanisms relating obesity and increased risk of nutrient deficiencies

The aforementioned evidence indicates that an association between obesity and multiple micronutrient deficiencies exists. With the bulk of studies cross-sectional in nature, it remains unclear whether this relationship is causal and if obesity precedes the development of the deficiency, or if in some cases, the deficiency may contribute to obesity (as may be the case for calcium). Numerous hypotheses have been proposed to explain the link between obesity and micronutrient deficiencies.

Diet quality

Obesity may be associated with poor micronutrient status because of poor dietary intake. In two studies, pregnant women with high pre-pregnancy BMI were shown to have poorer quality diets than those who were leaner [21,22]. Laraia *et al.* observed a dose–response relationship between pre-pregnancy BMI and inadequate servings of grains, vegetables, iron, and folate in mid-pregnancy among 2394 lower- to middle-income North Carolina women [22]. Further, pregravid obesity was associated with increased odds of low-quality diet, even when controlling for potential confounders such as education, pre-pregnancy vitamin use, and physical activity. Likewise, in another cohort study of 1777 Massachusetts women in their first trimester of pregnancy, women with high pre-pregnancy BMI had significantly poorer diet quality, as measured by the Alternate Health Eating Index modified for pregnancy [21]. In the NHANES III and 1999–2000, a dataset of cross-sectional nationally representative surveys of 8369 non-pregnant, reproductive-age women in the United States, Mojtabai also observed that women of higher BMI had significantly lower intakes of folate compared with leaner women [3]. Yet it is critical to note that because these investigators observed that higher BMI is associated with a lower serum folate concentration even after controlling for folate intake, decreased intake relative to overall increased body mass may not entirely explain the micronutrient deficiencies described among obese pregnant women.

Altered metabolic processes

Obesity-specific distribution and utilization of micronutrients and obesity-related metabolic changes such as oxidative stress may also contribute to the relationship between obesity and micronutrient deficiencies.

Distribution/utilization

It is well established that plasma volume directly correlates with BMI [23]. Therefore, observed decreases in micronutrient concentrations among those individuals with increased BMI could be due, in part, to their increased plasma volume. Furthermore, carotenoids, which are partially fat soluble, are sequestered in fat tissue and therefore may be reduced in obese individuals as a relatively smaller quantity of carotenoids are distributed in blood and plasma [24].

In addition, obese persons may have an impaired ability to use the micronutrients taken in through diet and supplements. For example, Wortsman *et al.* demonstrated that compared with lean individuals, non-pregnant overweight and obese adults have a reduced response in circulating 25(OH)D concentrations after oral vitamin D supplementation as well as exposure to ultraviolet irradiation [25]. These authors suggest that the lower concentration of 25(OH)D in obese persons is due to the reduced bioavailability of vitamin D as it is sequestered within adipose tissue. Another example of altered storage is the lack of association between BMI and RBC folate (a marker of long-term folate status), but a strong inverse relationship between BMI and serum folate [3,4]. Overweight or obese individuals may have adequate long-term folate storage but an inability to mobilize, circulate, and utilize these folate stores. Abnormal folate distribution and/or dysfunctional metabolism may cause maternal folate reserves to be less available to the growing embryo and, therefore, a potential contributing mechanism to increased NTD observed among obese pregnant women [1].

The relationship between adiposity and low iron is believed to be related to reduced iron intake, inadequate iron absorption, or iron sequestration [2]. Adiposity predicts lower iron absorption in reproductive-age women [13]. Iron absorption can be inhibited by other dietary factors including eggs, coffee, tea, and zinc as well as by the intrinsic peptide hormone hepcidin. Hepcidin, considered the master regulator of iron homeostasis, sequesters iron within intestinal enterocytes by its inhibition of ferroportin. Its expression is increased by pro-inflammatory cytokines such as interleukin 6 and tumor necrosis factor alpha, levels of which are amplified in chronic inflammatory states such as obesity [26].

Oxidative stress

Obese individuals exhibit increased systemic and adipose tissue-specific oxidative stress [27], causing the production of reactive oxygen species. The production of these reactive oxygen species may lead to heightened oxidative consumption of antioxidants such as vitamin C, vitamin E, carotenoids, selenium, and zinc. For example, the enzyme superoxide dismutase (SOD), which contains and is therefore dependent on zinc, is an important antioxidant defense against free radicals. The enzymatic activity of SOD in overweight/obese persons, and specifically in obese pregnant women, is significantly reduced compared to that in individuals of normal weight [28]. Likewise, serum gamma-glutamyltransferase (GGT) is an enzyme that plays an important role in antioxidant defense systems, may be a marker of oxidative stress, and has been implicated in the pathogenesis of diabetes. Body mass index appears to be positively associated with current and future

serum GGT [24]. In a longitudinal evaluation of 3146 men and women enrolled in the Coronary Artery Risk Development in Young Adults (CARDIA) study, serum vitamin C, ß-carotene, and folate concentrations were inversely associated with serum GGT [29]. Subsequent analysis of these patients revealed that serum antioxidants (specifically ß-carotene) inversely predicted ten-year future serum GGT [30].

Leptin alteration

Leptin, a protein hormone synthesized by adipocytes, plays a key role in regulating energy intake and expenditure. This pleiotropic molecule is implicated in insulin resistance and inflammation, as well as poor pregnancy outcomes such as pre-eclampsia and intrauterine growth restriction [31]. Multiple micronutrient deficiencies affect leptin expression and its serum concentrations. Adequate intakes of B vitamins, vitamin E, and ß-carotene are associated with lower leptin serum levels, and vitamin A and D supplementation have been separately demonstrated to reduce leptin expression [2].

Anatomic changes

Bariatric surgery poses a unique situation with regards to micronutrient deficiencies. A recent systematic review suggests that after surgery, these patients are at risk for deficiencies in multiple micronutrients, including folate, vitamin C, vitamin D, iron, selenium, and zinc [32]. In addition, over-the-counter multivitamin and mineral supplements may not provide adequate amounts of certain nutrients, making additional supplementation necessary for postbariatric surgery patients to maintain optimal micronutrient status. The type of bariatric surgery directly affects the etiology of which deficiencies occur: banding procedures are restrictive in nature thereby limiting food consumption and overall intake, while bypass procedures lead to malabsorption as altered anatomy ultimately decreases secretory and absorptive surface area [32]. The effect of pre-pregnancy bariatric surgery on pregnancy outcome is described in Chapter 19.

Should dietary recommendations differ for obese women?

Given the potential for obesity to impair absorption, transport, utilization, bioavailability, and storage of micronutrients, an argument could be made that nutrient needs are higher in obese pregnancy. Several researchers have addressed the issue of modifying dietary recommendations among obese individuals. Folate is one nutrient that has received some attention in this regard. Women with high BMI may require more than the recommended dose of 400 µg of folic acid daily to obtain the same level of protection against NTD as leaner women. Mojtabai used data from NHANES 1999–2000 and a proposed model formula to predict the association between folic acid intake and serum levels. The authors projected that women with a BMI $\geq 30 \, kg/m^2$ would need to consume an additional 350 µg of folate daily to achieve the same serum folate level as women with a BMI $<20 \, kg/m^2$ [3].

Others have demonstrated that obese individuals may require supplemental vitamin C to achieve the same plasma ascorbic acid levels as those who are leaner [33]. After depleting 68 men of vitamin C for one month and subsequently repleting their vitamin C status, these authors found that body weight was inversely associated with lower attained plasma ascorbic acid level. It is possible that this difference is due to an alteration in distribution and plasma volume in obese persons, as described above. Unfortunately, we are unaware of other nutrients that have been explored in this fashion.

The Royal College of Obstetricians and Gynaecologists (RCOG), together with the Centre for Maternal and Child Enquiries (CMACE), recommends that women desiring conception with a BMI ≥ 30 should be advised to consume 5 mg of folic acid supplementation daily, starting at least one month prior to conception and continuing throughout the first trimester [34]. This guideline also recommends that women with a pre-pregnancy BMI ≥ 30 should be counseled to consume 10 µg of supplemental vitamin D daily during pregnancy and while breastfeeding. In obese women who have undergone bariatric surgery and are pregnant or planning pregnancy, the American Congress of Obstetricians and Gynecologists (ACOG) recommends assessment of folate, vitamin B_{12}, iron, and calcium with possible supplementation [35].

Micronutrient interventions to improve birth outcomes among obese women

With the poor micronutrient status of obese women of childbearing age, and potentially the same relationship in obese pregnant women, it is critical to understand whether micronutrient interventions could positively impact birth outcomes in obese pregnancy.

Randomized controlled trials

We are unaware of any randomized controlled trials (RCTs) designed to test the hypothesis that supplementation with single or multiple micronutrients prevents adverse birth or pregnancy outcomes among obese women. The inferences we can draw from micronutrient RCTs are limited to the few studies that have presented subanalyses by maternal BMI.

Fall et al. conducted a 2009 review and meta-analysis of birth outcomes from 12 recent, high-quality randomized, double-blinded controlled trials among pregnant women in developing countries [36]. In all studies, pregnant women were randomized to treatment with multiple micronutrients providing approximately the recommended dietary allowance of a wide range of vitamins and minerals or placebo, iron–folic acid, iron–folic acid–vitamin A, or iron alone as the comparison group. In their analysis, the authors found that supplementation caused small but statistically significant increases in infant birthweight and the frequency of large for gestational age (LGA) birth, as well as reductions in low birthweight and SGA birth. Importantly, they observed that the impact of supplementation varied by maternal BMI. In pooled analyses of all 12 studies, multiple micronutrient supplementation led to a 39.0 g increase in birthweight among mothers with a BMI $\geq 20 \, kg/m^2$, but had essentially no impact in mothers with a BMI $<20 \, kg/m^2$. The authors noted that several of the 12 studies noted particularly strong effect modification, with the intervention leading to a 7.6 g (95% CI: 1.9–3.3 g) increase in birthweight for every one unit (kg/m^2) increase in maternal BMI. It is notable that maternal BMIs ranged from 15 to 30 kg/m^2 in these trials, with a near absence of obese women by Western standards. Therefore, the effect modification observed may have been driven by underweight women, and whether the small but statistically significant benefit of multiple micronutrient supplementation on birthweight is generalizable to obese women remains unknown. Furthermore, because these studies were limited to low-income countries, the application of their findings to developed countries is also uncertain.

In the Vitamins in Pre-eclampsia (VIP) trial, Poston et al. [7] enrolled 2410 pregnant women from the United Kingdom who were at high risk for pre-eclampsia, including 804 primiparous obese (BMI $\geq 30 \, kg/m^2$) mothers, to test whether concomitant supplementation with vitamin C and vitamin E prevented pre-eclampsia. Women were randomized to receive either daily supplements of 1000 mg vitamin C and 400 IU vitamin E or matched placebo from the second trimester until delivery. In the full cohort, there was no difference in the frequency of pre-eclampsia between groups. In subanalyses of primiparous obese women, the incidence of pre-eclampsia in the supplemented group (40/394, 10%) was not different from the placebo group (47/405, 12%; risk ratio 0.97; 95% CI: 0.59–1.30). Neither risk of low birthweight nor SGA varied by treatment group among the obese mothers.

Using a nearly identical protocol as the VIP trial, the WHO Maternal and Perinatal Research Network conducted a multicenter RCT of vitamins C and E supplementation in women at high risk of pre-eclampsia who resided in countries with low socioeconomic status and overall poor nutrition [37]. Of the 1381 women randomized, 249 had a BMI $\geq 30 \, kg/m^2$ (n = 128 and n = 121 were randomized to receive vitamins and placebo, respectively). As in the Poston trial, there was no benefit of supplementation with vitamins C and E on pre-eclampsia risk in the whole cohort. However, in the subanalyses performed for this trial, the investigators observed that the incidence of pre-eclampsia was reduced among obese women in the treatment group (12.5%) compared with women in the placebo group (22.3%). The difference was of borderline statistical significance (risk ratio 0.6; 95% CI: 0.3–1.0), likely because of the overall small sample size of women with a BMI $\geq 30 \, kg/m^2$. A trend toward a reduction in very low birthweight (<1500 g) due to the treatment was also noted among obese women (risk ratio 0.4; 95% CI: 0.1–1.0).

Goldenberg et al. conducted a randomized, double-blinded, placebo-controlled trial to determine if zinc supplementation increased birthweight [38]. African American women with relatively low plasma zinc concentrations (n = 580) were randomized at <23 weeks gestation. In the entire cohort, the researchers noted a benefit of the treatment on birthweight and several key anthropometric measures in the infants at birth. However, the protective effect of zinc appeared to be limited to women with a BMI $<26 \, kg/m^2$. Treatment with zinc caused statistically significant improvements in infant birthweight, head circumference, and arm length, as well as borderline significant increases in gestational age, preterm birth <32 weeks, very low birthweight

(<1500 g), subscapular skinfold thickness, neonatal hospital stay, and neonatal sepsis among women with a BMI $<26 \, kg/m^2$. In heavier women, no significant differences in these measures were noted.

Observational studies

Several high-quality observational studies of birth defects, pre-eclampsia, and SGA birth may provide additional insight into whether micronutrient supplementation may reduce the likelihood of poor outcomes among obese pregnant women.

In a large population-based case-control study in California, intake of $\geq 400 \, \mu g$ of folic acid from diet and supplements was associated with a 40% reduction in the risk of NTD among women weighing less than 70 kg. Yet folic acid intake did not incur a protective effect among heavier women [39]. Other investigators evaluated the association between maternal weight and NTD before and after mandatory folic acid fortification of grain products in Canada [40], and found that elevated maternal weight was associated with a slight increase in odds of NTD before mandatory folic acid fortification of grain products (adjusted OR 1.4; 95% CI: 1.0–1.8). After fortification, the risk associated with high maternal weight strengthened (adjusted OR 2.8; 95% CI: 1.2–6.6). This finding suggests that mandatory folic acid fortification may have had little impact on NTD rates among overweight and obese women in this region.

Watkins and Botto conducted a large case-control study in the southeastern United States and found that among mothers who were average weight, regular use of periconceptional multivitamins reduced the risk of a congenital heart defect in the offspring (OR 0.61; 95% CI: 0.36–0.99) [41]. However, no protective effect of multivitamin use was observed among overweight women (BMI $>26 \, kg/m^2$) (OR 1.69; 95% CI: 0.69–3.84). Dietary zinc intakes have also been associated with a reduced risk of NTD among lean, but not overweight, women [42]. In another study, Carmichael et al. studied 454 cases of NTD and 462 controls from California and reported that mothers with poor diet quality in the preconception period (as indicated by low intakes of iron, vitamin B_6, vitamin A, calcium, and folate, and high intakes of fat and sweets) had an elevated risk of NTD. In subanalyses, the elevated risk appeared to be limited to non-obese women [43].

Other investigators have observed similar trends in associations between multivitamin use and risk of pre-eclampsia and SGA birth. In a cohort of 1835 women in Pittsburgh, Pennsylvania, women who reported regular use of multivitamins in the six months around conception had a 45% reduction in the risk of pre-eclampsia [44]. Pre-pregnancy overweight modified this effect. Among lean women, multivitamin use was highly protective against pre-eclampsia (adjusted OR 0.29; 95% CI: 0.12–0.65), but no relation was observed among overweight mothers (adjusted OR 1.08; 95% CI: 0.52–2.25). To test the robustness of this study's findings, researchers used data from the Danish National Birth Cohort, including 18 551 periconceptional multivitamin users, 2468 folic acid-only users, and 7582 non-users [45]. The lower the pre-pregnancy BMI, the stronger the association between regular multivitamin use and pre-eclampsia. Finally, similar results were found in a cohort study of SGA birth, where multivitamins were associated with a reduced risk in lean but not obese women [46].

Taken together, the randomized trial data and the observational data suggest that while risk of pregnancy and birth outcomes among lean women may be reduced with dietary or supplemental intake of specific micronutrients, obese pregnant women may not benefit at the same doses.

Summary

There are major gaps in knowledge regarding whether micronutrient supplements may provide an effective intervention for preventing adverse pregnancy and birth outcomes among obese mothers. No RCTs have been conducted to evaluate this important public health question. Subanalyses of trial data and observational data point to the likelihood that some micronutrient exposures will not have a beneficial impact on adverse outcomes in obese women. The growing body of evidence illustrating that obese women of childbearing age are at higher risk of poor micronutrient status than lean women supports these conclusions. Thus obese pregnant women may require higher doses of micronutrients to see the same protective effect as their leaner counterparts.

Well-designed RCTs of micronutrient supplementation in populations of obese pregnant women are needed to establish the causal link between micronutrients and birth outcomes in this at-risk group, and to assist clinical and public health decision-making. Future rigorous observational studies exploring a wide range of micronutrients and risk of poor outcomes

in large samples of women with high pre-pregnancy BMIs will add to the evidence base. Moreover, additional research into the specific nutrients that may be adversely affected by high fat mass before and during pregnancy will help pinpoint the aspects of nutritional status that are of greatest concern in obese mothers and help focus intervention research.

References

1. Bodnar L M. Maternal obesity and adverse pregnancy outcomes: the role of nutrition and physical activity. In Baker P, Balen A H, Poston L & Sattars N (eds.) *Obesity and Reproductive Health.* (London: RCOG Press, 2007), pp. 145–62.

2. Garcia O P, Long K Z & Rosado J L. Impact of micronutrient deficiencies on obesity. *Nutr Rev* 2009;**67**(10):559–72.

3. Mojtabai R. Body mass index and serum folate in childbearing age women. *Eur J Epidemiol* 2004;**19**(11):1029–36.

4. Kimmons J E, Blanck H M, Tohill B C, Zhang J & Khan L K. Associations between body mass index and the prevalence of low micronutrient levels among US adults. *Med Gen Med* 2006;**8**(4):59.

5. Ortega R M, Lopez-Sobaler A M, Andres P, *et al.* Folate status in young overweight and obese women: changes associated with weight reduction and increased folate intake. *J Nutr Sci Vitaminol (Tokyo)* 2009;**55**(2):149–55.

6. Han Y S, Ha E H, Park H S, Kim Y J & Lee S S. Relationships between pregnancy outcomes, biochemical markers and pre-pregnancy body mass index. *Int J Obes (Lond)* 2010;**35**(4):570–7.

7. Poston L, Briley A L, Seed P T, Kelly F J, Shennan A H. Vitamin C and vitamin E in pregnant women at risk for pre-eclampsia (VIP trial): randomised placebo-controlled trial. *Lancet* 2006;**367**(9517):1145–54.

8. Rajasingam D, Seed P T, Briley A L, Shennan A H & Poston L. A prospective study of pregnancy outcome and biomarkers of oxidative stress in nulliparous obese women. *Am J Obstet Gynecol* 2009;**200**(4):395e1–9.

9. Bates C J, Mishra G D & Prentice A. Gamma-tocopherol as a possible marker for nutrition-related risk: results from four national diet and nutrition surveys in Britain. *Br J Nutr* 2004;**92**(1):137–50.

10. Hahn S, Haselhorst U, Tan S, *et al.* Low serum 25-hydroxyvitamin d concentrations are associated with insulin resistance and obesity in women with polycystic ovary syndrome. *Exp Clin Endocrinol Diabetes* 2006;**114**(10):577–83.

11. Bodnar L M, Catov J M, Roberts J M & Simhan H N. Prepregnancy obesity predicts poor vitamin

D status in mothers and their neonates. *J Nutr* 2007;**137**(11):2437–42.

12. Chambers E C, Heshka S, Gallagher D, *et al.* Serum iron and body fat distribution in a multiethnic cohort of adults living in New York City. *J Am Diet Assoc* 2006;**106**(5):680–4.

13. Zimmermann M B, Zeder C, Muthayya S, *et al.* Adiposity in women and children from transition countries predicts decreased iron absorption, iron deficiency and a reduced response to iron fortification. *Int J Obes (Lond)* 2008;**32**(7):1098–104.

14. Bodnar L M, Siega-Riz A M, Arab L, Chantala K & McDonald T. Predictors of pregnancy and postpartum iron status in low-income women. *Public Health Nutr* 2004;**7**(6):701–11.

15. Garn S M & Petzold A S. Fatness and hematological levels during pregnancy. *Am J Clin Nutr* 1982;**36**:729–30.

16. Bodnar L M, Siega-Riz A M & Cogswell M E. High prepregnancy BMI increases the risk of postpartum anemia. *Obes Res* 2004;**12**(6):941–8.

17. Tamura T, Goldenberg R L, Johnston K E & Chapman V R. Relationship between pre-pregnancy BMI and plasma zinc concentrations in early pregnancy. *Br J Nutr* 2004;**91**(5):773–7.

18. Major G C, Chaput J P, Ledoux M, *et al.* Recent developments in calcium-related obesity research. *Obes Rev* 2008;**9**(5):428–45.

19. Zemel M B, Shi H, Greer B, Dirienzo D & Zemel P C. Regulation of adiposity by dietary calcium. *FASEB J* 2000;**14**(9):1132–8.

20. Major G C, Alarie F P, Dore J & Tremblay A. Calcium plus vitamin D supplementation and fat mass loss in female very low-calcium consumers: potential link with a calcium-specific appetite control. *Br J Nutr* 2009;**101**(5):659–63.

21. Rifas-Shiman S L, Rich-Edwards J W, Kleinman K P, Oken E & Gillman M W. Dietary quality during pregnancy varies by maternal characteristics in Project Viva: a US cohort. *J Am Diet Assoc* 2009;**109**(6):1004–11.

22. Laraia B A, Bodnar L M & Siega-Riz A M. Pregravid body mass index is negatively associated with diet quality during pregnancy. *Public Health Nutr* 2007;**10**(9):920–6.

23. Pearson T C, Guthrie D L, Simpson J, *et al.* Interpretation of measured red cell mass and plasma volume in adults: Expert Panel on Radionuclides of the International Council for Standardization in Haematology. *Br J Haematol* 1995;**89**(4):748–56.

24. Andersen L F, Jacobs D R, Jr., Gross M D, *et al.* Longitudinal associations between body mass index

and serum carotenoids: the CARDIA study. *Br J Nutr* 2006;**95**(2):358–65.

25. Wortsman J, Matsuoka L Y, Chen T C, Lu Z & Holick M F. Decreased bioavailability of vitamin D in obesity. *Am J Clin Nutr* 2000;**72**(3):690–3.

26. McClung J P & Karl J P. Iron deficiency and obesity: the contribution of inflammation and diminished iron absorption. *Nutr Rev* 2009;**67**(2):100–4.

27. Vincent H K, Innes K E & Vincent K R. Oxidative stress and potential interventions to reduce oxidative stress in overweight and obesity. *Diabetes Obes Metab* 2007;**9**(6):813–39.

28. Al-Saleh E, Nandakumaran M, Al-Harmi J, Sadan T & Al-Enezi H. Maternal–fetal status of copper, iron, molybdenum, selenium, and zinc in obese pregnant women in late gestation. *Biol Trace Elem Res* 2006;**113**(2):113–23.

29. Lee D H, Steffen L M, Jacobs D R, Jr. Association between serum gamma-glutamyltransferase and dietary factors: the coronary artery risk development in young adults (CARDIA) study. *Am J Clin Nutr* 2004;**79**(4):600–5.

30. Lee D H, Gross M D, Jacobs D R, Jr. Association of serum carotenoids and tocopherols with gamma-glutamyltransferase: the cardiovascular risk development in young adults (CARDIA) study. *Clin Chem* 2004;**50**(3):582–8.

31. Henson M C & Castracane V D. Leptin in pregnancy. *Biol Reprod* 2000;**63**(5):1219–28.

32. Shankar P, Boylan M & Sriram K. Micronutrient deficiencies after bariatric surgery. *Nutrition* 2010;**26**(11/12):1031–7.

33. Block G, Mangels A R, Patterson B H, *et al.* Body weight and prior depletion affect plasma ascorbate levels attained on identical vitamin C intake: a controlled-diet study. *J Am Coll Nutr* 1999;**18**(6):628–37.

34. Modder J & Fitzsimons K J. *CMACE/RCOG Joint Guideline: Management of Women with Obesity in Pregnancy*. (London: Centre for Maternal and Child Enquiries and the Royal College of Obstetricians and Gynaecologists, March 2010).

35. American College of Obstetricians and Gynecologists. ACOG Committee Opinion number 315, September 2005. Obesity in pregnancy. *Obstet Gynecol* 2005;**106**(3):671–5.

36. Fall C H, Fisher D J, Osmond C & Margetts B M. Multiple micronutrient supplementation during pregnancy in low-income countries: a meta-analysis of effects on birth size and length of gestation. *Food Nutr Bull* 2009;**30**(4 Suppl):S533–46.

37. Villar J, Purwar M, Merialdi M, *et al.* World Health Organisation multicentre randomised trial of

supplementation with vitamins C and E among pregnant women at high risk for pre-eclampsia in populations of low nutritional status from developing countries. *BJOG* 2009;**116**(6):780–8.

38. Goldenberg R L, Tamura T, Neggers Y, *et al.* The effect of zinc supplementation on pregnancy outcome. [see comment]. *JAMA* 1995;**274**(6):463–8.

39. Werler M M, Louik C, Shapiro S & Mitchell A A. Prepregnant weight in relation to risk of neural tube defects. *JAMA* 1996;**275**(14):1089–92.

40. Ray J G, Wyatt P R, Vermeulen M J, Meier C & Cole D E. Greater maternal weight and the ongoing risk of neural tube defects after folic acid flour fortification. *Obstet Gynecol* 2005;**105**(2):261–5.

41. Watkins M L & Botto L D. Maternal prepregnancy weight and congenital heart defects in offspring. *Epidemiology* 2001;**12**(4):439–46.

42. Velie E M, Block G, Shaw G M, *et al.* Maternal supplemental and dietary zinc intake and the occurrence of neural tube defects in California. *Am J Epidemiol* 1999;**150**(6):605–16.

43. Carmichael S L, Shaw G M, Selvin S & Schaffer D M. Diet quality and risk of neural tube defects. *Med Hypotheses* 2003;**60**(3):351–5.

44. Bodnar L M, Tang G, Ness R B, Harger G & Roberts J M. Periconceptional multivitamin use reduces the risk of preeclampsia. *Am J Epidemiol* 2006;**164**(5):470–7.

45. Catov J M, Nohr E A, Bodnar L M, *et al.* Association of periconceptional multivitamin use with reduced risk of preeclampsia among normal-weight women in the Danish national birth cohort. *Am J Epidemiol* 2009;**169**(11):1304–11.

46. Catov J M, Bodnar L M, Ness R B, Markovic N & Roberts J M. Association of periconceptional multivitamin use and risk of preterm or small-for-gestational-age births. *Am J Epidemiol* 2007;**166**(3):296–303.

Pre-pregnancy bariatric surgery: improved fertility and pregnancy outcome?

Roland G. Devlieger and Isabelle Guelinckx

Introduction

Ideally interventions to improve pregnancy outcome in obese women should start in the preconceptional period. Lifestyle changes leading toward a negative energy balance (energy intake < energy expenditure) and consequently to weight loss are advisable as a first step. However, the effectiveness of these lifestyle interventions in non-pregnant adults to maintain the induced weight loss in the long term is low, even if these conventional actions are supported by pharmacotherapy. In relation to morbid obesity, bariatric surgery, also known as obesity surgery, offers a more effective treatment: it results in a substantial weight loss that is sustainable in the long term and in improvement of obesity-associated co-morbidities [1,2]. A surgical intervention is therefore increasingly being considered when conventional interventions have failed in patients with a body mass index (BMI) of more than $40 \, \text{kg/m}^2$ and for those with a BMI of over $35 \, \text{kg/m}^2$ with co-morbidities such as sleep apnea, diabetes, joint disease, and cardiopulmonary problems [3].

As obesity rates rise worldwide, so have the number of bariatric operations and in the number of practicing bariatric surgeons [4,5]. In 2008 approximately 220 000 people with morbid obesity underwent bariatric surgery in the USA and Canada [6]. About 85% of all bariatric surgery patients are women of reproductive age [5]. Additionally, an increasing number of adolescents, predominantly female, are having bariatric surgery [7]. Consequently, health care providers will increasingly be confronted with pregnant women with a medical history of bariatric surgery.

The following section summarizes the most commonly performed bariatric operations. We further review the impact of pre-pregnancy bariatric surgery

on the female reproductive functions most appropriate to the theme of this book and the relevant pregnancy outcome parameters. Finally, we formulate recommendations for clinical care of these patients for both the postoperative as well as the prenatal period.

Bariatric surgery

Bariatric surgery results in weight loss through different mechanisms depending on the type of surgery performed. The procedures are classified as restrictive, malabsorptive, or a combination of both (Figure 17.1). The first type leads to a restricted energy intake by reducing gastric storage capacity. A small gastric pouch is created at the proximal part of the stomach by the use of staples or a band. The amount of food that can be consumed at one time will decrease since an early feeling of satiety will be induced. Procedures of this type include the vertical banded gastroplasty, sleeve gastrectomy, and the laparoscopic adjustable gastric band. For the laparoscopic adjustable gastric band, a silicon inflatable gastric band is placed horizontally around the proximal part of the stomach. Through a subcutaneous port, the band is inflated or deflated with fluid, creating a small or larger opening to the gastric pouch. The second type includes the malabsorptive procedures such as the biliopancreatic diversion or Scopinaro procedure, and biliopancreatic diversion with duodenal switch and jejuno-ileal bypass. A large section of the small intestine is bypassed reducing nutrient uptake. At present the jejuno-ileal bypass is rarely used due to substantial long-term complications of hepatic failure, calcium oxalate kidney stones, renal failure, arthritis, and malnutrition [8]. The mixed procedures limit both energy intake and uptake. The Roux-en-Y gastric bypass also involves the creation

Maternal Obesity, ed. Matthew W. Gillman and Lucilla Poston. Published by Cambridge University Press. © Cambridge University Press 2012.

Procedure type	Restrictive procedures	Malabsorptive procedures	Mixed procedures
Operation examples	Laparoscopic adjustable gastric banding (LAGB)	Biliopancreatic diversion (BPD)	Roux-en-Y gastric bypass (RYGB)
	Sleeve gastrectomy	Biliopancreatic diversion with duodenal switch (BPD-DS)	
	Vertical banded gastroplasty	Jejuno-ileal bypass	
Mechanism of weight loss	Reduced food intake • reduced gastric capacity • early satiety	Reduced nutritient absorbtion • small intestine bypassed	Reduced intake and uptake
Schematic examples	LAGB	BPD-DS	RYGB

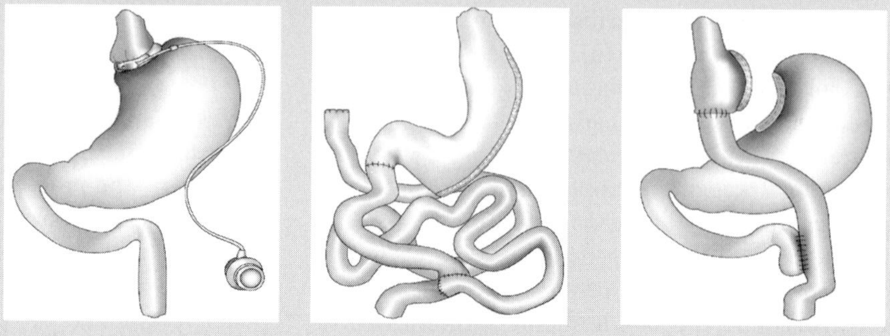

Figure 17.1. Classification of bariatric surgery procedures.

of a gastric pouch; however, in this case the pouch is separated from the remaining stomach by stapling or transection. The gastric pouch empties directly into the distal jejunum, bypassing the remaining stomach, duodenum, and most of the proximal jejunum. Nowadays, over 90% of procedures are performed laparoscopically [6]. According to the Bariatric Surgery Registry the proportion of bariatric surgery that is of mixed restrictive–malabsorptive type increased from 33% in 1987 to 94% in 2004, while the restrictive procedures decreased correspondingly [5]. However, in 2008 another international survey reported a different profile: the most commonly performed procedures were laparoscopic adjustable gastric banding (42.3%), laparoscopic standard Roux-en-Y gastric bypass (39.7%), and total sleeve gastrectomies (4.5%) [6]. Moreover, the trends differ in Europe vs. the United States [6]. The discrepancy between the results of both surveys could be due to the difference in countries studied, the time of registration (2004 vs. 2008) and the registration method. The Bariatric Surgery Registry is a dataset

that was continuously completed by surgeons, whereas the survey by Buchwald *et al.* was an email survey to surgeons.

The Swedish obese subjects study included 3505 non-pregnant participants who were followed for two years after bariatric surgery. The weight loss among the surgery patients was substantial compared to the control group receiving conventional treatment in whom there was a slight gain in weight (23.4% loss vs. 0.1% gain; $p < 0.001$). After ten years of follow-up the weight loss was greater in the gastric bypass group (25%, SD 11) compared to vertical banded gastroplasty (16%, SD 11), or the gastric banding group (14%, SD 14). Besides weight loss, the improvement of co-morbidities or even the resolution of chronic conditions after surgery was notable, independently of the type of bariatric surgery. Compared to conventional obesity treatment, patients who underwent surgery were more likely to recover from diabetes, hypertension, dyslipidemia, obstructive sleep apnea, and hyperuricemia [9,10]. As a result, life expectancy is extended and the quality of life related to general health perception, social interaction, anxiety, and depression is enhanced [1,10].

Reported adverse events following surgery vary according to the type of procedure. The operative mortalities after laparoscopic adjustable gastric band and Roux-en-Y gastric bypass are approximately 0.1% and 0.5%, respectively [11]. Frequent long-term complications following laparoscopic adjustable gastric band may include hyperemesis, gastric prolapse, stomal obstruction, esophageal and gastric pouch dilatation, gastric erosion and necrosis, and access port problems or infection [11]. Roux-en-Y gastric bypass can be complicated in the long term by dumping stomal stenosis, marginal ulcers, staple line disruption, and internal hernias [11,12]. Patients with a history of bariatric surgery are at risk of nutrient deficiencies including vitamins B_{12}, B_1, C, folate, A, D, and K along with deficiencies in calcium, iron, selenium, zinc, and copper [13]. Nutritional deficiencies after laparosopic adjustable gastric band are less common than after Roux-en-Y gastric bypass [14]. However, they can occur because of the restricted dietary intake or intolerance to certain foods and therefore a limited intake of nutrients. Nutritional deficiencies after Roux-en-Y gastric bypass can arise through different mechanisms: first, the induced dietary restriction induced by the operation leads to insufficient intake and an intolerance to certain food items (meat, milk, fiber), that can result in a diet with limited variation [15]; second, the inferior part of the stomach is relatively inactive leading to decreased gastric acid secretion, necessary to absorb vitamins and minerals (vitamin B_{12} and iron); third, the absorption sites for several specific nutrients are bypassed; finally, asynergia between the bolus and the biliopancreatic secretions may result in decreased absorptive capacity of the common part of the small intestine. This last mechanism can specifically lead to fat malabsorption, and consequently to malabsorption of the fat-soluble vitamins [16,17].

The consensus among bariatric surgeons is that long-term success not only depends on the type of bariatric surgery and the skills of the surgeon, but also – for both restrictive and malabsorptive procedures – on the patient's psychological stability, motivation, and knowledge regarding the operation and its consequences [11]. The patient should also be aware that lifelong adjustments to eating behavior and physical activity are required to obtain weight loss and weight maintenance and to prevent long-term complications [18–21]. Screening and follow-up for these factors by a multidisciplinary team is therefore not an expensive luxury, but a clinical necessity. This applies especially for women of reproductive age: pregnancy is a state of increased nutritional demands and complications affect not only the woman but also the fetus.

Fertility after bariatric surgery

Several authors have recently reviewed the impact of bariatric surgery on female reproductive function [22,23]. In general, the weight loss as a result of the surgery reverses the adverse effects of obesity on fertility (Figure 17.2).

Hormonal alterations in non-pregnant woman after bariatric surgery are the result of decreased adipose

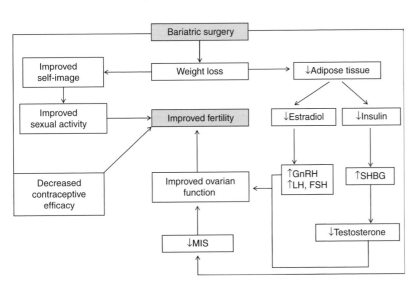

Figure 17.2. Effects of bariatric surgery on fertility. Abbreviations: FSH: follicular stimulating hormone; GnRH: gonadotropin releasing hormone; LH: lutenising hormone; MIS: Müllerian inhibiting substance; SHBG: sex hormone binding globulin.

tissue mass, resulting in lower estradiol levels, stimulating the hypothalamic release of gonadotropin releasing hormone (GnRH) and luteinising hormone (LH), and of follicular stimulating hormone (FSH) secretion by the pituitary gland. Weight loss also lowers insulin levels, resulting in increased sex hormone binding globulin (SHBG) and decreased peripheral testosterone concentrations. Finally, Müllerian inhibiting substance (MIS) levels are decreased after bariatric surgery.

As a result, almost all parameters of reproductive function are improved. Most cohort studies or case series comparing the pre- and postoperative fertility status, report an improvement in spontaneous pregnancy rates after bariatric surgery. In anovulatory obese women, up to 71% regained cyclicity of menstrual blood loss after surgery, in proportion to the amount of weight loss [24].

Sexual interest, activity, and function also appear to improve after weight loss, independent of the modality used to obtain this reduction in weight [22]. These improvements may represent an important incentive to undergo the operation in a proportion of women. Clinicians are therefore encouraged to routinely evaluate sexual function in women who plan to undergo bariatric surgery.

Pregnancy after bariatric surgery

Attempts to review the literature on pregnancy after bariatric surgery are limited by the quality of the available studies [16,39]. All studies so far are observational and have a varying design, different control groups, and, globally, small study groups (Table 17.1). This may lead to an underestimation of the complication rates. Mixing the different types of bariatric surgery might lead to unreliable conclusions since a different outcome can be expected after the restrictive type than after the malabsorptive types [16]. Conclusions about the consequences of pre-pregnancy bariatric surgery on maternal health and pregnancy outcome therefore need to be drawn with necessary caution.

Maternal nutritional deficiencies

The safety of a postoperative pregnancy after bariatric surgery has been questioned, since malnutrition and, more specifically, nutritional deficiencies during pregnancy may potentially lead to fetal complications (Table 17.2). The risks for complications such as preterm birth and neural tube defects (NTD) due to respectively maternal iron-deficient anemia and folic acid deficiency are well known [17]. More specific complications due

to nutritional deficiencies have been reported in pregnant women who underwent bariatric surgery, independently of the time between surgery and conception: fetal growth retardation, oligohydramnios, electrolyte imbalances, and cerebral hemorrhage (vitamin K deficiency), bilateral micropthalmia and permanent retinal damage (vitamin A deficiency), and even fetal deaths [25–32]. Vitamin B_{12} deficiency can be expected after all surgical procedures since vitamin B_{12} uptake requires intrinsic factor, the production of which is reduced after surgery. Vitamin B_{12} deficiency can also cause maternal anemia. This maternal deficit is, however, also reflected in the concentration in the breast milk and can therefore result in Vitamin B_{12} insufficiency in the baby causing pancytopenia and physical and neurological developmental delay [33–36]. Other nutrients that require attention are proteins, calcium, and vitamin D [16]. Maternal vitamin D insufficiency is associated with neonatal hypocalcemia or rickets. The woman might even develop a symptomatic maternal osteomalacia in case of a severe deficit [17]. The general nutritional status of a pregnant woman after bariatric surgery can be compromised to such a degree that parenteral nutrition is required during pregnancy. A cohort study reported that parenteral nutrition was necessary in 21% of the pregnant women with a biliopancreatic diversion [37]. Screening and treatment of these deficiencies during pregnancy is therefore an integral part of the clinical care in these patients.

Pregnancy outcomes

The weight loss after bariatric surgery results in a lower incidence of obesity-related maternal morbidities such as gestational diabetes, pre-eclampsia, and gestational hypertension [38]. The incidences of these outcomes after bariatric surgery are lower than in obese women without bariatric surgery, or approach those of non-obese controls. Based on the current evidence a history of bariatric surgery does not seem to be an indication for cesarean delivery. Some studies report lower rates of cesarean delivery, but others report higher or comparable rates [39].

The question whether pregnancy jeopardizes the aim of bariatric surgery, namely long-term weight loss, has been largely ignored in the literature. Investigators have addressed this topic by examining gestational weight gain (GWG) and postpartum weight retention (PPWR) in these patients. Bariatric surgery seems to protect against excessive GWG: three studies, including two that

Table 17.1 Observational studies on pregnancy following bariatric procedures by type of procedure: study population, comparison group, and main maternal and neonatal outcomes

Author, year	Study population	Comparison group	Most relevant maternal findings in study population	Most relevant neonatal findings in study population
Laparoscopic adjustable gastric banding				
Ducarme *et al.* 2007 [41]	13 consecutive pregnancies	414 consecutive obese	Less GDM (0% vs. 22%) p < 0.05 Less PET (0% vs. 3.1%) p < 0.05 Less CS (15.3% vs. 34.4%) p < 0.01 Band complications NR	Less LBW (7.7% vs. 10.6%) p < 0.05 Less macrosomia (7.7% vs. 14.6%) p < 0.05
Dixon *et al.* 2005 [40]	79 consecutive first postoperative pregnancies	(1) 40 consecutive preoperative pregnancies (2) 79 BMI-matched controls	Less PET (5% vs. 28%) p < 0.05 Less PIH (10% vs. 45%) p < 0.05 Less GDM (6.3% vs. 19%) p < 0.05 Less PET (5% vs. 25%) p < 0.05 Less PIH (10% vs. 38%) p < 0.05 Band complications 5%	NR Less PMD (6.3% vs. 12.7%) p = 0.08
Dixon *et al.* 2001 [78]	22 selected pregnancies	264 preoperative pregnancies	Less PIH (4.5% vs. 37%) p < 0.05 Band complications 9%	NR
Skull *et al.* 2004 [56]	49 consecutive pregnancies	31 consecutive preoperative pregnancies	Less GDM (8% vs. 27%) p < 0.05 Band complications 4.1%	NR
Bar-Zohar *et al.* 2006 [79]	81 postoperative pregnancies	none	GDM 7.4% PIH 16% CS 20% Band complications 2.4%	NR
Martin *et al.* 1998 [61]	23 postoperative pregnancies	none	GDM 0% PIH 0% CS 22% Band complications NR	NR
Weiss *et al.* 2001 [53]	7 unexpected postoperative pregnancies	none	Band complications 29%	High rate of LBW (40%)
Vertical banded gastroplasty				
Bilenka *et al.* 1995 [80]	14 postoperative pregnancies in 9 patients	18 preoperative pregnancies in same 9 patients	Less miscarriages (7% vs. 39%) p < 0.05 Less GDM (0% vs. 16.7%) p = 0.06 More PIH (15.3% vs. 5.6%) p < 0.05	Normal birthweights
Roux-en-Y gastric bypass				
Richards *et al.* 1987 [81]	57 postoperative pregnancies	57 matched preoperative pregnancies	Less PIH (8.8% vs. 45.6%) p < 0.05	Less macrosomia (15.8% vs. 36.8%) p < 0.05 Perinatal mortality 3.5% in study group and controls
Wittgrove *et al.* 1998 [42]	17 selected postoperative patients	Preoperative pregnancies from same 17 patients	Less GDM (0% vs. 23.5%) p < 0.05 Less PIH (0% vs. 41%) p < 0.001	Less macrosomia (5.6% vs. 30.4%) p < 0.05
Landsberger *et al.* 2006 [82]	19 patients	19 matched controls for preoperative BMI 19 matched controls for postoperative BMI	More PET (p = 0.05)	NR

Table 17.1 (*cont.*)

Author, year	Study population	Comparison group	Most relevant maternal findings in study population	Most relevant neonatal findings in study population
Wax *et al.* 2008 [69]	38 consecutive pregnancies	76 matched controls	More PET (29% vs. 7.9%) p < 0.05	High PMD in study group (26%) and controls (22%)
Patel *et al.* 2008 [55]	26 consecutive pregnancies	254 controls (1) 188 non-obese (2) 39 obese (3) 27 severely obese	More CS (61.5% vs. 36.2%) p < 0.05	High PMD in study group (27%) and controls (20%) Less macrosomia (0% vs. 18.5%) p < 0.05
Nomura *et al.* 2011 [83]	17 pregnancies <4 yr postoperative conception	13 pregnancies >4 yr postoperative conception	Overall PIH 30% Less anemia (1st trimester) and Fe replacement therapy p < 0.05	Overall SGA 23.3%
Biliopancreatic diversion/duodenal switch				
Friedman *et al.* 1995 [37]	152 consecutive pregnancies	77 preoperative pregnancies	More CS (44% vs. 31.2%) p < 0.05	Perinatal mortality 2.6% in study group and controls
Marceau *et al.* 2004 [62]	251 full-term pregnancies from 783 questionnaires	1236 full-term preoperative pregnancies	High miscarriage rates in study group (26%) and controls (21.6%)	High LBW (27.4%) in study group (NR in controls) Less macrosomia (7.7% vs. 34.8%) p < 0.001
Kral *et al.* 2006 [84]	79 children from primigravid postoperative pregnancies	34 children from primigravid preoperative pregnancies	Less CS (19% vs. 34%) p = 0.08	NR
Mixed bariatric procedures				
Deitel *et al.* 1988 [85]	9 selected pregnancies	274 selected preoperative pregnancies	Less GDM (0% vs. 7%) p < 0.05 Less PET (0 %vs. 12.8%) p < 0.001 Less PIH (0% vs. 26.7%) p < 0.001 Less CS (0% vs. 11.2%) p < 0.01	NR
Sheiner *et al.* 2004 [58]	298 consecutive deliveries	158 912 consecutive deliveries (population registry)	More GDM (9.4% vs. 5.0%) p < 0.001 More CS (25.2% vs. 12.2%) p < 0.001	More macrosomia (9.4% vs. 4.6%) p < 0.001
Weintraub *et al.* 2008 [59]	507 postoperative deliveries	301 preoperative deliveries	Less GDM (11.0% vs. 17.3) p < 0.05 Less PET (1.0% vs. 4.0%) p <0.001 Less PIH (11.2% vs. 23.6%) p < 0.001	Less macrosomia (3.2% vs. 7.6%) p < 0.005
Sheiner *et al.* 2011 [68]	104 pregnancies conceived during the first postoperative year	385 pregnancies conceived after the first postoperative year	Surgical complications 7% No difference in PIH, GDM	Congenital malformations 1.9%

Abbreviations: CS: cesarean section; GDM: gestational diabetes; LBW: low birthweight (<2.5 kg); NR: not reported; PET: pre-eclamptic toxemia; PIH: pregnancy-induced hypertension; PMD: premature delivery (<37 weeks).

Table 17.2 Most common nutritional deficiencies and related maternal and fetal/neonatal complications after bariatric surgery

Nutritional deficiencies	Maternal complications	Fetal/neonatal complications
Iron	Anemia	IUGR
Proteins	Odema, weight loss	IUGR
Vitamin B$_{12}$	Anemia	Pancytopenia, developmental delay
Folic acid	Anemia	Neural tube defects
Vitamin D	Osteomalacia	Hypocalcemia, rickets
Vitamin A		Microphthalmia, retinal damage
Vitamin K	Coagulation disorders	Cerebral hemorrhage, IUD
Calcium	Hypocalcemia	Hypocalcemia

Abbreviations: IUD: intrauterine demise; IUGR: intrauterine growth restriction.

compared pregnancies before and after bariatric surgery in the same women, found lower GWG in those who had undergone surgery [40–42]. However, just like the GWG of obese women without bariatric surgery, weight gain in postoperative pregnancies can vary widely [16]. The time between the surgery and the time of conception probably influences GWG. Dao *et al.* found a large difference in GWG between a group of women who became pregnant early after surgery compared to a late group: 1.81 kg (range –31.75 kg to 20.41 kg) vs. 15.42 kg (range 5.90 kg to 34.02 kg) (p =.002) [43].

Furthermore, the rate of postpartum weight loss in women who had pre-pregnancy bariatric surgery is similar to the rate of postoperative weight loss in non-pregnant women [44]. The effect of pregnancy on long-term weight loss after bariatric surgery has not yet been studied.

During pregnancy, the most commonly reported complication of pre-pregnancy bariatric surgery is internal hernia. In 2008, the literature contained already 11 case reports of intestinal herniations or obstructions in pregnant women with a Roux-en-Y gastric bypass. Recently six more case series were published [45–50]. The reported incidence of intestinal obstruction after Roux-en-Y gastric bypass in a non-pregnant population is up to 5% [51]. Internal hernias in pregnancy are believed to be created by the increased intra-abdominal

pressure. The most common timing for bowel obstruction is mid-pregnancy when the uterus puts pressure on the intestine, at term when the fetal head descends, and in the postpartum period with rapid involution of the uterus [52]. The three specific locations for hernia formation are the transverse mesocolon defect, the Petersen's space, and the jejuno–jejunostomy mesenteric defect. Early recognition and intervention are crucial since the internal hernia could have a tragic outcome including maternal and fetal death [16]. An obstruction could progress to bowel strangulation, anastomotic disruption, dilation of the bypassed stomach, necrosis, and perforation. Immediate recognition of an internal hernia is difficult since patients will present with non-specific abdominal complaints and diagnostic and therapeutic interventions are often delayed. Other reported surgical complications during pregnancy are band migration resulting in vomiting, severe dehydration and electrolyte disturbances, gastric ulceration, and strictures [53–56].

Fetal and infant morbidities

Even though a literature review published in 2007 concluded that the effect of weight loss by bariatric surgery on miscarriage rate was insufficiently studied [57], the most recent reports suggest a decline in miscarriage rates after bariatric surgery [22,23].

Few studies report on perinatal mortality or congenital malformations in pregnancies after bariatric surgery. Theoretically there is an increased risk to develop fatal congenital malformations after bariatric surgery since vitamin and mineral deficiencies are common postoperatively. However, one of the largest studies by Sheiner *et al.* (2004) observed no difference between the postsurgery group consisting of both restrictive and malabsorptive procedures and the obese control group (5% vs. 4%, p = 0.36) [58]. In 2008, the same group published another retrospective study indicating a higher rate of fetal malformations after bariatric surgery than in pregnancies before surgery [59]. This association, however, was no longer significant when controlling for age (OR 1.9; 95% CI: 0.88–4.1; p = 0.089) but on the other hand, the high OR suggests a larger sample size is required to assess more accurately the influence of surgery. Another indication came from two case series published in the late 1980s. Unexpectedly high rates of NTD were observed after bariatric surgery, but the mothers in these cases were all non-adherent with recommended vitamin supplementation [60,61].

Regarding perinatal mortality, the few studies that have reported on this outcome have seen no increase after laparosopic adjustable gastric band, Roux-en-Y gastric bypass, or even biliopancreatic diversion, although the total numbers of outcomes is very small [39]. To make a solid conclusion on any of the less common outcomes such as congenital malformation or perinatal mortality, the study population needs to be large enough. Unfortunately, most knowledge in this area of research is limited to small, often uncontrolled series that lack power to detect uncommon outcomes such as congenital malformations.

Although one study reported an increased incidence of preterm deliveries in pregnancies conceived within the first year after bariatric surgery [55], this observation was not confirmed by others [16,39,40,43].

Babies born from mothers who underwent pre-pregnancy bariatric surgery have a lower mean birthweight. Bariatric surgery also reduces the prevalence of macrosomia and large for gestational age (LGA) babies compared to obese and non-obese controls [16,39]. The incidence of intrauterine growth restriction (IUGR) and small for gestational age (SGA) babies appears to be increased [16]. However, there is some disagreement in the literature. A systematic review found no difference in the incidence of low birthweight after both restrictive and malabsorptive type of surgery, but only four articles included in the review reported on low birthweight [39]. Since there are case series and cohort studies mentioning high incidences of growth restriction, this aspect certainly requires more attention and dedicated studies to evaluate fetal growth and altered fetal body composition in this population [26,37,55,62].

Clinical recommendations

Women experiencing pregnancy after bariatric surgery have important reproductive health care needs. The specific needs of these high-risk pregnancies are best addressed by a multidisciplinary team including obstetricians, surgeons, endocrinologists, pediatricians, psychiatrists, and nutritionists. Recommendations regarding preconceptional, prenatal, and postpartum follow-up are summarized in Table 17.3 [16].

Time between bariatric surgery and conception

All women of reproductive age should be advised on the reproductive repercussions of bariatric surgery before and after the procedure. The American College of Obstetricians and Gynecologists (ACOG) advises to wait at least 12 months before becoming pregnant [63], as this is approximately the mean time period before a stabilization of body weight is achieved. Rapid weight loss (relative starvation phase) may be deleterious to mother and fetus [64]. Moreover, one study has suggested that after a laparoscopic adjustable band, pregnancy shortly postsurgery may predispose to band revisions [65]. Also, a trend towards more miscarriages and preterm delivery was reported in a group conceiving soon after surgery compared to a group conceiving later [43,55]. However, delaying pregnancy too long may also incur risks. The need for intravenous iron therapy or packed red cell transfusion, for instance, was more frequent among women who became pregnant after four years compared to less than four years after Roux-en-Y gastric bypass (30.8% vs. 0%, p = 0.026) [66]. In a non-pregnant population major nutritional complications following bariatric surgery have lasted more than 20 years after surgery [67].

In contrast to studies favoring postponement of conception, two studies found similar obstetrical and neonatal outcomes in women conceiving during vs. after the period of maximal weight loss following bariatric surgery [68,69]. The study of Sheiner *et al.* [68] was, however, biased by the overrepresentation of restrictive procedures in the group pregnant early after the surgery [68].

At this point no conclusive evidence exists to suggest that pregnancy during the first postoperative year is safe. Until more research is performed, clinicians should advise their postoperative patients to delay pregnancy until a stable weight is reached.

Contraception

The recommendation to postpone conception until after the rapid weight loss phase due to bariatric surgery implies that the patients are advised on safe and effective contraceptive use during that period. However, unintended pregnancies after bariatric surgery are frequently reported and are at the highest risk for nutritional deficiencies during the critical period of embryogenesis. Especially among adolescents counseling is important since the pregnancy rates after bariatric surgery are double the rate compared to the general adolescent population (12.8% vs. 6.4%) [70]. Previously obese women with anovulatory cycles not requiring contraception before surgery should be informed that fertility will likely be improved after

Table 17.3 Management recommendations for pregnancy after bariatric surgery

Stage	Management
Preconception	Postoperative detection and correction of nutritional deficiencies.
	Supplementation tailored to type of bariatric procedure performed with specific attention for folic acid, vitamin B_{12}, iron, and fat-soluble vitamins.
	Visits to a nutritionist/lifestyle coach to ensure a healthy and varied diet and healthy level of physical activity.
	Fertility counseling, advice on reliable contraception to delay pregnancy for 12 months after surgery. Non-oral administration of hormonal contraception should be considered.
Prenatal care	Early prenatal consultation to determine baseline nutritional status, followed by regular check-ups.
	Nutritional supplementation tailored to the individual patient and the type of bariatric procedure performed. A standard prenatal vitamin daily is the minimum requirement.
	Serial ultrasound examination with specific attention for correct dating and detection of fetal growth restriction and malformations.
	Advise gestational weight gain within IOM patient guidelines for preconceptional BMI.
	For an adjustable gastric banding procedure active band management is advisable according to gestational weight gain and individual health status.
	Awareness for possible intestinal obstruction during pregnancy.
	Fasting and 2 h postprandial glucose level monitoring instead of glucose challenge test or oral glucose tolerance test to detect gestational diabetes mellitus among pregnant women with gastric bypass.
Postpartum care	Recommend and support breastfeeding.
	Inform pediatrician of maternal bariatric surgery history and possible effects on the newborn.
	Postoperative follow-up and correction of nutritional deficiencies.
	Visits to a nutritionist to ensure a healthy and varied diet, and to guide further weight loss if required.

surgery. They may need to be started on a contraceptive regime for the first time in their lives. As many postoperative patients are still obese, safety concerns may rise regarding the possibility of increased post-surgery risk of venous thromboembolism when using combined oral contraceptives. Summarizing the limited evidence on contraceptive use in this population, Paulen *et al.* found this risk to be largely theoretical [71]. The World Health Organization's *Medical Eligibility Criteria for Contraceptive Use* recommends that obese women planning major surgery involving prolonged immobilization should not use combined oral contraceptives, the combined hormonal patch, or the vaginal ring but no specific recommendations are available for postbariatric women wanting to delay pregnancy [72]. Concerns also exist around the effectiveness of oral contraception in postsurgical patients [71]. Effectiveness could be decreased by the surgically-induced gastrointestinal malabsorption, but also by postoperative complications such as sustained diarrhea and/or vomiting. Second, there could be a potential of fracture risk due to bone loss with the use of depot medroxyprogesterone acetate in a population already losing bone mass as a consequence of

weight loss and nutritional deficiencies [73]. A recent systematic review, however, did not find any evidence for substantial decrease in effectiveness of oral contraceptive, nor of failure rates, or for any other more reliable contraceptive method [71]. This conclusion nevertheless was necessarily based on limited data: one prospective non-comparative study, one descriptive study, one case report, and two pharmacokinetic studies, which reported on contraceptive hormone levels and absorption following a single dose of contraceptive hormones in women after jejuno-ileal bypass. Until more evidence is available, physicians should recommend oral contraception with prudence after bariatric surgery and should consider non-oral administration of hormonal contraception.

Prenatal care

Some aspects of prenatal care in women with a history of bariatric surgery require specific attention.

Ultrasound examination

In view of the increased risk for unplanned and unexpected pregnancies, fetal malformations and growth restriction, we advise a detailed sonographic follow-up for these pregnancies [16]. As many of these women are still obese, the acquisition of high-quality images can be hampered and referral to specific expertise centers is often necessary.

Screening for gestational diabetes

Alternatives for the glucose challenge test or the oral glucose tolerance test are suggested by the American Diabetes Association (ADA) since these tests to detect gestational diabetes can cause dumping symptoms in a patient with malabsorptive type of surgery. One proposed alternative is home glucose monitoring (fasting and two-hour postprandial blood sugar) for approximately one week during the 24th to 28th weeks of gestation [74,75].

Gestational weight gain

There is no evidence to support any specific GWG recommendations for women pregnant following bariatric surgery, but it may be considered advisable for the patient to gain weight within the range recommended for all women by the US Institute of Medicine. The recommendations depend on the woman's preconception BMI. In case of a normal preconception weight, she should gain 11.5 to 16 kg (25 to 35 lbs). In case of preconceptional overweight or obesity, the recommended ranges are respectively 7.0 to 11.5 kg (15 to 25 lbs) and 5.0 to 9.0 kg (11 to 20 lbs) [76]. In patients with a laparoscopic adjustable gastric band, active band management may reduce adverse outcomes. This includes the removal of all band fluid as early as possible in the pregnancy to minimize the effect on emesis. After 14 weeks gestation or later, fluid can be inserted again in cases of excessive GWG. To minimize the impact of delivery on the gastric band and vice versa, the fluid is removed again at 36 weeks of gestation [16].

Nutritional advice

Ideally a woman with bariatric surgery starts off with a good nutritional status preconceptionally, meaning a healthy varied diet with or without necessary supplementation. During pregnancy prevention of nutritional deficiencies remains an indisputable priority. No controlled trials exist to determine the type of supplements and the dosages to be prescribed during pregnancy after bariatric surgery, so no consensus regarding nutritional management of pregnant women after bariatric surgery exists. A pregnancy-specific multivitamin supplement is a minimal recommendation for pregnant women with bariatric surgery. However, one does not know the proportion absorbed of each constituent, especially in patients with a malabsorptive type of surgery. Therefore, it is reasonable to assess nutritional status every trimester and adapt a prescription to the patient's plasma micronutrient profile. In case of a proven deficiency, a monthly check-up for overdoses and to adapt doses is required. Overdoses of vitamin A need to be avoided since an excess is associated with birth defects. When prescribing a supplement, the pharmaceutical formulation needs to be taken into consideration. A patient with a gastric band could prefer a tablet, syrup, or drinkable solution, or even an intramuscular injection, rather than a capsule, since capsules can cause dysphagia at the level of the band. A dose of 400 μg folate daily is recommended as for all reproductive-age women. Prescribing a higher dose could be considered in cases where the woman after bariatric surgery is still obese, since maternal obesity is a risk factor for malformations such as NTD or cleft palate [77]. Prescribing supplements needs to be accompanied by an explanation of the relationship between gastric bypass surgery, nutrient deficiencies, and associated consequences. Although not supported by scientific evidence, we believe that such an explanation may contribute to the women's compliance with daily multivitamin consumption during pregnancy especially in view of the fact that less than 60% of postoperative, non-pregnant bariatric surgery patients continue to take multivitamin supplements for a prolonged period of time [78].

Concluding remarks

Bariatric surgery is the most reliable way to sustain weight loss in the morbidly obese. In women of reproductive age, fertility is often enhanced after bariatric surgery. Pregnancy after surgery improves many pregnancy outcomes but adds new risks related to nutritional deficiencies and surgical complications, thus requiring a specialized multidisciplinary approach. As most clinical recommendations are largely based on limited or inconsistent scientific evidence or consensus expert opinion, further large prospective trials and registries are urgently needed.

References

1. Picot J, Jones J, Colquitt J L, *et al.* The clinical effectiveness and cost-effectiveness of bariatric

(weight loss) surgery for obesity: a systematic review and economic evaluation. *Health Technol Assess* 2009;**13**(41):1–190.

2. Colquitt J L, Picot J, Loveman E, *et al.* Surgery for obesity. *Cochrane Database Syst Rev* 2009;**2**:CD003641.

3. Anon. NIH conference. Gastrointestinal surgery for severe obesity. Consensus Development Conference Panel. *Ann Intern Med* 1991;**115**:956–61.

4. World Health Organization. *Overweight and Obesity. Fact sheet No.311.* (Geneva: World Health Organization, 2006).

5. Samuel I, Mason E E, Renquist K E, *et al.* Bariatric surgery trends: an 18-year report from the International Bariatric Surgery Registry. *Am J Surg* 2006;**192**(5):657–62.

6. Buchwald H & Oien D M. Metabolic/bariatric surgery worldwide 2008. *Obes Surg* 2009;**19**(12):1605–11.

7. Schilling P L, Davis M M, Albanese C T, *et al.* National trends in adolescent bariatric surgical procedures and implications for surgical centers of excellence. *J Am Coll Surg* 2008;**206**(1):1–12.

8. Livingston E H. Obesity and its surgical management. *Am J Surg.* 2002;**184**(2):103–13.

9. Sjostrom L, Narbro K, Sjostrom C D, *et al.* Effects of bariatric surgery on mortality in Swedish obese subjects. *N Engl J Med* 2007;**357**(8):741–52.

10. Buchwald H, Avidor Y, Braunwald E, *et al.* Bariatric surgery: a systematic review and meta-analysis. *JAMA* 2004;**292**(14):1724–37.

11. Buchwald H. Consensus conference statement. Bariatric surgery for morbid obesity: health implications for patients, health professionals, and third-party payers. *Surg Obes Relat Dis* 2005;**1**(3):371–81.

12. Woodard C B. Pregnancy following bariatric surgery. *J Perinat Neonatal Nurs* 2004;**18**(4):329–40.

13. Shankar P, Boylan M & Sriram K. Micronutrient deficiencies after bariatric surgery. *Nutrition* 2010;**26**(11/12):1031–7.

14. Stocker D J. Management of the bariatric surgery patient. *Endocrinol Metab Clin North Am* 2003;**32**(2):437–57.

15. Avinoah E, Ovnat A & Charuzi I. Nutritional status seven years after Roux-en-Y gastric bypass surgery. *Surgery* 1992;**111**(2):137–42.

16. Guelinckx I, Devlieger R & Vansant G. Reproductive outcome after bariatric surgery: a critical review. *Hum Reprod Update* 2009;**15**(2):189–201.

17. Poitou Bernert C, Ciangura C, Coupaye M, *et al.* Nutritional deficiency after gastric bypass: diagnosis, prevention and treatment. *Diabetes Metab* 2007;**33**(1):13–24.

18. Apovian C M, Baker C, Ludwig D S, *et al.* Best practice guidelines in pediatric/adolescent weight loss surgery. *Obes Res* 2005;**13**(2):274–82.

19. Colles S L, Dixon J B & O'Brien P E. Hunger control and regular physical activity facilitate weight loss after laparoscopic adjustable gastric banding. *Obes Surg* 2008;**18**(7):833–40.

20. Hwang K O, Childs J H, Goodrick G K, *et al.* Explanations for unsuccessful weight loss among bariatric surgery candidates. *Obes Surg* 2009;**19**(10):1377–83.

21. Tucker O N, Szomstein S & Rosenthal R J. Nutritional consequences of weight-loss surgery. *Med Clin North Am* 2007;**91**(3):499–514.

22. Merhi Z O. Impact of bariatric surgery on female reproduction. *Fertil Steril* 2009;**92**(5):1501–8.

23. Shah D K & Ginsburg E S. Bariatric surgery and fertility. *Curr Opin Obstet Gynecol* 2010;**22**(3):248–54.

24. Teitelman M, Grotegut C A, Williams N N, *et al.* The impact of bariatric surgery on menstrual patterns. *Obes Surg* 2006;**16**(11):1457–63.

25. Cools M, Duval E L & Jespers A. Adverse neonatal outcome after maternal biliopancreatic diversion operation: report of nine cases. *Eur J Pediatr* 2006;**165**(3):199–202.

26. Adami G F, Friedman D, Cuneo S, *et al.* Intravenous nutritional support in pregnancy. Experience following biliopancreatic diversion. *Clin Nutr* 1992;**11**(2):106–9.

27. Granstrom L, & Backman L. Fetal growth retardation after gastric banding. *Acta Obstet Gynecol Scand* 1990;**69**(6):533–6.

28. Gurewitsch E D, Smith-Levitin M & Mack J. Pregnancy following gastric bypass surgery for morbid obesity. *Obstet Gynecol* 1996;**88**(4 Pt 2):658–61.

29. Martens W S, 2nd, Martin L F & Berlin C M, Jr. Failure of a nursing infant to thrive after the mother's gastric bypass for morbid obesity. *Pediatrics* 1990;**86**(5):777–8.

30. Weissman A, Hagay Z, Schachter M, *et al.* Severe maternal and fetal electrolyte imbalance in pregnancy after gastric surgery for morbid obesity. A case report. *J Reprod Med* 1995;**40**(11):813–16.

31. Eerdekens A, Debeer A, Van Hoey G, *et al.* Maternal bariatric surgery: adverse outcomes in neonates. *Eur J Pediatr* 2009;**169**(2):191–6.

32. Van Mieghem T, Van Schoubroeck D, Depiere M, *et al.* Fetal cerebral hemorrhage due to vitamin K deficiency after complicated bariatric surgery. *Obstet Gynecol* 2008;**112**:434–6.

33. Campbell C D, Ganesh J & Ficicioglu C. Two newborns with nutritional vitamin B12 deficiency: challenges in newborn screening for vitamin B12 deficiency. *Haematologica* 2005;**90**(12 Suppl):45.

34. Celiker M Y & Chawla A. Congenital B12 deficiency following maternal gastric bypass. *J Perinatol* 2009;**29**(9):640–2.

35. Grange D K & Finlay J L. Nutritional vitamin B12 deficiency in a breastfed infant following maternal gastric bypass. *Pediatr Hematol Oncol* 1994;**11**(3):311–18.

36. Wardinsky T D, Montes R G, Friederich R L, *et al.* Vitamin B12 deficiency associated with low breast-milk vitamin B12 concentration in an infant following maternal gastric bypass surgery. *Arch Pediatr Adolesc Med* 1995;**149**(11):1281–4.

37. Friedman D, Cuneo S, Valenzano M, *et al.* Pregnancies in an 18-year follow-up after biliopancreatic diversion. *Obes Surg* 1995;**5**(3):308–13.

38. Bennett W L, Gilson M M, Jamshidi R, *et al.* Impact of bariatric surgery on hypertensive disorders in pregnancy: retrospective analysis of insurance claims data. *BMJ* 2010;**340**:c1662.

39. Maggard M A, Yermilov I, Li Z, *et al.* Pregnancy and fertility following bariatric surgery: a systematic review. *JAMA* 2008;**300**(19):2286–96.

40. Dixon J B, Dixon M E & O'Brien P E. Birth outcomes in obese women after laparoscopic adjustable gastric banding. *Obstet Gynecol* 2005;**106**(5 Pt 1):965–72.

41. Ducarme G, Revaux A, Rodrigues A, *et al.* Obstetric outcome following laparoscopic adjustable gastric banding. *Int J Gynaecol Obstet* 2007;**98**(3):244–7.

42. Wittgrove A C, Jester L, Wittgrove P, *et al.* Pregnancy following gastric bypass for morbid obesity. *Obes Surg* 1998;**8**(4):461–4; discussion 5–6.

43. Dao T, Kuhn J, Ehmer D, *et al.* Pregnancy outcomes after gastric-bypass surgery. *Am J Surg* 2006;**192**(6):762–6.

44. Printen K J & Scott D. Pregnancy following gastric bypass for the treatment of morbid obesity. *Am Surg* 1982;**48**(8):363–5.

45. Efthimiou E, Stein L, Court O, *et al.* Internal hernia after gastric bypass surgery during middle trimester pregnancy resulting in fetal loss: risk of internal hernia never ends. *Surg Obes Relat Dis* 2009;**5**(3):378–80.

46. Torres-Villalobos G M, Kellogg T A, Leslie D B, *et al.* Small bowel obstruction and internal hernias during pregnancy after gastric bypass surgery. *Obes Surg* 2009;**19**(7):944–50.

47. Gagne D J, DeVoogd K, Rutkoski J D, *et al.* Laparoscopic repair of internal hernia during pregnancy after Roux-en-Y gastric bypass. *Surg Obes Relat Dis* 2010;**6**(1):88–92.

48. Gazzalle A, Braun D, Cavazzola L T, *et al.* Late intestinal obstruction due to an intestinal volvulus in a pregnant patient with a previous Roux-en-Y gastric bypass. *Obes Surg* 2010;**20**(12):1740–2.

49. Naef M, Mouton W G & Wagner H E. Small-bowel volvulus in late pregnancy due to internal hernia after laparoscopic Roux-en-Y gastric bypass. *Obes Surg* 2010;**20**(12):1737–9.

50. Rosenkrantz A B, Kurian M & Kim D. MRI appearance of internal hernia following Roux-en-Y gastric bypass surgery in the pregnant patient. *Clin Radiol* 2010;**65**(3):246–9.

51. Wax J R, Wolff R, Cobean R, *et al.* Intussusception complicating pregnancy following laparoscopic Roux-en-Y gastric bypass. *Obes Surg* 2007;**17**(7):977–9.

52. Kakarla N, Dailey C, Marino T, *et al.* Pregnancy after gastric bypass surgery and internal hernia formation. *Obstet Gynecol* 2005;**105**(5 Pt 2):1195–8.

53. Weiss HG, Nehoda H, Labeck B, *et al.* Pregnancies after adjustable gastric banding. *Obes Surg* 2001;**11**(3):303–6.

54. Gaudry P, Mognol P, Fortin A, *et al.* Reflection on one case of acute peritonitis due to adjustable gastric banding during pregnancy. *Gynecol Obstet Fertil* 2006;**34**(5):407–9.

55. Patel J A, Patel N A, Thomas R L, *et al.* Pregnancy outcomes after laparoscopic Roux-en-Y gastric bypass. *Surg Obes Relat Dis* 2008;**4**(1):39–45.

56. Skull A J, Slater G H, Duncombe J E, *et al.* Laparoscopic adjustable banding in pregnancy: safety, patient tolerance and effect on obesity-related pregnancy outcomes. *Obes Surg* 2004;**14**(2):230–5.

57. Merhi Z O & Pal L. Effect of weight loss by bariatric surgery on the risk of miscarriage. *Gynecol Obstet Invest* 2007;**64**(4):224–7.

58. Sheiner E, Levy A, Silverberg D, *et al.* Pregnancy after bariatric surgery is not associated with adverse perinatal outcome. *Am J Obstet Gynecol* 2004;**190**(5):1335–40.

59. Weintraub A Y, Levy A, Levi I, *et al.* Effect of bariatric surgery on pregnancy outcome. *Int J Gynaecol Obstet* 2008;**103**(3):246–51.

60. Haddow J E, Hill LE, Kloza E M, *et al.* Neural tube defects after gastric bypass. *Lancet* 1986;**1**(8493):1330.

61. Martin L, Chavez G F, Adams M J, Jr., *et al.* Gastric bypass surgery as maternal risk factor for neural tube defects. *Lancet* 1988;**1**(8586):640–1.

62. Marceau P, Kaufman D, Biron S, *et al.* Outcome of pregnancies after biliopancreatic diversion. *Obes Surg* 2004;**14**(3):318–24.

63. American College of Obstetricians and Gynecologists. ACOG practice bulletin no. 105: bariatric surgery and pregnancy. *Obstet Gynecol* 2009;**113**(6):1405–12.

64. Painter R C, Roseboom T J & Bleker O P. Prenatal exposure to the Dutch famine and disease in later life: an overview. *Reprod Toxicol* 2005;**20**(3):345–52.

65. Haward R N, Brown W A & O'Brien P E. Does pregnancy increase the need for revisional surgery after laparoscopic adjustable gastric banding? *Obes Surg* 2011;**21**(9):1362–9.

66. Nomura R M, Dias M C, Igai A M, *et al.* Anemia during pregnancy after silastic ring Roux-en-Y gastric bypass: influence of time to conception. *Obes Surg* 2011;**21**(4):479–84.

67. Bal B S, Finelli F C & Koch T R. Origins of and recognition of micronutrient deficiencies after gastric bypass surgery. *Curr Diab Rep* 2011;**11**(2):136–41.

68. Sheiner E, Edri A, Balaban E, *et al.* Pregnancy outcome of patients who conceive during or after the first year following bariatric surgery. *Am J Obstet Gynecol* 2011;**204**(1):50e1–6.

69. Wax J R, Cartin A, Wolff R, *et al.* Pregnancy following gastric bypass for morbid obesity: effect of surgery-to-conception interval on maternal and neonatal outcomes. *Obes Surg* 2008;**18**(12):1517–21.

70. Roehrig H R, Xanthakos S A, Sweeney J, *et al.* Pregnancy after gastric bypass surgery in adolescents. *Obes Surg* 2007;**17**(7):873–7.

71. Paulen M E, Zapata L B, Cansino C, *et al.* Contraceptive use among women with a history of bariatric surgery: a systematic review. *Contraception* 2010;**82**(1):86–94.

72. World Health Organization. *Medical Eligibility for Contraceptive Use: 2008 Update.* (Geneva: World Health Organization, 2008). www.who.int/reproductivehealth/topics/family_planning/updates/en/ [Accessed January 11, 2012].

73. Coates P S, Fernstrom J D, Fernstrom M H, *et al.* Gastric bypass surgery for morbid obesity leads to an increase in bone turnover and a decrease in bone mass. *J Clin Endocrinol Metab* 2004;**89**(3):1061–5.

74. Wax J R, Heersink D, Pinette M G, *et al.* Symptomatic hypoglycemia complicating pregnancy following Roux-en-Y gastric bypass surgery. *Obes Surg* 2007;**17**(5):698–700.

75. American Diabetes Association. Gestational diabetes mellitus. Practice guideline. *Diabetes Care* 2004;**27**(Suppl 1):s88–90.

76. Institute of Medicine. *Weight Gain During Pregnancy: Reexamining the Guidelines.* (Washington, DC: The National Academies Press, 2009).

77. Centers for Disease Control and Prevention. CDC Grand Rounds: additional opportunities to prevent neural tube defects with folic acid fortification. *MMWR Morb Mortal Wkly Rep* 2010;**59**(31):980–4.

78. Dixon J B, Dixon M E & O'Brien P E. Elevated homocysteine levels with weight loss after Lap-Band surgery: higher folate and vitamin B12 levels required to maintain homocysteine level. *Int J Obes Relat Metab Disord* 2001;**25**(2):219–27.

79. Bar-Zohar D, Azem F, Klausner J, & Abu-Abeid S. Pregnancy after laparoscopic adjustable gastric banding: perinatal outcome is favorable also for women with relatively high gestational weight gain. *Surg Endosc* 2006;**20**(10):1580–3.

80. Bilenka B, Ben-Shlomo I, Cozacov C, Gold C H, & Zohar S. Fertility, miscarriage and pregnancy after vertical banded gastroplasty operation for morbid obesity. *Acta Obstet Gynecol Scand* 1995;**74**(1):42–4.

81. Richards D S, Miller D K, & Goodman G N. Pregnancy after gastric bypass for morbid obesity. *J Reprod Med* 1987;**32**(3):172–6.

82. Landsberger E, Ankrah Y, Segal-Isaacson CJ, *et al.* Should severely obese women complete childbearing prior to bariatric surgery? *Am J Obstet Gynecol* 2006;**195**:S93.

83. Nomura R M, Dias M C, Igai A M, Paiva L V & Zugaib M. Anemia during pregnancy after silastic ring Roux-en-Y gastric bypass: influence of time to conception. *Obes Surg* 2011;**21**(4):479–84.

84. Kral J G, Biron S, Simard S, *et al.* Large maternal weight loss from obesity surgery prevents transmission of obesity to children who were followed for 2 to 18 years. *Pediatrics* 2006;**118**(6):e1644–9.

85. Deitel M, Stone E, Kassam H A, Wilk E J & Sutherland D J. Gynecologic–obstetric changes after loss of massive excess weight following bariatric surgery. *J Am Coll Nutr* 1988;**7**(2):147–53.

Chapter 18

Clinical management of obesity in pregnancy

Carolyn Chiswick and Fiona C. Denison

Introduction

Obesity is now the commonest antenatal co-morbidity. With one in five of the antenatal population in both the US and the UK being obese, maternal obesity will inevitably be encountered by all obstetricians, from those with a special interest in high-risk obstetrics, to those covering the delivery suite out of hours. Therefore it is essential that all clinicians have the knowledge and expertise to manage obese women during pregnancy and labor.

As reviewed in Chapter 4 pregnant women who are obese are at greater risk of a wide range of pregnancy complications from pre-pregnancy, throughout the antenatal period, intrapartum, and postnatally (Table 18.1). The offspring of obese mothers are also at greater risk of perinatal morbidity and long-term health problems. There are also technical challenges such as the availability of appropriate equipment and moving and handling problems.

This chapter aims to provide a summary of the clinical management of obesity in pregnancy, based on evidence where it exists, and highlighting areas where further research is needed.

Pre-pregnancy care

Primary care services have a responsibility to ensure that all women of childbearing age are aware of the excess risks associated with obesity in pregnancy [1]. Any visit to a health care provider by a young woman who is overweight should be viewed as an opportunity to advise about the benefits of weight loss and strategies to achieve this [2]. Overweight women planning a pregnancy should be given the opportunity and encouragement to optimize their pre-pregnancy weight. Losing 5% to 10% of their body weight prior

Table 18.1 Risks of obesity in pregnancy

Problem	Level of increased risk
Miscarriage [99]	One- to three-fold
Fetal abnormality (spina bifida, heart defect, omphalocele) [100]	Two- to four-fold
Iatrogenic preterm birth [101]	One-and-a-half- to two-fold
Pre-eclampsia [102]	Two-fold
Venous thromboembolism [103]	Three- to four-fold
Gestational diabetes [61,71]	Four-fold
Induction of labor [61,71]	Two-fold
Cesarean section [61,71]	Two-fold
Postpartum hemorrhage [61]	One- to two-fold
Infection (wound, urinary tract, genital tract) [61]	Two-fold
Stillbirth [104]	One- to five-fold
Maternal death [73]	Increased

to conception has significant health benefits [3,4]. For example, minimal weight loss in women with polycystic ovarian syndrome and anovulation can result in ovulation induction, restoration of fertility, and spontaneous conception. Rapid weight loss immediately prior to pregnancy should not be encouraged as it is associated with poorer outcomes [2].

In women seeking a pregnancy it is also important to optimize treatment of common obesity co-morbidities, such as hypertension and diabetes [1]. Current medications should be reviewed and adjusted to suit pregnancy, e.g., potential teratogens, such as sulphonylureas and angiotensin converting enzyme inhibitors [5], should be discontinued and substituted with

Maternal Obesity, ed. Matthew W. Gillman and Lucilla Poston. Published by Cambridge University Press. © Cambridge University Press 2012.

alternatives with an established safety profile during pregnancy [6].

Folic acid

As reviewed in Chapters 6 and 17, obese women are at greater risk of having a fetus affected with a neural tube defect (NTD). A meta-analysis of 12 observational cohort studies reported an unadjusted odds ratio for a NTD-affected pregnancy rising from 1.22 (95% CI: 0.99–1.49) in overweight women to 1.70 (95% CI: 1.34–2.15) and 3.11 (95% CI: 1.75–5.46) in obese, and severely obese women compared with normal weight women [7]. Various mechanisms have been proposed including undiagnosed type 2 diabetes at conception [8], lower serum folate levels in obese women [9], and decreased ultrasound detection of anomalies in obese women [10] leading to the continuation of pregnancies that would otherwise have been terminated.

The benefits of preconceptual folic acid in reducing the risk of NTD are well established in the general pregnancy population [11], thus all women trying to conceive are encouraged to take periconceptual folic acid at the standard 400 µg dose [12]. In those women identified as being at higher risk, e.g., women with a previously affected pregnancy, a higher dose of folate supplementation reduces the risk of having a fetus affected by an NTD in a subsequent pregnancy [13]. However, the protective effects of periconceptual folic acid do not appear to benefit obese women. A Canadian study demonstrated no benefit, in terms of reduction in incidence of NTD, following introduction of flour fortification with folic acid in women with increased body mass index (BMI) [14]. Whether higher dose supplementation of folic acid effects a reduction in risk of NTD in obese women remains to be established in clinical trials. Despite this lack of evidence, the Royal College of Obstetricians and Gynaecologists (RCOG) in the UK recommends obese women should receive higher dose supplementation (Centre for Maternal and Child Enquiries (CMACE)/ RCOG Joint Guideline) [15] and the American College of Obstetricians and Gynecologists (ACOG) advises this should be considered [16].

Vitamin D

High pre-pregnancy BMI is associated with low serum vitamin D levels during pregnancy and as reviewed in Chapter 17 women with a BMI >30kg/m^2 are at increased risk of vitamin D deficiency compared to healthy weight controls [17]. The main source of vitamin D is synthesis on skin exposure to sunlight. In countries where there is limited sunlight of appropriate wavelength, for example the UK, skin exposure alone may not be sufficient to achieve optimal vitamin D status for pregnancy [18]. The UK RCOG recommends vitamin D supplementation of 10 µg/400 IU per day for women with a BMI >30kg/m^2 (CEMACE/RCOG joint guideline). However, there are no randomized clinical trials (RCTs) to support these recommendations, and limited evidence regarding the safety of higher dose antenatal vitamin D regimes [19].

Antenatal care

Obese women who are pregnant are recognized as a high-risk group by both the ACOG and RCOG and should therefore be referred for appropriate antenatal care [1]. With the worldwide prevalence of obesity so high, and expected to continue to rise, dedicated clinics are unlikely to be feasible for the majority of units and so care should be integrated into all antenatal clinics with clear guidance available.

Both the ACOG in the USA [16] and the National Institute for Health and Clinical Excellence (NICE) in the UK recommend all women have their weight and height accurately measured and recorded at booking, and BMI calculated in order to identify those at risk. Self-reported height is often overestimated and weight underestimated, particularly in the obese [20]. Appropriate equipment must be available to record these measurements accurately, including weighing scales capable of accurate measurement in heavier women. Weighing throughout pregnancy is controversial and discussed further below. However, for women with a BMI >35 kg/m^2, weight should always be remeasured and BMI recalculated in the third trimester to allow planning for any special equipment required at delivery.

While preconceptual counseling for women with obesity is the ideal scenario, most women will present for the first time already pregnant. A full and frank discussion must take place with the woman to inform her of the potential risks and the management strategies for her pregnancy [1]. If discussion takes place in a sensitive way it may encourage her to engage positively with the services available. A multidisciplinary team approach to care is helpful with input from obstetricians, obstetric anesthetists, endocrinologists, dieticians, and midwives.

Weight management in obese pregnancies and recommendations for gestational weight gain

All obese women should receive a dietary assessment and nutritional counseling. Input from a dietician can be invaluable in this regard. There is some evidence that significant weight loss during pregnancy in obese women may be harmful to the fetus. A recent retrospective cohort study demonstrated that the benefits of gestational weight loss in reducing the risk of pre-eclampsia and non-elective cesarean section were outweighed by increased risk of preterm birth and small for gestational age (SGA) in all but women with Class III obesity (defined as a BMI ≥40kg/m²) [21]. The recent UK NICE guidelines [4] therefore emphasize that pregnancy is not the time to commence a weight loss program and that the emphasis should be on weight maintenance, rather than weight loss.

It is debated whether women need to be routinely weighed (or not) during pregnancy with clinical practice varying widely. In the UK, NICE do not advocate repeated weighing of women throughout pregnancy, citing insufficient evidence of any benefit. Routine weighing has a very low positive predictive power to detect SGA, and indeed may cause psychological distress [22,23]. However, as reviewed in Chapter 19, repeated weighing is standard practice throughout pregnancy in the USA, with the Institute of Medicine (IOM) recently revising their guidance on recommendations for weight gain in pregnancy, adding more specific guidelines for those who are obese at booking (see Table 18.2) [24]. These guidelines for GWG are not universally accepted, with research from a large Swedish cohort recommending a smaller weight gain in all BMI categories compared to the IOM (see Table 18.2) [25]. Furthermore, as discussed in Chapter 19 neither of these guidelines provides recommendations for those with BMI >40 kg/m², and an increasing number of women fall into this category. Despite several similar studies, many of which informed the new IOM guidelines, a universally accepted consensus about optimal weight gain during pregnancy remains to be established, particularly among women with a BMI >40 kg/m². It must also be borne in mind that recommendations for one particular population may not be applicable to another, for example, with a different ethnic mix.

Table 18.2 Institute of Medicine recommendations for weight gain during pregnancy, by pre-pregnancy BMI

Pre-pregnancy BMI	BMI, kg/m² (WHO)	Total weight gain range, kg/lbs[a]
Underweight	<18.5	12.5–18.0/28–40
Normal weight	18.5–24.9	11.5–16.0/25–35
Overweight	25.0–29.9	7.0–11.5/15–25
Obese (includes all classes)	≥30.0	5.0–9.0/11–20

[a] *Weight Gain During Pregnancy: Reexamining the Guidelines.* 2009. Institute of Medicine [24].

Ever since the release of the original IOM guidelines in 1990, studies have shown that weight gain within the recommended ranges has the potential to influence pregnancy outcome [26]. An early study showed that gaining weight within the IOM guidelines reduced the risk of adverse neonatal and delivery outcomes by the same amount as when using population-specific weight gain ranges [27]. A meta-analysis of 150 studies concluded that weight gain below these ranges was associated with a significant increase in the risk of low birthweight (<2500 g), SGA infants (birthweight < 10th percentile for their gestational age), a failure to initiate breastfeeding, and an increase in spontaneous preterm birth [28]. Gaining more weight than recommended led to a higher prevalence of large for gestational age (LGA) babies (birthweight > 90th percentile for their gestational age), a three-fold increase in the risk of macrosomia (birthweight >4000 g) [29], an increased risk of future childhood obesity [30], and complications for the mother such as cesarean delivery and postpartum weight retention (PPWR) [31,32]. A retrospective cohort study of over 20 000 births found that gestational weight gain above the guidelines was associated with an increased risk of seizure, hypoglycemia, polycythemia, meconium aspiration syndrome, and LGA infants [33]. Despite these findings, only 30% to 40% of women achieve weight gain within the recommended ranges [30,34]. Most women exceed the guidelines – 40% to 50% of women compared to 20% to 25% who have inadequate weight gain [33], and overweight/obese women are more likely to exceed guidelines than normal/underweight women [35]. This may be because a large proportion of women are receiving inaccurate weight gain guidance or none at all [36]. There is therefore a need to educate service providers on optimal weight gain during pregnancy, and provide interventions to assist women to reach their target weight gain.

A recent Cochrane review (confirmed as being up to date in 2010) concluded that regular aerobic exercise during pregnancy appears to improve physical fitness [37]. Women should therefore be encouraged by their health care provider to participate in regular moderate exercise throughout their pregnancy and be reassured that this is not harmful (www.rcog.org.uk/womens-health/clinical-guidance/exercise-pregnancy) [4,38]. Whether the benefits of exercise extend to improvements in other maternal and fetal outcomes, for example a reduction in risk of pre-eclampsia, gestational diabetes, or decreased fetal fat mass is, however, less clear. Although some studies suggest wider health benefits of exercise [39,40], the same Cochrane review concluded that current evidence is insufficient to infer important risks or benefits for the mother or baby [37]. The optimal combination of exercise with/without other lifestyle interventions in overweight or obese pregnant women to achieve maximal health benefit remains to be established and is currently the subject of a number of multicenter clinical trials. The reader is referred to Chapters 14, 15, and 16, which review interventional strategies.

Ultrasound and anomaly screening

Obstetric ultrasound is used widely in the developed world for pregnancy dating, detection of higher order pregnancies and fetal anomaly, and estimation of fetal growth. Obese women are more likely to book late, have a fetus affected with a congenital abnormality [7], and also have a macrosomic baby [41]. Thus ultrasound is an invaluable tool in the care of obese women in pregnancy. However, by absorbing the associated energy, adipose tissue can significantly attenuate the ultrasound signal. The high-frequency, high-resolution signal used for detection of fetal anomaly is significantly absorbed at a lesser depth, sacrificing image quality. Scans performed on women with a BMI greater than the 90th centile during the second and third trimester have a 14.5% reduction in visualization of organs compared to lean women [42]. It is important to inform women of the reduced sensitivity of ultrasound as a screening tool for fetal anomaly in the presence of obesity and that repeat visits are more likely to be required to obtain all the necessary images [43]. Magnetic resonance imaging (MRI) is not affected by maternal obesity and may be a helpful adjunct if there is suspicion of an anomaly on ultrasound.

Screening for aneuploidy

There are numerous screening tests for aneuploidy involving either blood tests alone or in combination with ultrasound measurement of nuchal translucency. Both of these are subject to reduced accuracy in obese women. Nuchal translucency imaging, which requires specialist training, can be difficult to perform and its validity as a screening tool relies on accuracy of measurement. Maternal obesity is associated with a longer time to perform the first-trimester ultrasound examination for aneuploidy risk assessment, increased need for transvaginal ultrasound examination for nuchal translucency visualization, and a lower likelihood of obtaining an adequate nasal bone image [44]. Furthermore, Rode *et al.* report that compared to non-obese women, obese women are at increased risk of having a nuchal translucency >95th centile (1.7 (95% CI: 1.2–2.6) in otherwise healthy fetuses [45]. This has the potential to affect screening performance and cause unnecessary anxiety in women.

Serum markers used for the detection of aneuploidy include pregnancy-associated plasma protein A (PAPP-A), free beta human chorionic gonadotropin (hCG), and alphafetoprotein (aFP). These are fetally or placentally derived and subject to dilution in larger women with increased blood volumes [46]. Maternal weight is routinely incorporated into risk calculations and must therefore be recorded accurately on the sample request card.

Growth scans

Estimation of fetal size is an important part of antenatal care for all women. The NICE guidelines in the UK recommend serial measurement of symphysiofundal height in centimeters with a tape measure. Plotting these measurements on growth charts may help identify the small or large for dates baby. However, these simple, non-invasive measurements in obese women can be unreliable and indeed sometimes impossible. The alternative is to perform serial ultrasound scans to measure growth but these too may be inaccurate, particularly in women with a high BMI [47,48].

Diabetes

Obesity is a well-recognised risk factor for gestational diabetes mellitus and pre-gestational diabetes is more prevalent in obese women. There is no doubt that appropriate treatment of diabetes in pregnancy significantly

Table 18.3 Diagnostic criteria for the 75 g oral glucose tolerance test (OGTT)

Time	WHO [54] Plasma glucose	HAPO [106] Plasma glucose	ADA [53] Plasma glucose
Fasting	≥7.0 mmol/l	>5.1 mmol/l	>5.1 mmol/l
2 hours	>7.8 mmol/l	>8.5 mmol/l	>8.5 mmol/l

reduces the risk of serious adverse perinatal outcome (e.g., death, shoulder dystocia, bone fracture, nerve palsy) [49].

There is no international consensus on when, how, and whom to screen for gestational diabetes. Both NICE [50] in the UK and ACOG [51] in the USA recommend screening for gestational diabetes mellitus (GDM) at 24 to 28 weeks gestation in women with a BMI >30 kg/m². Consideration may be given to screening earlier in pregnancy if a woman has had GDM in a previous pregnancy. Diagnostic criteria vary around the world with recommendations from the Hyperglycemia and Adverse Pregnancy Outcomes (HAPO) study [52] being the same as the American Diabetes Association (ADA) [53] but different from the World Health Organization (WHO) [54]. Even within the UK there is discordance in practice. The NICE guideline is used in England, which adopts the WHO criteria, while in Scotland, the Scottish Intercollegiate Guideline Network (SIGN; www.sign.ac.uk) [55] has adopted the HAPO recommendations. Table 18.3 summarizes these various criteria.

Once a diagnosis has been made, tight glycemic control must be achieved. Treatment with dietary modification may be sufficient but obese women are more likely to need insulin therapy than lean women [56]. Following the Metformin in Gestational Diabetes (MIG) trial [57], the oral hypoglycemic agent metformin is now widely used as a first-line treatment for gestational diabetes. This study demonstrated it to be effective, safe, and preferable to patients. The use of metformin is now endorsed by NICE in the UK [50].

The immediate aim of therapy is to prevent fetal macrosomia and consequent birth trauma. Diagnosis also allows identification of women who require post-pregnancy follow up to try to modify risk for development of diabetes and cardiovascular disease in later life. The children of these women may also be followed up to assess the impact of maternal hyperglycemia on their long-term risk of obesity and altered glucose metabolism. Given the increasing population of obese women, the newer guidance for screening and stricter diagnostic criteria will clearly identify greater numbers of women with gestational diabetes. This will inevitably have cost implications. However, if it presents the opportunity to prevent a significant burden of disease in later life in both mothers and their offspring, then it may prove cost-effective.

Hypertension

It has long been recognized that hypertensive disorders are more prevalent in the obese population [58]. During pregnancy, this same elevated risk applies. Obese women are at greater risk of having pre-existing hypertension and of developing pregnancy-induced hypertensive disorders, including pre-eclampsia [25,59–61].

Routine antenatal care should include a measurement of blood pressure at the initial and every subsequent visit. This in itself can be difficult and is subject to error in obese women. An appropriate size of cuff must be used to achieve an accurate measurement. Too small a cuff will overestimate blood pressure, too large a cuff is associated with less error [62]. The Pre-eclampsia Community Guidelines (PRECOG) advise a different size of cuff depending on arm circumference (Table 18.4) [63] (www.apec.org.uk/precog.htm). The ACOG guidance suggests the cuff be at least 1.5 times the upper arm circumference, or the cuff bladder encircles at least 80% of the arm [64].

Treatment of hypertension in pregnancy is indicated if the systolic pressure exceeds 150 mmHg or the diastolic exceeds 110 mmHg. Methyldopa, nifedipine, and labetalol are all commonly used in pregnancy [65]. ACE inhibitors should be avoided as they are associated with congenital abnormalities and fetal death [5].

Identification of risk factors and vigilant screening is essential for the early recognition and appropriate treatment of pre-eclampsia. Antiplatelet therapy with low-dose aspirin is of mild to moderate benefit in prevention of pre-eclampsia in women at high risk of developing the disease [66]. Data for the benefits of aspirin in obese women are lacking and "moderate risk factors" are ill defined. Despite this, it is the opinion of the NICE guideline development group that women with more than one moderate risk factor may benefit from 75 mg of aspirin from 12 weeks gestation [67]. There is no evidence of any benefit from nutritional supplements such as calcium, fish oils, and vitamins C and E [68].

Table 18.4 Arm circumference and blood pressure cuff size

Arm circumference	Appropriate cuff	Cuff size
Up to 33 cm	Standard	13 × 23 cm
33–41 cm	Large	15 × 33 cm
≥41 cm	Thigh cuff	18 × 36 cm

Pre-eclampsia Community Guidelines (PRECOG) www.apec. org.uk.

To enable appropriate screening, women with a BMI greater than 35 kg/m² should be seen more frequently in pregnancy than lean women. There is no consensus on the frequency of these visits. The UK RCOG guideline suggests three-weekly intervals from 24 to 32 weeks and two-weekly intervals from 32 weeks until delivery [15]. Urinalysis for protein should be checked on each occasion with quantification of proteinuria by 24-hour urine collection or albumin/creatinine ratio.

Treatment of elevated blood pressure is the same as for pregnancy-induced hypertension. However, the cure is of course delivery of the baby and placenta, and multidisciplinary team input is invaluable in planning delivery.

Preterm birth

There has been uncertainty regarding the risk of preterm birth among overweight and obese women. A recent meta-analysis of 84 studies, totaling over a million women, concludes that obese women do have an increased risk of preterm birth before 32 weeks and induced preterm birth before 37 weeks [69]. Clearly in many cases there will be a definite medical need for preterm induction. However, clinicians must be mindful to resist the temptation to induce labor for softer reasons.

Other illnesses

Obesity is associated with an increased incidence of common minor morbidities of pregnancy [70]. Overweight women are significantly more likely to suffer heartburn, carpel tunnel syndrome, symphysis pubis dysfunction, and chest infection. Moreover, they are more likely to require medications to treat these conditions than women of normal weight, for example alginate reflux suppressants for heartburn. This has significant cost implications for society [71].

Of more serious concern is the recent emergence of the H1N1 strain of the influenza A virus, which reached pandemic status in 2009. Pregnant women were identified as a group at high risk of severe influenza-related complications. A prospective national cohort study in the UK identified maternal obesity to be associated with both admission to hospital with confirmed infection and critical illness from H1N1 infection [72]. This serves to highlight the importance of offering vaccination to this vulnerable group. Women must be reassured that the vaccine is not contraindicated at any stage of pregnancy and is still beneficial in the postnatal period when women are still at greater risk of complications.

Venous thromboembolism

Thromboembolic disease remains a leading cause of maternal mortality worldwide and obesity is the most important risk factor for thromboembolism. In the UK, 18 women died from thrombosis in the triennium 2006 to 2008 (CEMACE) [73]. Fourteen of these women were overweight (BMI >25 kg/m²), of whom 11 had a BMI ≥30 kg/m². The postpartum period is the time of greatest risk, secondary to vascular damage at the time of delivery. This will be attenuated by a period of immobility, particularly following surgical delivery. Care providers, including those working in the community and the emergency department, should have an awareness of the increased risk to this group of patients and a low threshold for initiating investigation of possible thromboembolism.

The antenatal period is also a time of increased thrombotic risk, particularly for the obese individual. The RCOG in the UK recommends antenatal thromboprophylaxis with low molecular weight heparin (LMWH) be considered for any woman who has a BMI greater than 30 kg/m² plus two or more additional risk factors and this should commence as early as practically possible in pregnancy [74]. All women receiving antenatal prophylaxis should usually continue for six weeks following delivery, regardless of mode of delivery. As a minimum precaution, obese women admitted to hospital in the antenatal period should be kept adequately hydrated and wear properly fitting graduated elastic compression stockings [74].

It should be routine practice to give thromboprophylaxis with LMWH to all women following cesarean delivery, regardless of BMI. However, consideration should be given to treatment with LMWH even after vaginal birth for women with a BMI >30 kg/m² and should be initiated in all women with a BMI >40 kg/m²

Table 18.5 Suggested dosing regimen for prophylactic dose low molecular weight heparin (LMWH)

Weight (kg)	Dose
91–130	60 mg Enoxaparin; 7500 units Dalteparin; 7000 units Tinzaparin daily
131–170	80 mg Enoxaparin; 10 000 units Dalteparin; 9000 units Tinzaparin daily
>170	0.6 mg/kg/day Enoxaparin; 75 units/kg/day Dalteparin; 75 units/kg/day Tinzaparin

RCOG Clinical Green Top Guideline No.37a. 2009 [74]

for a period of seven days [74]. The appropriate dose of LMWH is weight dependent and a suggested regime is illustrated in Table 18.5. However, the target range of anti-Xa of 0.2 to 0.4 units/ml for thromboprophylaxis is based on the recommendations of a consensus report, which has not been validated in clinical trials [75]. There is therefore a need for adequately powered trials so that dosing regimes for LMWH thromboprophylaxis during pregnancy are evidence based.

Anesthetics

The anesthetist plays an important role in the care of the obese parturient. A meeting with the patient during the antenatal period is helpful to discuss the possible complications and mechanisms in place for reducing potential harm. Specialist anesthetic obstetric clinics exist in some areas but these may need to be focused on those at the extreme end of the obesity spectrum, depending on local prevalence of obesity and resources.

Commonly cited problems include difficulties with venous access, unsuccessful epidural siting, difficulty with tracheal intubation, and increased risk of aspiration [76]. Difficult tracheal intubation should be anticipated and senior experienced assistance should be available. Failed intubation in the obstetric population may be as high as 1 in 250, compared with 1 in 2000 in the general population [77]. This risk is further exaggerated in the obese parturient due to anatomical differences. A "ramped" position to align the external auditory meatus with the sternal notch may provide an improved view at laryngoscopy. This may be achieved using pillows or blankets under the upper body or purpose-made, commercially available wedges.

Once intubated, obese women are more difficult to ventilate due to the weight of the chest wall from large breasts and cephalad displacement of the abdominal pannus during cesarean section. High positive airway pressures are required to achieve adequate tidal volumes. It is the responsibility of all staff to ensure the use of a left lateral tilt or wedge to minimize aortocaval compression.

Many anesthetists would advocate siting an epidural early in labor to try to reduce the risk of requiring regional or general anesthetic administration in an emergency situation [76]. Imaging of the back with ultrasound may be helpful to identify the landmarks, which are hidden by subcutaneous fat [78].

Intravenous access should be established early to avoid difficulties with this should an emergency situation arise. Where difficulty is anticipated, many anesthetists would prefer to have the first attempt at obtaining intravenous access, rather than repeated failed attempts by less experienced staff. Indeed, this is a recommendation from the most recent Confidential Enquiry into Maternal Deaths report in the UK [1]. The use of an intraosseous needle is also now recommended, for immediate access where peripheral access is not possible in an emergency, by resuscitation councils in the UK. Easy to use, impact-driven needles are commercially available (for example EZ-IO, Vidacare®).

Intrapartum care

Obese women should be encouraged to deliver in a consultant-led maternity unit where there is ready access to experienced anesthetic and obstetric staff. These patients face a higher risk of intrapartum complications such as inadequate progress in labor, shoulder dystocia, and cesarean section. There is also an increased risk of postpartum hemorrhage. Given the increased risk of aspiration of stomach contents, obese women should be discouraged from eating during labor and regular ranitidine should be prescribed to reduce the risk of aspiration should the need for general anesthesia arise [79].

Abdominal palpation can be challenging and if there is any doubt then ultrasound should be used to confirm fetal presentation in early labor. External continuous fetal monitoring can be difficult given the abdominal pannus and the use of a fetal scalp electrode is helpful in such situations. Mobilizing in early labor may be encouraged to promote progress and reduce risk of venous thromboembolism. Adequate hydration should be maintained and graduated elastic compression stockings may be worn throughout labor.

Assisted vaginal delivery

As has previously been mentioned, obese women are more likely to have a macrosomic fetus. This increases the likelihood of shoulder dystocia, postpartum hemorrhage, and failed instrumental delivery. Consideration should be given to all of these factors when deciding on optimal management to expedite delivery. It is essential that an obstetrician with the expertise to manage all of these complications is present for the delivery. It may be more difficult to assess the position and station of the vertex in an obese patient and also to perform additional maneuvers to manage a shoulder dystocia. This should all be borne in mind when making the decision to assist vaginal delivery.

Cesarean section

The risk of cesarean section is increased in the obese parturient, approaching 50% in the morbidly obese group [80]. Surgery is challenging and best performed by those with experience [81]. Any facility offering care to obese women in labor should have appropriate equipment readily available. Standard modern operating tables support a body weight of 130 to 160 kg, with newer tables supporting weights of 225 kg, or in some cases up to 360 kg. If the maternal weight cannot be supported by the operating table, then it may occasionally be necessary to operate with the woman on a bed. However, operating on a bed is suboptimal, with access being more uncomfortable and awkward for the obstetrician, anesthetists, and assistants. Longer surgical instruments and retractors may be required. Postoperatively, high dependency and intensive care facilities are more likely to be required [81].

Preoperative planning is desirable but may not be feasible in the emergency situation. The obstetrician must bear in mind the extra time that may be required to perform regional or general anesthesia and the impact this may have, for example, on a fetus with suspected compromise.

Wound asepsis is very important, as maternal obesity is associated with increased risk of wound infection and subsequent complications. Particular attention must be given to the skin folds beneath the panniculus and in the groins. Where time allows, there may be some value in attempting to reduce skin colonization and subsequent wound infection by cleansing the skin prior to anesthetic administration and then again immediately prior to commencing the procedure. Although the effectiveness of this regime has been demonstrated in other surgical specialities [82], its clinical effectiveness has not to date been demonstrated in obstetrics. There is some evidence, however, that a reduction in wound infections is possible if meticulous pre- and postoperative wound hygiene is followed, with a recent study reporting a reduction in wound infection rates after cesarean section from 7.5% to 1.2% after introduction of a quality improvement initiative (including educational intervention, comprehensive preoperative skin preparation, and revised instrument sterilization methods) [83].

There is a paucity of evidence to guide the surgeon as to the best incision for abdominal delivery with both advantages and disadvantages to midline and transverse suprapubic incisions. Most obstetricians are more familiar with a low transverse incision beneath the panniculus. This has a cosmetic advantage for the patient. Moreover, a transverse incision has a superior closed strength and is less prone to wound breakdown. It is also associated with less postoperative pain and therefore allows easier respiratory effort and earlier mobilization of the patient with obvious advantages. However, the transverse incision may not provide sufficient surgical exposure. Also, the necessary cephalad displacement of the pannus can contribute further to cardiorespiratory embarrassment. The necessary division of the fascial and muscle layers may increase the risk of hematoma formation. Furthermore, the wound will invariably lie in the folds beneath the panniculus and be prone to infection.

A vertical midline incision provides the optimal exposure to the abdominal cavity. It does not necessitate division of the rectus muscles from the fascia, generally allowing quicker access and less blood loss. However, there is greater postoperative pain contributing to a higher likelihood of respiratory complications, longer period of immobility, and it is also cosmetically less acceptable to women. Vertical midline incisions are also associated with increased risk of scar dehiscence and hernia formation; however, the risk of both can be minimized by optimizing surgical technique [84]. With either approach, closure of the sheath should be with a delayed absorbable suture (e.g., polydioxanone; PDS, Johnson & Johnson Medical Ltd, UK or polyglycolide-trimethylene carbonate; Maxon, Mansfield, MA). Both invoke little tissue reaction and maintain their tensile strength at four weeks.

There is evidence that closure of the fat layer reduces the risk of subsequent wound dehiscence [85]; however, it is not certain whether the use (or otherwise) of a fat drain at cesarean section provides added benefit. A recent Cochrane review concluded that, from the limited evidence available (seven small trials), there was no evidence that routine use of wound drains at cesarean section conferred any benefit, but recommended that larger trials should be undertaken, with blinded outcomes, to justify the use of wound drains in women with different degrees of obesity, or having their first or repeat cesarean sections [86]. This finding has been supported by a more recent meta-analysis, which reached similar conclusions [87].

Abdominal adiposity is a strong risk factor for postoperative complication. The most common cause of postoperative morbidity is wound complications, including infection, seroma, and hematoma formation. In one study of 969 women, Tran *et al.* [88] demonstrated that for every five unit (kg/m^2) increase in BMI, the risk of postoperative infection doubles. The fatty tissue has a poor vascular supply and this increases susceptibility to infection. Both the American and UK colleges of obstetricians and gynecologists advocate the use of intraoperative antibiotic prophylaxis with a single dose of narrow spectrum antibiotic, such as first-generation cephalosporin. There is strong evidence that antibiotic prophylaxis for cesarean delivery given before skin incision, rather than after cord clamping, decreases the incidence of postpartum endometritis and total infectious morbidities, without affecting neonatal outcomes [89]. Standard dosing is usually appropriate but in the morbidly obese a higher dose may be required [90] and repeat doses may be required where there has been a prolonged operation or excessive blood loss.

Vaginal birth after cesarean section

Encouraging women to have a vaginal birth after a cesarean section (VBAC) is one of the strategies for reducing the high rates of cesarean section in the developed world. Several groups have examined the success rates of VBAC and these overwhelmingly demonstrate a reduced success rate in women with a high BMI compared to those of normal weight [91,92]. In addition, among morbidly obese women (BMI >40 kg/m^2), a trial of labor carries a greater than five-fold risk of uterine rupture/dehiscence and neonatal injury (fractures, brachial plexus injuries, and lacerations) (2.1% vs. 0.4%, and 7.2% vs. 3.8%, respectively), and almost a two-fold increase in composite maternal morbidity (1.1% vs. 0.2%). Obstetricians need to consider this evidence carefully when planning mode of delivery and counsel women appropriately to allow an informed decision to be made regarding trial of VBAC vs. an elective repeat cesarean section.

Postpartum hemorrhage

Several groups have demonstrated an association between increasing BMI and risk of postpartum hemorrhage [59,60]. In light of this, obstetricians and midwives must be vigilant in their management of the third stage of labor and anticipate postpartum hemorrhage. Intravenous access should be established during labor. There should be early use of ergometrine and oxytocin and cross-matched blood should be available if required. The usual maneuvers employed for the control of postpartum hemorrhage such as fundal massage and bimanual compression are challenging in the obese and may well be ineffectual. There should be early recourse to examination under anesthetic to facilitate the management of hemorrhage.

Postnatal care

The particular needs of the obese new mother should not be forgotten once her baby is delivered. She remains at greater risk of morbidity compared to lean mothers. We have already discussed infective morbidity and vigilance must be maintained to observe for signs of sepsis. Input from tissue viability nurse specialists can be invaluable in wound care. Wound hygiene should be taught and assistance given to clean and dry beneath the pannus in women who are unable to do this for themselves. Fat necrosis of the abdominal pannus at sites separate from the wound has recently been reported and carries significant morbidity [93].

Early mobilization should be encouraged to reduce the risk of venous thromboembolism and basal atelectasis. As previously discussed, thromboprophylaxis is advisable regardless of the mode of delivery.

Breastfeeding

The current WHO recommendation is that babies be exclusively breastfed for the first six months of life. However, as reviewed in Chapter 8, breastfeeding rates in the Western world are extremely poor, particularly among women who are overweight [94]. This may be due to the mechanical difficulties of larger breasts, poor positioning, and self-consciousness about breastfeeding "modestly." As we have discussed, this group are also more likely to have delivered by cesarean section and have had excessive bleeding after delivery, both of which can impact negatively on breastfeeding. There may also be a physiological contribution. Rasmussen *et al.* demonstrated a diminished prolactin response to suckling in the first week postpartum [95]. They postulate this may contribute to early lactation failure and premature cessation of breastfeeding. Whatever the reason, clearly cessation of breastfeeding leads to higher rates of formula feeding, which in turn may be associated with increased rates of childhood obesity, thus potentially perpetuating the cycle of disadvantage to the next generation [96]. Overweight women must be supported by health care professionals in their decision to breastfeed, with ongoing support until breastfeeding is well established. There has been longstanding controversy regarding the benefit of breastfeeding and postpartum weight loss but it seems that breastfeeding for the recommended six months is associated with lower post-pregnancy weight retention in women who have gained a normal amount of weight during pregnancy [97,98].

Contraception

All of the progesterone-only methods of contraception are safe in the postpartum period, whether the woman is breastfeeding or not, and regardless of her BMI. The choice of method is entirely dependent on the woman's preference for mode of delivery, duration of use, and possible effect on bleeding. Current evidence does not support the practice of prescribing a double dose of progesterone-only pill for women weighing over 70 kg. The use of the combined oral contraceptive pill is not recommended for breastfeeding women. It may be used from 21 days postpartum in non-breastfeeding women. There are no specific restrictions on combined oral contraceptive use in obese women in the postnatal period but clinical judgment should be exercised in the presence of other risk factors for venous thromboembolism. Women should be reassured that no method of contraception is associated with weight gain, other than depot-medroxyprogesterone acetate (Depo-Provera). The importance of contraception should be emphasized in obese women to enable time for inter-pregnancy weight loss.

Summary

The global obesity epidemic presents a major challenge for health care providers in obstetrics. Obese women must be recognized as a high-risk group and as such

should receive individualized specialist care before, during, and after their pregnancy. They should be made aware of the risks pregnancy poses to them and their baby, and informed of the strategies available to manage those risks to enable them to make informed decisions regarding their management.

References

1. Cantwell R, Clutton-Brock T, Cooper G, *et al.* Saving Mothers' Lives: reviewing maternal deaths to make motherhood safer: 2006–2008. The Eighth Report of the Confidential Enquiries into Maternal Deaths in the United Kingdom. *BJOG* **118**(Suppl 1):1–203.

2. Nelson S M & Fleming R F. The preconceptual contraception paradigm: obesity and infertility. *Hum Reprod* 2007;**22**:912–15.

3. NICE. NICE clinical guideline 43. Obesity: guidance on the prevention, identification, assessment and management of overweight and obesity in adults and children. (London: National Institute for Health and Clinical Excellence, 2006). www.nice.org.uk/nicemedia/pdf/CG43NICEGuideline.pdf [Accessed January 11, 2012]

4. NICE. NICE Public health guidance 27. Dietary interventions and physical activity interventions for weight management before, during and after pregnancy. (London: National Institute for Health and Clinical Excellence, 2010). http://guidance.nice.org.uk/PH27 [Accessed January 11, 2012]

5. Friedman J M. ACE inhibitors and congenital anomalies. *N Engl J Med* 2006;**354**:2498–500.

6. Rubin P C & Ramsey M (eds). *Prescribing in Pregnancy*, 4th edn. (Blackwell Publishing, 2008).

7. Rasmussen S A, Chu S Y, Kim S Y, *et al.* Maternal obesity and risk of neural tube defects: a metaanalysis. *Am J Obstet Gynecol* 2008;**198**:611–19.

8. Jovanovic L. Definition, size of the problem, screening and diagnostic criteria: who should be screened, cost-effectiveness, and feasibility of screening. *Int J Gynaecol Obstet* 2009;**104**(Suppl 1):s17–19.

9. Mojtabai R. Body mass index and serum folate in childbearing age women. *Eur J Epidemiol* 2004;**19**:1029–36.

10. Dashe J S, McIntire D D & Twickler D M. Effect of maternal obesity on the ultrasound detection of anomalous fetuses. *Obstet Gynecol* 2009;**113**:1001–7.

11. Scholl T O & Johnson W G. Folic acid: influence on the outcome of pregnancy. *Am J Clin Nutr* 2000;**71**:1295S–303S.

12. De-Regil L M, Fernandez-Gaxiola A C, Dowswell T, *et al.* Effects and safety of periconceptional folate

supplementation for preventing birth defects. *Cochrane Database Syst Rev* **10**:CD007950. www.thecochranelibrary.com/view/0/index.html [Accessed January 11, 2012].

13. Anon. Prevention of neural tube defects: results of the Medical Research Council Vitamin Study. MRC Vitamin Study Research Group. *Lancet* 1991;**338**:131–7.

14. Ray J G, Wyatt P R, Vermeulen M J, *et al.* Greater maternal weight and the ongoing risk of neural tube defects after folic acid flour fortification. *Obstet Gynecol* 2005;**105**:261–5.

15. Modder J & Fitzsimons K J. CMACE/RCOG Joint Guideline: Management of women with obesity in pregnancy. (London: Centre for Maternal and Child Enquiries and the Royal College of Obstetricians and Gynaecologists, 2010). www.rcog.org.uk/womens-health/clinical-guidance/management-women-obesity-pregnancy [Accessed January 11, 2012].

16. American College of Obstetricians and Gynecologists. ACOG Committee Opinion number 315, September 2005. Obesity in pregnancy. *Obstet Gynecol* 2005;**106**:671–5.

17. Bodnar L M, Catov J M, Roberts J M, *et al.* Prepregnancy obesity predicts poor vitamin D status in mothers and their neonates. *J Nutr* 2007;**137**:2437–42.

18. Swan G. Findings from the latest National Diet and Nutrition Survey. *Proc Nutr Soc* 2004;**63**:505–12.

19. Roth D E. Vitamin D supplementation during pregnancy: safety considerations in the design and interpretation of clinical trials. *J Perinatol* 2011;**31**:449–59.

20. Gorber S C, Tremblay M, Moher D, *et al.* A comparison of direct vs. self-report measures for assessing height, weight and body mass index: a systematic review. *Obes Rev* 2007;**8**:307–26.

21. Beyerlein A, Schiessl B, Lack N, *et al.* Associations of gestational weight loss with birth-related outcome: a retrospective cohort study. *BJOG* **118**:55–61.

22. Dawes M G & Grudzinskas J G. Patterns of maternal weight gain in pregnancy. *Br J Obstet Gynaecol* 1991;**98**:195–201.

23. Dawes M G & Grudzinskas J G. Repeated measurement of maternal weight during pregnancy. Is this a useful practice? *Br J Obstet Gynaecol* 1991;**98**:189–94.

24. Institute of Medicine. Weight gain during pregnancy: reexamining the guidelines. 2009. www.iom.edu/Reports/2009/Weight-Gain-During-Pregnancy-Reexamining-the-Guidelines.aspx [Accessed January 12, 2012].

25. Cedergren M I. Optimal gestational weight gain for body mass index categories. *Obstet Gynecol* 2007;**110**:759–64.

26. Abrams B, Altman S L & Pickett K E. Pregnancy weight gain: still controversial. *Am J Clin Nutr* 2000;**71**:1233S–41S.

27. Parker J D & Abrams B. Prenatal weight gain advice: an examination of the recent prenatal weight gain recommendations of the Institute of Medicine. *Obstet Gynecol* 1992;**79**:664–9.

28. Viswanathan M, Siega-Riz A M, Moos M K, *et al.* Outcomes of maternal weight gain. *Evid Rep Technol Assess* 2008;**168**:1–223.

29. Hedderson M M, Weiss N S, Sacks D A, *et al.* Pregnancy weight gain and risk of neonatal complications: macrosomia, hypoglycemia, and hyperbilirubinemia. *Obstet Gynecol* 2006;**108**:1153–61.

30. Oken E, Taveras E M, Kleinman K P, *et al.* Gestational weight gain and child adiposity at age 3 years. *Am J Obstet Gynecol* 2007;**196**:322e1–8.

31. Artal R, Lockwood C J & Brown H L. Weight gain recommendations in pregnancy and the obesity epidemic. *Obstet Gynecol* 2010;**115**:152–5.

32. Amorim A R, Rossner S, Neovius M, *et al.* Does excess pregnancy weight gain constitute a major risk for increasing long-term BMI? *Obesity (Silver Spring)* 2007;**15**:1278–86.

33. Stotland N E, Cheng Y W, Hopkins L M, *et al.* Gestational weight gain and adverse neonatal outcome among term infants. *Obstet Gynecol* 2006;**108**:635–43.

34. Schieve L A, Cogswell M E & Scanlon K S. Trends in pregnancy weight gain within and outside ranges recommended by the Institute of Medicine in a WIC population. *Matern Child Health J* 1998;**2**:111–16.

35. Haakstad L A, Voldner N, Henriksen T, *et al.* Physical activity level and weight gain in a cohort of pregnant Norwegian women. *Acta Obstet Gynecol Scand* 2007;**86**:559–64.

36. Cogswell M E, Scanlon K S, Fein S B, *et al.* Medically advised, mother's personal target, and actual weight gain during pregnancy. *Obstet Gynecol* 1999;**94**:616–22.

37. Kramer M S & McDonald S W. Aerobic exercise for women during pregnancy. *Cochrane Database Syst Rev* 2006;**3**:CD000180. www.thecochranelibrary.com/view/0/index.html [Accessed January 12, 2012].

38. Davies G A, Wolfe L A, Mottola M F, *et al.* Exercise in pregnancy and the postpartum period. *J Obstet Gynaecol Can* 2003;**25**:516–29.

39. Tobias D K, Zhang C, van Dam R M, *et al.* Physical activity before and during pregnancy and risk of gestational diabetes mellitus: a meta-analysis. *Diabetes Care* **34**:223–9.

40. Melzer K, Schutz Y, Boulvain M, *et al.* Physical activity and pregnancy: cardiovascular adaptations,

recommendations and pregnancy outcomes. *Sports Med* **40**:493–507.

41. Jolly M C, Sebire N J, Harris J P, *et al.* Risk factors for macrosomia and its clinical consequences: a study of 350,311 pregnancies. *Eur J Obstet Gynecol Reprod Biol* 2003;**111**:9–14.

42. Wolfe H M, Sokol R J, Martier S M, *et al.* Maternal obesity: a potential source of error in sonographic prenatal diagnosis. *Obstet Gynecol* 1990;**76**:339–42.

43. Phatak M & Ramsay J. Impact of maternal obesity on procedure of mid-trimester anomaly scan. *J Obstet Gynaecol* **30**:447–50.

44. Gandhi M, Fox N S, Russo-Stieglitz K, *et al.* Effect of increased body mass index on first-trimester ultrasound examination for aneuploidy risk assessment. *Obstet Gynecol* 2009;**114**:856–9.

45. Rode L, Ekelund C, Pedersen N G, *et al.* Maternal smoking, obesity and male fetal sex predispose to a large nuchal translucency thickness in healthy fetuses. *Fetal Diagn Ther* 2011;**29**:201–7.

46. Wald N, Cuckle H, Boreham J, *et al.* The effect of maternal weight on maternal serum alpha-fetoprotein levels. *Br J Obstet Gynaecol* 1981;**88**:1094–6.

47. Colman A, Maharaj D, Hutton J, *et al.* Reliability of ultrasound estimation of fetal weight in term singleton pregnancies. *N Z Med J* 2006;**119**:U2146.

48. Dudley N J. A systematic review of the ultrasound estimation of fetal weight. *Ultrasound Obstet Gynecol* 2005;**25**:80–9.

49. Crowther C A, Hiller J E, Moss J R, *et al.* Effect of treatment of gestational diabetes mellitus on pregnancy outcomes. *N Engl J Med* 2005;**352**:2477–86.

50. NICE. Clinical guidelines 63. Diabetes in pregnancy: management of diabetes and its complications from pre-conception to the postnatal period. (London: NICE 2008). www.nice.org.uk/CG63 [Accessed January 12, 2012].

51. American College of Obstetricians and Gynecologists Committee on Practice Bulletins – Obstetrics. Clinical management guidelines for obstetrician-gynecologists. Number 30, September 2001 (replaces Technical Bulletin Number 200, December 1994). Gestational diabetes. *Obstet Gynecol* 2001;**98**:525–38.

52. Metzger B E, Gabbe S G, Persson B, *et al.* International association of diabetes and pregnancy study groups recommendations on the diagnosis and classification of hyperglycemia in pregnancy. *Diabetes Care* **33**:676–82.

53. American Diabetes Association. Standards of medical care in diabetes – 2011. *Diabetes Care* 2011;**34**(Suppl 1):s11–61.

54. Alberti K G & Zimmet P Z. Definition, diagnosis and classification of diabetes mellitus and its complications.

Part 1: diagnosis and classification of diabetes mellitus provisional report of a WHO consultation. *Diabet Med* 1998;**15**:539–53.

55. Scottish Intercollegiate Guidelines Network. Management of diabetes. A national clinical guideline. Guideline No. 116. (Edinburgh: Scottish Intercollegiate Guidelines Network, 2010). www.sign.ac.uk/ guidelines/fulltext/116/index.html [Accessed January 12, 2012].

56. Comtois R, Seguin M C, Aris-Jilwan N, *et al.* Comparison of obese and non-obese patients with gestational diabetes. *Int J Obes Relat Metab Disord* 1993;**17**:605–8.

57. Rowan J A, Hague W M, Gao W, *et al.* Metformin versus insulin for the treatment of gestational diabetes. *N Engl J Med* 2008;**358**:2003–15.

58. Kannel W B, Brand N, Skinner J J, Jr., *et al.* The relation of adiposity to blood pressure and development of hypertension. The Framingham study. *Ann Intern Med* 1967;**67**:48–59.

59. Bhattacharya S, Campbell D M, Liston W A, *et al.* Effect of body mass index on pregnancy outcomes in nulliparous women delivering singleton babies. *BMC Public Health* 2007;**7**:168.

60. Denison F C, Price J, Graham C, *et al.* Maternal obesity, length of gestation, risk of postdates pregnancy and spontaneous onset of labour at term. *BJOG* 2008;**115**:720–5.

61. Sebire N J, Jolly M, Harris J P, *et al.* Maternal obesity and pregnancy outcome: a study of 287,213 pregnancies in London. *Int J Obes Relat Metab Disord* 2001;**25**:1175–82.

62. Maxwell M H, Waks A U, Schroth P C, *et al.* Error in blood-pressure measurement due to incorrect cuff size in obese patients. *Lancet* 1982;**2**:33–6.

63. PRECOG Development Group. The pre-eclampsia community guideline. Evidence based screening and detection of pre-eclampsia, 2004. www.apec.org.uk/ pdf/guidelinepublishedvers04.pdf [Accessed January 12, 2012].

64. ACOG Committee on Obstetric Practice. ACOG practice bulletin. Diagnosis and management of preeclampsia and eclampsia. Number 33, January 2002. American College of Obstetricians and Gynecologists. *Int J Gynaecol Obstet* 2002;**77**:67–75.

65. Nelson-Piercy C M. *Handbook of Obstetric Medicine*, 4th edn. (London: Informa Healthcare, 2010).

66. Duley L, Henderson-Smart D J, Knight M, *et al.* Antiplatelet agents for preventing pre-eclampsia and its complications. *Cochrane Database Syst Rev* 2004;CD004659. www2.cochrane.org/reviews/en/ ab004659.html [Accessed January 12, 2012].

67. NICE. Clinical Guidelines 107: Hypertension in pregnancy: the management of hypertensive disorders during pregnancy. (NICE, 2010). www.nice.org.uk/guidance/CG107 [Accessed January 12, 2012].

68. Sibai B, Dekker G, Kupferminc M. Pre-eclampsia. *Lancet* 2005;**365**:785–99.

69. McDonald S D, Han Z, Mulla S, *et al.* Overweight and obesity in mothers and risk of preterm birth and low birth weight infants: systematic review and meta-analyses. *BMJ* 2010;**341**:c3428.

70. Denison F C, Norrie G, Graham B, *et al.* Increased maternal BMI is associated with an increased risk of minor complications during pregnancy with consequent cost implications. *BJOG* 2009;**116**:1467–72.

71. Denison F C, Norrie G, Graham B, *et al.* Increased maternal BMI is associated with an increased risk of minor complications during pregnancy with consequent cost implications. *BJOG* 2009;**116**:1467–72.

72. Yates L, Pierce M, Stephens S, *et al.* Influenza A/H1N1v in pregnancy: an investigation of the characteristics and management of affected women and the relationship to pregnancy outcomes for mother and infant. *Health Technol Assess* **14**:109–82.

73. Lewis G (ed.). The Confidential Enquiry into Maternal and Child Health (CEMACH). Saving Mothers' Lives: reviewing maternal deaths to make motherhood safer – 2003–2005. The Seventh Report on Confidential Enquiries into Maternal Deaths in the United Kingdom. (CEMACH: London, 2007).

74. Royal College of Obstetricians and Gynaecologists. Reducing the risk of thrombosis and embolism during pregnancy and the puerperium. (Green-top guideline No37a). (RCOG, 2009).

75. Duhl A J, Paidas M J, Ural S H, *et al.* Antithrombotic therapy and pregnancy: consensus report and recommendations for prevention and treatment of venous thromboembolism and adverse pregnancy outcomes. *Am J Obstet Gynecol* 2007;**197**:457e1–21.

76. Saravanakumar K, Rao S G & Cooper G M. The challenges of obesity and obstetric anaesthesia. *Curr Opin Obstet Gynecol* 2006;**18**:631–5.

77. Barnardo P D & Jenkins J G. Failed tracheal intubation in obstetrics: a 6-year review in a UK region. *Anaesthesia* 2000;**55**:690–4.

78. Balki M, Lee Y, Halpern S, *et al.* Ultrasound imaging of the lumbar spine in the transverse plane: the correlation between estimated and actual depth to the epidural space in obese parturients. *Anesth Analg* 2009;**108**:1876–81.

79. Abera A B, Sales K J, Catalano R D, *et al.* EP2 receptor mediated cAMP release is augmented by PGF 2 alpha activation of the FP receptor via the calcium-calmodulin pathway. *Cell Signal* **22**:71–9.

80. Homer C S, Kurinczuk J J, Spark P, *et al.* Planned vaginal delivery or planned caesarean delivery in women with extreme obesity. *BJOG* **118**:480–7.

81. Alexander C I & Liston W A. Operating on the obese woman – a review. *BJOG* 2006;**113**:1167–72.

82. Zywiel M G, Daley J A, Delanois R E, *et al.* Advance pre-operative chlorhexidine reduces the incidence of surgical site infections in knee arthroplasty. *Int Orthop* 2011;**35**(7):1001–6.

83. Rauk P N. Educational intervention, revised instrument sterilization methods, and comprehensive preoperative skin preparation protocol reduce cesarean section surgical site infections. *Am J Infect Control* **38**:319–23.

84. Cliby W A. Abdominal incision wound breakdown. *Clin Obstet Gynecol* 2002;**45**:507–17.

85. Naumann R W, Hauth J C, Owen J, *et al.* Subcutaneous tissue approximation in relation to wound disruption after cesarean delivery in obese women. *Obstet Gynecol* 1995;**85**:412–16.

86. Gates S, Anderson E R. Wound drainage for caesarean section. *Cochrane Database Syst Rev* 2005;CD004549.

87. Hellums E K, Lin M G & Ramsey P S. Prophylactic subcutaneous drainage for prevention of wound complications after cesarean delivery – a metaanalysis. *Am J Obstet Gynecol* 2007;**197**:229–35.

88. Tran T S, Jamulitrat S, Chongsuvivatwong V, *et al.* Risk factors for postcesarean surgical site infection. *Obstet Gynecol* 2000;**95**:367–71.

89. Costantine M M, Rahman M, Ghulmiyah L, *et al.* Timing of perioperative antibiotics for cesarean delivery: a metaanalysis. *Am J Obstet Gynecol* 2008;**199**:301e1–6.

90. Cheymol G. Effects of obesity on pharmacokinetics implications for drug therapy. *Clin Pharmacokinet* 2000;**39**:215–31.

91. Hibbard J U, Gilbert S, Landon M B, *et al.* Trial of labor or repeat cesarean delivery in women with morbid obesity and previous cesarean delivery. *Obstet Gynecol* 2006;**108**:125–33.

92. Durnwald C P, Ehrenberg H M & Mercer B M. The impact of maternal obesity and weight gain on vaginal birth after cesarean section success. *Am J Obstet Gynecol* 2004;**191**:954–7.

93. Chiswick C, Cooper E S, Norman J E, *et al.* Fat necrois of the abdominal pannus following caesarean section in patients with morbid obesity. *Eur J Gynecol Reprod Biol* 2012;**160**:118–19.

94. Amir L H & Donath S. A systematic review of maternal obesity and breastfeeding intention, initiation and duration. *BMC Pregnancy Childbirth* 2007;7:9.

95. Rasmussen K M & Kjolhede C L. Prepregnant overweight and obesity diminish the prolactin response to suckling in the first week postpartum. *Pediatrics* 2004;**113**:e465–71.

96. Armitage J A, Poston L & Taylor P D. Developmental origins of obesity and the metabolic syndrome: the role of maternal obesity. *Front Horm Res* 2008;**36**:73–84.

97. Baker J L, Gamborg M, Heitmann B L, *et al.* Breastfeeding reduces postpartum weight retention. *Am J Clin Nutr* 2008;**88**:1543–51.

98. HAPO Study Cooperative Research Group. Hyperglycemia and Adverse Pregnancy Outcome (HAPO) Study: associations with maternal body mass index. *BJOG* 2010;**117**(5):575–84.

99. Lashen H, Fear K & Sturdee D W. Obesity is associated with increased risk of first trimester and recurrent miscarriage: matched case-control study. *Hum Reprod* 2004;**19**:1644–6.

100. Watkins M L, Rasmussen S A, Honein M A, *et al.* Maternal obesity and risk for birth defects. *Pediatrics* 2003;**111**:1152–8.

101. McDonald S D, Han Z, Mulla S, *et al.* Overweight and obesity in mothers and risk of preterm birth and low birth weight infants: systematic review and meta-analyses. *BMJ* 2010;**341**:c3428.

102. O'Brien T E, Ray J G, Chan W S. Maternal body mass index and the risk of preeclampsia: a systematic overview. *Epidemiology* 2003;**14**:368–74.

103. Jacobsen A F, Skjeldestad F E, Sandset P M. Ante- and postnatal risk factors of venous thrombosis: a hospital-based case-control study. *J Thromb Haemost* 2008;**6**:905–12.

104. Chu S Y, Kim S Y, Lau J, *et al.* Maternal obesity and risk of stillbirth: a metaanalysis. *Am J Obstet Gynecol* 2007;**197**:223–8.

105. Metzger B E, Lowe L P, Dyer A R, *et al.* Hyperglycemia and adverse pregnancy outcomes. *N Engl J Med* 2008;**358**:1991–2002.

Chapter

19

Public health policies relating to obesity in childbearing women

Kathleen M. Rasmussen

The development of obesity is more complex in women than in men because, in addition to the usual reasons for becoming obese, the vast majority of women become pregnant at some point in their life (85% by age 44 yr) [1], and substantial weight gain is recommended for each pregnancy. Depending on a woman's pre-pregnancy body mass index (BMI), the latest American guidelines [2] recommend that women be weighed during each routine prenatal care visit and gain as little as 5 kg or as much as 18 kg during pregnancy (Table 19.1). Unfortunately, the weight gained during pregnancy may be difficult to lose postpartum [3]. Women who are too heavy when they conceive have a high risk for complications of pregnancy and difficulties with labor and delivery (reviewed in [2,4]), so it is important for women to conceive at a normal BMI, gain weight appropriately while pregnant, and then return to their pre-pregnancy weight postpartum before becoming pregnant again [2].

Within the American context, national public health policies and programs related to helping women to conceive at a healthy weight, gain weight appropriately during pregnancy, and limit weight retention postpartum will be covered in this chapter. In addition, the specific challenges involved in developing guidelines for gestational weight gain (GWG) among the heaviest women will be considered.

The United States does not have an official policy related to nutrition in general or the prevention of maternal obesity more specifically. Instead it has developed a variety of norms, standards, and targets that serve as the foundation for action by individuals, organizations, and local, state and federal agencies. Among other possibilities, they may be derived from the deliberations of expert committees, whose work is often commissioned by the federal government. For example, since 1970, three such committees have

Table 19.1 Recommended total weight gain during pregnancy by pre-pregnancy body mass index (BMI) [2]

Pre-pregnancy BMI (kg/m²)	Total weight gain, kg (lb)
Underweight (<18.5)	12.5–18 (28–40)
Normal weight (18.5–24.9)	11.5–16 (25–35)
Overweight (25.0–29.9)	7–11.5 (15–25)
Obese (≥30)	5–9 (11–20)

published guidelines for GWG [2,5,6]. This guidance not only informs the development of various federal- and state-level policy instruments, as discussed below, but it can also be influential in changing the recommended practices or standards of care used by health care providers (e.g., the adoption of guidelines for GWG by the American Congress of Obstetricians and Gynecologists) as happened recently [7].

Preconceptional weight

The primary policy instrument related to beginning pregnancy at a healthy weight is *Healthy People 2020*, which is prepared by the US Department of Health and Human Services (HHS) once each decade. This document provides a framework for public health action and a set of goals for improving the public's health in accord with this framework. Within the framework of these goals, public health policies and programs are developed by appropriate organizations or agencies at every level of government. *Healthy People 2020* includes a goal (MICH-16.5) that by 2020 53.4% of women should have a healthy weight (defined as a BMI of 18.5–24.9 kg/m²) before pregnancy [8]. If achieved, this would represent a 10% improvement over the

Maternal Obesity, ed. Matthew W. Gillman and Lucilla Poston. Published by Cambridge University Press. © Cambridge University Press 2012.

2007 baseline of 48.5% of women of childbearing age. Unfortunately, since that baseline, a still higher proportion of women are not at a healthy weight [9] (Figure 19.1). Moreover, this target is far from the recommendation that "[all] women should enter pregnancy with a BMI in the normal weight category" made by the expert committee of the Institute of Medicine (IOM)/National Research Council (NRC) that recently revised the American guidelines for GWG [2].

To help women to begin pregnancy at a healthy weight, *Healthy People 2020* includes two developmental goals: by 2020 women should have discussed "preconception health with a health care worker prior to pregnancy" (MICH-16.1) and "used contraception to plan pregnancy" (MICH-16.6) [8]. Potential sources of data to ascertain how many women engage in these behaviors are specified for these development goals, but no numerical targets are provided, so these are weaker goals. Nonetheless, they are an important indication of the importance of these actions, which could become goals in a subsequent edition of *Healthy People*. These goals are in accord with the recommendation of the IOM/NRC committee [2] that "those who provide health care or related services to women of childbearing age should include preconceptional counseling in their care." One of the purposes of this preconceptional care is to assist women who are not at a healthy weight (the 59.5% of American women of 20 to 39 years old who are overweight or heavier (BMI ≥25 kg/m²) [9]) to achieve a healthy weight before conceiving. This is unlikely to be possible among women who fail to plan their pregnancies.

Other groups have also issued recommendations for the improvement of preconceptional care, including the IOM (*Nutrition Services in Perinatal Care*) [10] and, more recently, the US Centers for Disease Control and Prevention (CDC) [1]. In particular, the CDC recommends that (a) as a part of primary care visits, all women of childbearing age should receive risk assessment and educational and health promotion counseling, (b) as a component of maternity care, one pre-pregnancy visit should be offered to couples and persons planning a pregnancy, and (c) components of preconceptional care should be integrated into existing local public health and related programs [1]. The CDC provides information to consumers about preconceptional care on its website [11].

There is also support for these initiatives in practice guidelines [12], which call for including "counseling on appropriate medical care and behavior to optimize

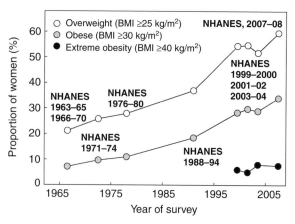

Figure 19.1. Prevalence of overweight, obesity, and extreme obesity among 20- to 39-year-old women (20- to 35-years-old through NHANES 1988–94), United States, 1963 to 2009. Data graphed from references [9,49,50].

pregnancy outcomes" in "all health encounters during a woman's reproductive years" and provide guidance for the content of nutrition counseling in preconceptional care. However, these kinds of medical services typically are passive in the US, waiting for women to request care. Moreover, such services are difficult to access for the millions of American women of childbearing age who lack health insurance [1]. Given that about half of the pregnancies in the US are unintended [13], in part because of inadequate access to and use of contraception [14], the US is far from having the services necessary to help the high proportion of women of childbearing age who are not at a healthy weight [9] (Figure 19.1) reach it before conceiving.

Weight during pregnancy

To help women to gain an appropriate amount of weight during pregnancy, *Healthy People 2020* includes a developmental goal (MICH-13) to "increase the proportion of mothers who achieve a recommended weight gain during their pregnancies" [8]; this is a reprise of a similar developmental goal [16–12] from *Healthy People 2010* [15]. The 2009 IOM/NRC report provided data that indicate that a minority of women in 2002–03 gained within the 1990 guidelines for GWG [2] (Figure 19.2). These data were not part of routine surveillance and, in fact, were based on information from only eight states. To remedy this situation, the IOM/NRC committee recommended that "the Department of Health and Human Services conduct routine surveillance of GWG… on a nationally representative sample of

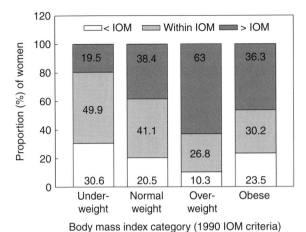

Figure 19.2. Distribution of GWG by pre-pregnancy BMI category among singleton, term deliveries, PRAMS data, 2002–3. Pre-pregnancy BMI categories are from the 1990 IOM guidelines for GWG [6]: underweight, <19.8 kg/m²; normal weight, 19.8–26.0 kg/m²; overweight, 26.1–29.0 kg/m², and obese, >29.0 kg/m². Adapted from Figure 2.7 in reference [2] with permission.

women" [2]. Achievement of this goal would provide the data necessary to establish a baseline value for the proportion of women who gain as recommended and then a target for future action.

This goal for appropriate weight gain during pregnancy is difficult for American women to achieve because it requires that they have access to prenatal care, choose to access it, and, once in prenatal care, receive counseling about their weight. Access to prenatal care is provided under the provisions of Title V of the Social Security Act, which is executed as a block grant to states and jurisdictions. It provides "gap-filling" prenatal services to more than 2 million women, especially those who have a low income or limited access to services [16]. In addition, states may choose to offer additional assistance to low-income women.

Guidance on implementing weight gain guidelines was developed for prenatal care providers [17] after the release of the 1990 GWG guidelines [6]. Current practice guidelines for prenatal care state that "Each pregnant woman should be provided with information about balanced nutrition, as well as ideal caloric intake and weight gain" and, more specifically, that "Nutritional consultation should be offered to all obese women" [12]. Nonetheless, research indicates that there is a discrepancy between the guidance about weight gain that physicians say that they are giving [18] and women say they are receiving [19,20]. Indeed, prenatal care providers perceive many barriers to providing adequate advice about GWG, including insufficient training, concern about the sensitivity of the topic, and the perception that counseling is ineffective [21].

Women who meet eligibility criteria related to income and nutritional need may also receive advice about GWG from the Special Supplemental Nutrition Program for Women, Infants, and Children (WIC), which is run by the US Department of Agriculture. In 2008, it served 1.02 million pregnant women, and 50.6% of these women enrolled in the WIC Program during their first trimester [22], when weight gain targets are often set. The WIC Program was developed at a time when inadequate GWG was a concern among low-income mothers; the food package that women received then was designed to provide additional food. And, indeed, participating in this program has been associated with reversal of low GWG [23]. At the state level, WIC Programs around the country have produced user-friendly versions of GWG charts based on the new IOM/NRC guidelines (e.g., [24]). Abnormal (low or high) GWG is a nutrition risk criterion used to establish program eligibility. There is reason to expect that low GWG may continue to be an issue among WIC participants and also that excessive GWG is now quite common among them. For example, food-insecure women, who had incomes low enough to qualify for the WIC Program, were more likely to be obese before conception and to gain excessively during pregnancy than food-secure women [25]. However, data to test these expectations are not available because the program does not report this information in their participation data. The new WIC food package, implemented in 2009, includes a wider choice of foods and emphasizes foods of higher nutrient density.

In summary, the policy framework for healthy weight gain during pregnancy exists and is supported by both expert committee reports and practice guidelines in the US. Access to prenatal care is available to low-income women through several government programs, but access for women with somewhat higher incomes may be restricted by lack of health insurance. Once in prenatal care, the advice about GWG appears to be variable. Assistance in gaining within the GWG guidelines, in the form of nutrition counseling, is available to low-income women who qualify for the WIC Program.

Postpartum weight

That American women may need assistance in losing weight postpartum has been recognized since at least 1992, with the publication of the second edition of *Nutrition Services in Perinatal Care* [10]. Although *Healthy People 2020* does not include an explicit goal for women to return to their pre-pregnancy weight postpartum, it does include goals related to breastfeeding that would assist women to do so. These include the goal to "increase the proportion of infants who are breastfed" from the 73.9% who were ever breastfed in 2007–09 to 81.9% (MICH-21). This goal includes four subgoals about increasing the exclusivity and duration of breastfeeding. These goals are especially challenging for obese women to meet as research has shown that they breastfeed for a shorter duration than normal weight women in the US [26,27] and elsewhere [28,29]. There are also two goals to facilitate reaching these national breastfeeding goals, namely "increase the proportion of employers that have worksite lactation support programs" (MICH-22) and "increase the proportion of live births that occur in facilities that provide recommended care of lactating mothers and their babies" (MICH-24) [8].

Achieving these goals would help women to lose weight after birth because breastfeeding that lasts longer or is more intensive is associated with greater weight loss (i.e. lower postpartum weight retention) in the first six months postpartum [30] (Figure 19.3), although breastfeeding appears to be less important in preventing longer term postpartum weight retention [31]. In addition, *Healthy People 2020* includes "increase the proportion of women giving birth who attend a postpartum care visit with a health worker" (MICH-19) as a developmental goal [8]. Such a postpartum care visit is supported by practice guidelines [12], and data from 11 states and New York City show that 88.7% of women had a postpartum visit in 2004. A postpartum visit was less likely among women with lower use of or access to health care (e.g., those with eight years or fewer of education or those who did not receive prenatal care) [32]. At present, this visit usually occurs four to six weeks after delivery and is a time when a woman's health is reviewed and contraceptives are prescribed. It is not comprehensive enough to include counseling on diet and physical activity and is held too late to prevent early termination of breastfeeding. Together this collection of goals for the postpartum period falls far short of reaching the IOM/NRC committee's call to offer "services, such as counseling on diet and physical activity, to all postpartum women" so women would be able to "conceive again at a healthy weight as well as improve their long-term health" [2].

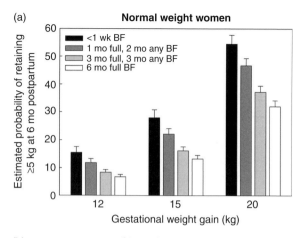

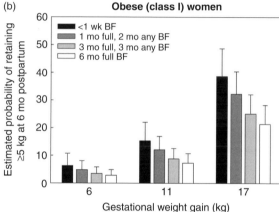

Figure 19.3. Estimated risk of retaining ≥5 kg at six months postpartum among 24 590 normal weight (a) or 7076 obese class 1 (BMI 30–34.9 kg/m²) (b) women from the Danish National Birth Cohort by breastfeeding patterns and percentiles of GWG (20th, 50th, and 80th). Data from reference [30].

The HHS supports breastfeeding, but does not provide services. Within HHS, the CDC issues an annual "Breastfeeding Report Card" [33] that is designed to draw attention to outcome indicators, such as progress toward the national goals for breastfeeding provided by the latest edition of *Healthy People*, as well as process indicators that represent elements of breastfeeding-friendly communities, such as support from birth facilities, health professionals, state legislation, and public facilities and services. To assist communities and states to improve their performance so as to meet the *Healthy People 2010* targets, the CDC has developed a guide to breastfeeding interventions [34]. This guide reviews evidence-based interventions in maternity care practices, support for breastfeeding in the workplace, peer support, educating mothers, professional support, and media and social marketing.

Also from within HHS, the Surgeon General periodically uses her "bully pulpit" to issue a "Call to Action to Support Breastfeeding" [35]. In her most recent "Call to Action," the Surgeon General [35] identified 20 key actions to improve support for breastfeeding that could be taken by mothers and their families, communities, the health care system, employers, and the scientific community. This "Call to Action" also recognizes the importance of providing paid maternity leave for all employed mothers and improving national leadership on the promotion and support of breastfeeding.

In summary, HHS has taken the lead in advocating for adoption of breastfeeding by American mothers, provided materials to support women in breastfeeding as well as employers and communities in making breastfeeding more feasible and normative, and has documented national progress toward these goals.

The WIC Program is an important policy instrument for the promotion of breastfeeding. In 2008, the WIC Program served 2.43 million infants [22], 57% of the 4.25 million babies born that year [36]. Federal regulations mandate that each state include a description of the methods that will be used to promote breastfeeding in the WIC Program [37]. These regulations explicitly permit WIC agencies to use food funds to purchase or rent breast pumps. This is important because providing WIC participants with pumps has been associated with prolonging breastfeeding (measured as a delay in requesting infant formula) [38]. Recently the WIC Program introduced a new food package for breastfeeding women to provide an incentive for them to increase the time that they breastfeed without supplementation [39]. Finally, the results of a recently completed implementation study indicate that *Loving Support* peer counseling to support breastfeeding has been adopted by all states and is widely available to pregnant participants [40].

Despite these many investments by the WIC Program, the proportion of WIC participants who choose to breastfeed or continue to 6 or 12 months remains lower than eligible women who chose not to participate [41] and the median duration of breastfeeding is quite short (13 wks) [22]. These discouraging breastfeeding statistics have been widely attributed to the distribution of large amounts of infant formula – more than half of that used in the US – by the program [42].

The WIC Program is the only federal program that addresses women's nutritional needs in the postpartum period and, of course, serves only those women who are eligible for the program, by criteria related to both low income (<185% of the Poverty Income Ratio) and nutritional risk. Women who do not choose to breastfeed can participate for only six weeks; those who breastfeed can participate for up to one year after delivery. The breastfeeding women receive food nutrition counseling at the time of recertification (every six months for a maximum of twice in this year) and breastfeeding support as needed. Women are referred elsewhere for contraceptive services.

Adequately intensive and prolonged breastfeeding may be a powerful means of reducing postpartum weight retention [30], but until it is nearly universal, other interventions, such as those outlined in the IOM/NRC report [2], are needed. Other interventions are especially important for obese women as their breastfeeding is likely to be short and they must lose the most weight if they are to reach a healthy weight before conceiving again. This review of current policies and programs reveals goals, rhetoric, and monitoring in support of breastfeeding for all new mothers. However, these goals will remain difficult to reach as long as the US continues to lack maternity leave of meaningful duration as well as workplace support for continued breastfeeding for all employed women. These kinds of policies are most important for low-income women, who are more likely than higher income women to have jobs without either maternity leave or workplace support for breastfeeding or breast pumping.

Developing guidelines for GWG for the heaviest women

Evidence is strong that women who are obese (BMI $\geq 30\,\text{kg/m}^2$) at the time of conception have a disproportionately high risk of adverse obstetric and neonatal outcomes [2,4]. Moreover, the heavier the woman is within the obese category, the higher is her risk of an adverse outcome. National data show that although obese women gain less weight during pregnancy than normal weight women, they are also more likely to exceed the recommended guidelines for GWG for their BMI category than are normal weight women [2]. In the latest national data for American women aged 20 to 39 years, 34.0%, 18.9%, and 7.6% had BMI values ≥ 30, ≥ 35, and $\geq 40\,\text{kg/m}^2$, respectively [9]. Although obese women are less likely to become pregnant than normal weight women, ~20% of pregnant women are obese at the time of conception, with much higher proportions in some population subgroups [43]. These figures add urgency to the need for GWG guidelines that are specific to these heavier women.

Evidence was available to the authors of the 2009 IOM/NRC report to support the development of a GWG guideline for obese women as a group, but not for specific, heavier subgroups of women within the obese category [2,44]. This was controversial as the need for such a guideline is great and some physicians have had success with their heaviest patients gaining very little or even losing weight while pregnant [45]. The expert committee process is an inherently conservative one: the committee must come to a consensus, its recommendation must be justified scientifically, and must survive extensive peer review. Moreover, because expert committee reports may be adopted as standards of care, the ethical duty to "do no harm" is taken seriously. For the heaviest pregnant women, this ethical duty was a particular challenge as anecdotal experiences of good outcomes with individual patients does not provide the level of evidence necessary to make well-informed, public health recommendations.

Since the latest GWG recommendations were issued in 2009, several large studies of the obstetric outcomes in obese women have been published. The trade-offs between lowering GWG and increasing the risks of such outcomes as preterm birth or small for gestational age newborns generally [46,47], but not always [48], remain. These studies have provided much needed additional data on large groups of women, but they did not contain the kind of information necessary to remove concerns, expressed in the 2009 IOM/NRC report, about the effects of very low weight gains or even weight losses during pregnancy on the short- and long-term health of the fetus [2].

In 2010, the American Congress of Obstetricians and Gynecologists adopted the IOM/NRC guidelines with a modification: for women with a pre-pregnancy BMI of $\geq 40\,kg/m^2$, they said that "a modest weight loss during pregnancy may be recommended. The weight loss should not be drastic, should be individualized for each woman, and should be done only under a health care provider's close supervision" [7].

Conclusions

The US has explicit public health targets to increase the proportion of women who begin pregnancy at a healthy weight and who gain weight during pregnancy within guidelines that are associated with good obstetric and neonatal outcomes. Although there is no explicit goal for women to return to their pre-pregnancy weight postpartum, there are goals related to increasing the duration of breastfeeding that could assist women to do this. However, these goals are operating in a difficult environment, one that is characterized by historically high rates of overweight and obesity among women of childbearing age and excessive GWG by the majority of pregnant women as well as inadequate support for breastfeeding in hospitals and workplaces, and inadequate maternity leave for optimal breastfeeding duration.

The IOM/NRC committee that recently revised the guidelines for GWG made recommendations that, if fully implemented, would represent a "radical change" in care offered to women of childbearing age [2], potentially leading to a reduction in obesity among women of childbearing age. These recommendations are in accord with current obstetric practice guidelines [7,12]. However, these recommendations and guidelines are not adequately supported by related policies and programs that would make them available to and affordable for all women of childbearing age.

Acknowledgments

The author thanks Drs. Barbara Abrams and David L. Pelletier for helpful comments on an earlier draft of this chapter.

References

1. Johnson K, Posner S F, Biermann J, et al. Recommendations to improve preconception health and health care – United States. A report of the CDC/ATSDR Preconception Care Work Group and the Select Panel on Preconception Care. *MMWR Recomm Rep* 2006;**55**(RR-6):1–23.

2. Institute of Medicine (US)/National Research Council (US) Committee to Reexamine IOM Pregnancy Weight Guidelines. Weight Gain During Pregnancy: Reexamining the Guidelines. (Washington, DC: National Academies Press; 2009).

3. Williamson D F, Madans J, Pamuk E, et al. A prospective study of childbearing and 10-year weight gain in US white women 25 to 45 years of age. *Int J Obes* 1994;**18**:561–9.

4. Viswanathan M, Siega-Riz A M, Moos M-K, et al. Outcomes of maternal weight gain. Evidence report/technology assessment, Number 168. (AHRQ Publication No. 08-E09). (Research Triangle Park, NC: RTI International – University of North Carolina Evidence-based Practice Center; 2008).

5. National Research Council (Committee on Maternal Nutrition, Food and Nutrition Board). *Maternal Nutrition and the Course of Pregnancy.* (Washington, DC: National Academy of Sciences, 1970).

6. Committee on Nutritional Status During Pregnancy and Lactation, Institute of Medicine. *Nutrition During Pregnancy: Part I, Weight Gain; Part II, Nutrient Supplements.* (Washington, DC: National Academy Press; 1990).

7. American College of Obstetricians and Gynecologists. Nutrition during pregnancy. Frequently asked questions, FAQ001, Pregnancy. (ACOG, 2011) www.acog.org/Search?Keyword=Nutrition During Pregnancy: Patient Education (Pamphlet AP001). [Accessed January 12, 2011].

8. Healthy People 2020. Maternal, infant, and child health objectives. http://healthypeople.gov/2020/topicsobjectives2020/objectiveslist.aspx?topicId=26 [Accessed January 12, 2012].

9. Flegal K M, Carroll M D, Ogden C L & Curtin L R. Prevalence and trends in obesity among US adults, 1999–2008. *JAMA* 2010;**303**:235–41.

10. Institute of Medicine (Committee on Nutritional Status During Pregnancy and Lactation). *Nutrition Services in Perinatal Care.* (Washington, DC: National Academy Press; 1992).

11. Centers for Disease Control and Prevention. Preconception care: frequently asked questions. www.cdc.gov/ncbddd/preconception/default.htm [Accessed January 12, 2011].

12. American Academy of Pediatrics, American College of Obstetricians and Gynecologists. *Guidelines for Perinatal Care*, 6th edn. (Elk Grove, IL and Washington, DC: American Academy of Pediatrics and American College of Obstetricians and Gynecologists; 2007).

13. Finer L B & Henshaw S K. Disparities in rates of unintended pregnancy in the United States, 1994 and 2001. *Perspect Sex Reprod Health* 2006;**38**:90–6.

14. O'Brien J. PRAMS and unintended pregnancy. (Centers for Disease Control and Prevention, 2012) http://www.cdc.gov/PRAMS/UP.htm [Accessed January 12, 2011].

15. US Department of Health and Human Services. *Healthy People 2010.* (Washington, DC: Department of Health and Human Services; 2000).

16. Maternal and Child Health Services. Title V Block Grant. http://mchb.hrsa.gov/programs/titlevgrants/index.html [Accessed January 20, 2012].

17. Institute of Medicine. *Nutrition During Pregnancy and Lactation: An Implementation Guide.* (Washington, DC: National Academy Press; 1992).

18. Power M L, Cogswell M E & Schulkin J. Obesity prevention and treatment practices of U.S. obstetrician-gynecologists. *Obstet Gynecol* 2006;**108**:961–8.

19. Cogswell M E, Scanlon K S, Fein S B & Schieve L A. Medically advised, mother's personal target, and actual weight gain during pregnancy. *Obstet Gynecol* 1999;**94**:616–22.

20. Stotland N E, Haas J S, Brawarsky P, *et al.* Body mass index, provider advice, and target gestational weight gain. *Am J Obstet Gynecol* 2005;**105**:633–8.

21. Stotland N E, Gilbert P, Bogetz Z, *et al.* Preventing excessive weight gain in pregnancy: how do prenatal care providers approach counseling? *J Womens Health (Larchmt)* 2010;**19**:807–14.

22. US Department of Agriculture, Food and Nutrition Service, Office of Research and Analysis. WIC participant and program characteristics 2008. Report No. WIC-08-PC. (Alexandria, VA: U.S. Department of Agriculture; 2010).

23. Rush D, Sloan N L, Leighton J, *et al.* Longitudinal study of pregnant women. *Am J Clin Nutr* 1988;**48**(Supp):439–83.

24. NC Department of Health and Human Services. Women's and Children's Health Section. Prenatal weight gain chart. www.nal.usda.gov/wicworks/Sharing_Center/NY/prenatalwt_charts.pdf 2011 [Accessed 27 January, 2012].

25. Laraia B A, Siega-Riz A M & Gundersen C. Household food insecurity is associated with self-reported pregravid weight status, gestational weight gain, and pregnancy complications. *J Am Diet Assoc* 2010;**110**:692–701.

26. Hilson J A, Rasmussen K M & Kjolhede C L. Maternal obesity and breastfeeding success in a rural population of white women. *Am J Clin Nutr* 1997;**66**:1371–8.

27. Li R, Jewell S & Grummer-Strawn L M. Maternal obesity and breast-feeding practices. *Am J Clin Nutr* 2003;**77**:931–6.

28. Baker J L, Michaelsen K F, Sørensen T I A & Rasmussen K M. High prepregnant body mass index is associated with early termination of full and any breastfeeding among Danish women. *Am J Clin Nutr* 2007;**86**:404–11.

29. Amir L H & Donath S. A systematic review of maternal obesity and breastfeeding intention, initiation and duration. *BMC Pregnancy Childbirth* 2007;**7**:9.

30. Baker J L, Gamborg M, Heitmann B L, *et al.* Breastfeeding reduces postpartum weight retention. *Am J Clin Nutr* 2008;**88**:1543–51.

31. Linné Y, Barkeling B & Rössner S. Long-term weight development after pregnancy. *Obesity Rev* 2002;**3**:75–83.

32. Centers for Disease Control and Prevention (CDC). Postpartum care visits – 11 states and New York City, 2004. *MMWR Morb Mortal Wkly Rep* 2007;**56**:1312–16.

33. Centers for Disease Control and Prevention. Breastfeeding report card – United States, 2011. www.cdc.gov/breastfeeding/data/reportcard.htm. [Accessed 12 January, 2012].

34. Shealy K R, Li R, Benton-Davis S, Grummer-Strawn L M. *The CDC Guide to Breastfeeding Interventions*. (Atlanta, GA: US Department of Health and Human Services; Centers for Disease Control and Prevention, 2005).

35. US Department of Health and Human Services. *The Surgeon General's Call to Action to Support Breastfeeding*. (Washington, DC: US Department of Health and Human Services, Office of the Surgeon General; 2011).

36. Hamilton B E, Martin J A & Ventura S J. Births: preliminary data for 2008. *Nat Vital Stat Rep* 2010;**58**(16):1–18.

37. USDA Food and Nutrition Service. Breastfeeding promotion in WIC: current federal requirements. www.fns.usda.gov/wic/Breastfeeding/bfrequirements.htm [Accessed January 12, 2012].

38. Meehan K, Harrison G G, Afifi A A, *et al.* The association between an electric pump loan program and the timing of requests for formula by working mothers in WIC. *J Hum Lact* 2008;**24**:150–8.

39. USDA Food and Nutrition Service. Providing quality nutrition services in implementing the breastfeeding promotion and support requirements of the new WIC food packages. www.fns.usda.gov/wic/policyandguidance/BreastfeedingFoodPackageGuidance.pdf [Accessed January 12, 2012].

40. USDA Food and Nutrition Service, Office of Research and Analysis. WIC Breastfeeding Peer Counseling Study: Final Implementation Report. Report No. WIC-10-BPC. (Alexandria, VA: US Department of Agriculture; 2010).

41. Scanlon K S, Grummer-Strawn L, Chen J & Molinari N. Racial and ethnic differences in breastfeeding initiation and duration, by state – National Immunization Survey, United States, 2004–2008. *MMWR Morb Mortal Wkly Rep* 2010;**59**:327–34.

42. Kent G. WIC's promotion of infant formula in the United States. *Int Breastfeeding J* 2006;**1**:8.

43. Chu S Y, Kim S Y & Bish C L. Prepregnancy obesity prevalence in the United States, 2004–2005. *Matern Child Health J* 2009;**13**:614–20.

44. Rasmussen K M, Abrams B, Bodnar L M, *et al.* Recommendations for weight gain during pregnancy in the context of the obesity epidemic. *Obstet Gynecol* 2010;**116**:1191–5.

45. Artal R, Lockwood C J & Brown H L. Weight gain recommendations in pregnancy and the obesity epidemic. *Obstet Gynecol* 2010;**115**:152–5.

46. Bodnar L M, Siega-Riz A M, Simhan H N, Himes K P & Abrams B. Severe obesity, gestational weight gain, and adverse birth outcomes. *Am J Clin Nutr* 2010;**91**:1642–9.

47. Beyerlein A, Schiessl B & von Kries R. Associations of gestational weight loss with birth-related outcome: a retrospecitve cohort study. *BJOG* 2011 ;**118**:55–61.

48. Hinkle S N, Sharma A J & Dietz P M. Gestational weight gain in obese mothers and associations with fetal growth. *Am J Clin Nutr* 2010;**92**:644–51.

49. US Department of Health and Human Services. Health, United States, 2005. www.cdc.gov/nchs/data/hus/hus05.pdf [Accessed January 12, 2012].

50. Ogden C L, Carroll M D, Curtin L R, *et al.* Prevalence of overweight and obesity in the United States, 1999–2004. *JAMA* 2006;**295**:1549–55.

Index